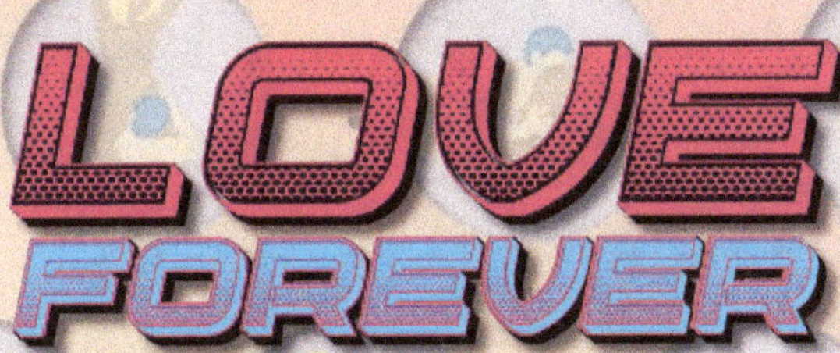

Sex Positions Calendar

365 Sex Positions

Kama Sutra

For the Modern Era

Written by Allison Eden

A Words Are Swords Publishing Book

Sex Positions Calendar: 365 Positions

Written by Allison Eden & Ryan Stabile

Published by Words Are Swords Publishing

2026 Edition.

This book is dedicated to all of my hot friends who let me take photos of them having sex. I'm disappointed we weren't able to get the entire 365, but it sure was fun trying, wasn't it?

Can you guess which ones I'm in?

Table of Contents

Introduction

When Words Are Swords asked me to do a sex position calendar, I must admit, I was pretty nervous. 365 seems like a lot of different sex positions, even for me a gal like me, who found a way to turn her debilitating hyper-sexual nymphomania into a full-time career writing about sex.

And then someone pointed out that, in every relationship I've ever been in, my number one rule is that **sex is mandatory at least once a day.** Being the professional slut that I am, I quickly embraced the challenge of coming up with exciting new positions. All I think about is sex all day anyway – who better to write a book of 365 sex positions?

Photo Credit

Taking high-quality photos is HARD! Some of the photos in this book are of my friends having sex. Thank you to Ryan Stabile, Steven Matthews, Jon C, Words Are Swords Pub, the L.A. FetLife community, and to my sweetheart darling, Bree, who was worried her mom would see the naked pictures of her in this book. Isn't that sweet? I'm even in a couple of the sex position photos, but I'll never tell which.

I did have to borrow a few with the permission of sexpositions.org. The rest are illustrations, which, I suppose, are good for educational purposes.

After this book was all said and done, I feel really inspired to do another 365 sex positions calendar using only photos of myself.

Using This Calendar

The first and most important parts of using this calendar are safety & consent. Consult your doctor before engaging in strenuous sexual activity. Make sure you're healthy enough to have sex and never do anything dangerous during sex.

Most of the content in this book will require a partner. If you've shown this book to your partner, and their reaction was, "Hell yeah! Let's do this!" then congrats on finding the perfect life partner and enjoy 365 days of awesome orgasms.

Although I don't personally subscribe to monogamy, I'm a firm believer that the cornerstone of all strong, healthy relationships is wild, hot, can-keep-my-hands-off-you sex. After 365 days of hot sex, 730 earth-shattering orgasms, and many bottles of lube, you're creating an unbreakable bond that will improve all facets of your life, and that of your partner's.

It's About the Journey, Not the Destination

Don't be overwhelmed by the idea of trying out 365 new positions. It may seem like a lot, but it's really not. To ease readers into it (no pub intended), I've listed easy positions that I hope everyone is familiar with at the very beginning. (If you have trouble with "Missionary", we need to have a chat)

You'll get the most out of the calendar by at least attempting every position in this book, marking down the ones you and your partner both enjoyed the most while forgetting about the rest. Positions like "Around the World" aren't for everyone, but they sure are fun to try out.

Also, your initial inclination may be to just skip entire sections that you find intimidating, but again, I urge you to at least try them out with a consenting partner. If you do decide to skip one or two, I've added a few extra bonus positions at the very end. Careful! They're challenging!

Ladies, I strongly recommend trying out a minimum of 2-3 positions from the anal section, even if that's something that you could never see yourself doing. Under the right conditions (Read: Lots of lube), you may find you really enjoy butt stuff. Once you realize that, it unlocks a whole new world of sexual exploration.

Honestly, I can't understand why so many women seem to have an aversion to putting stuff in their butts. All of my straight and bi female friends I convinced to try anal for the first time and now they all love it.

Lastly, as a bisexual single woman, I really wish I could have made this book more inclusive. Unfortunately, most of the positions in this book will require at least 1 penis and 1 vagina to successfully pull off. I'll be thinking about a follow up book just for the ladies.

Take it slow, but above all, have fun. One position a day is easy. If my dad can do it (Not my Daddy, but my actual father), so can you.

P.S. Please consider leaving a review for this book in the marketplace from which you purchased it. If you have any feedback on the content in this book, or if you want to send me your sex tapes for "constructive feedback", I wouldn't say no.

My email is: Yesdaddyally@gmail.com

- Allison Eden

Sexy Companion Books

Other book from the sex-crazed mind of Allison Eden.
Find them on Amazon or the reputable smut peddler near you.

Love Forever Sex Position Calendar: 365 Positions You've Never Tried

Nothing comes close to deepening the bond between two people when they commit to getting each other off in new & exciting ways every single day. Created with every body type in mind, *Love Forever* captures amateur couples demonstrating just how easy it is to turn up the heat of classic positions or challenge yourselves with advanced ones.

Sexy Games & More - Unlimited Sexploration: 10th Anniversary Edition

Revised for every type of relationship, sexual preference, & kink, *Sexy Games & More* is full of fun, spicy games that'll turn every night into date night. Explore the Kink & Fetish Index, Learn the Art of Erotic Massage, Master Dirty Talk, try out Role-Play Scenarios (*w/ $10 coupon for sexy costumes!*), Discover BDSM Around the World, Become an expert at Foreplay, Aftercare, & SO MUCH MORE! Whether you're looking for short-term fun or want to build erotic skills that last a lifetime, I personally guarantee *Sexy Games* will lead to better, hotter sex or your money back!

The Exhibitionist Bingo Challenge

An erotic fiction based entirely on real-life encounters, *The Exhibitionist Bingo Challenge*, follows a modern young couple living in Los Angeles as they explore the steamy world of public sex. The audiobook is out now!

Downright Dirty: A Sexy Raunchtastic Adult Coloring Book

Check all your stress, anxiety, & clothing at the door, break out the glitter pens, and drive into a world of 100+ decorative & debaucherous photos with *Downright Dirty: A Sexy Adult Coloring Book*. Paired with some of my personal favorite dirty phrases, positions, and body parts, *Downright Dirty* is both relaxing & stimulating.

Companion Toys & Tools

Make your sex life better with these toys & tools of the bedroom

1. **Coconut Oil -** https://amzn.to/4nZxPAm

I have been using this fractionated coconut oil for many years. I always keep a bottle of this stuff on my nightstand because it's an effective all-natural lube. Unlike most lube, coconut oil is great for your skin, has no smell, and is water-soluble, making it easy to wash out of bedsheets, easy-peasy.

But it's the convenience of the hand-pump is why I fell in love with this specific coconut oil. If it's dark enough in the bedroom, I can grab a handful of lube in a fraction of a second without anyone knowing I need lube. If you've ever tried to put the lid back on a bottle of Astro-Glide with oily, lubed-up fingers, then you know what a nightmare that is.

Best of all, it's $10 on Amazon!

2. **Hitachi Magic Wand -** https://amzn.to/46uJUYg

If you don't know what a Hitachi Magic Wand is for, ask literally any woman off the street (Just don't blame me if you get slapped).

If you own no other sex toys, the Magic Wand is really all you need. This baby can get any woman or man off in less than a minute. Hello, multiple orgasms.

3. **Cock Rings -** https://amzn.to/3UtdBBA

This variety multi-size cock ring set is built to help men last longer:

4. **Plug Trainer Set**

This is a good multi-size butt plug set for beginners: https://amzn.to/46thy0s

My personal favorite butt plug is this unicorn tail: https://amzn.to/4mcnYp8

5. **Penis Pumps -** https://amzn.to/3J5aIEs

I don't care what anyone says, I've SEEN penis pumps do some pretty spectacular things that defy the laws of physics. Anything that give a guy an extra 2 inches in a few minutes is okay by me.

January

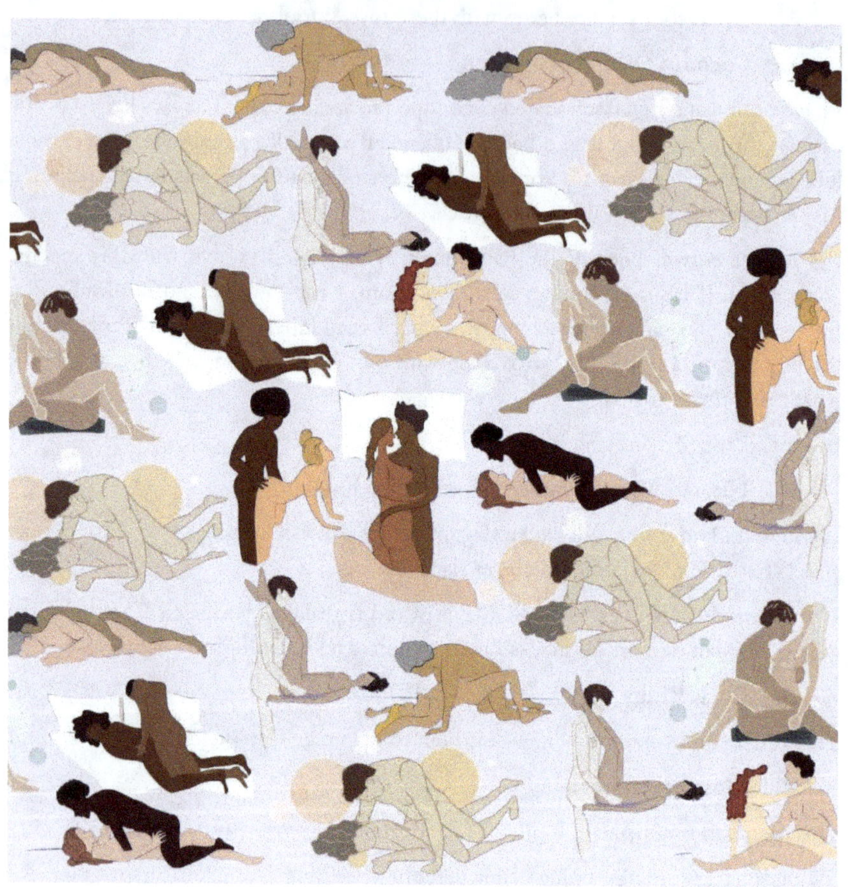

I want you thinking
of me.

I want your eyes
on me.

I want your hands
on me.

I want all of you.

January 1
The Folding Chair

While the woman may not be able to see how much pleasure she is giving her partner, she can feel the shivers of delight on his skin. Giving in completely to his pleasure, the man stands motionless and savours the moment.

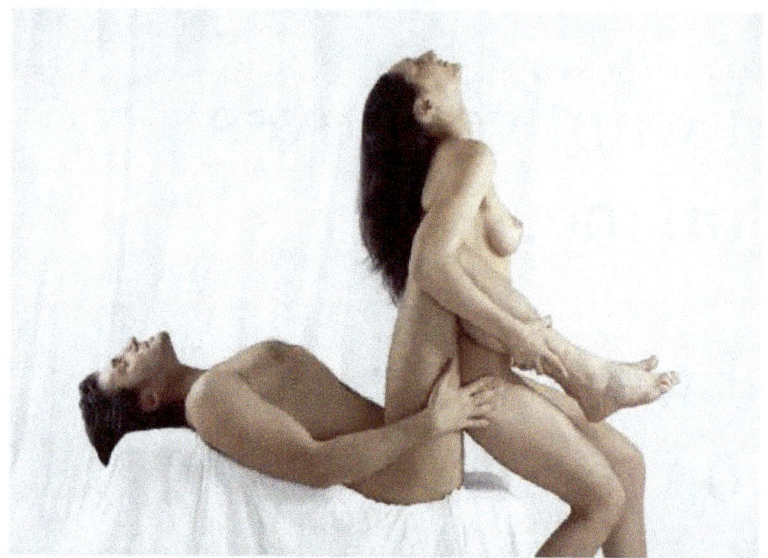

January 2

The Sleigh

On the road to amazing sensations, the oddly intertwined bodies are going in the same direction. The woman leads the team to new lands.

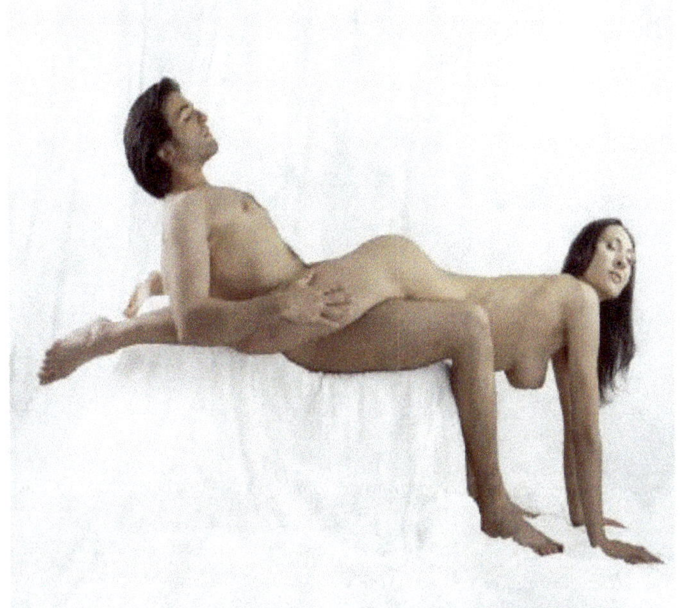

January 3

Sexecutive Woman

You have to be quite confident and enjoy a particular irony to confuse your partner with a desk. You also have to love your work… and what comes after work.

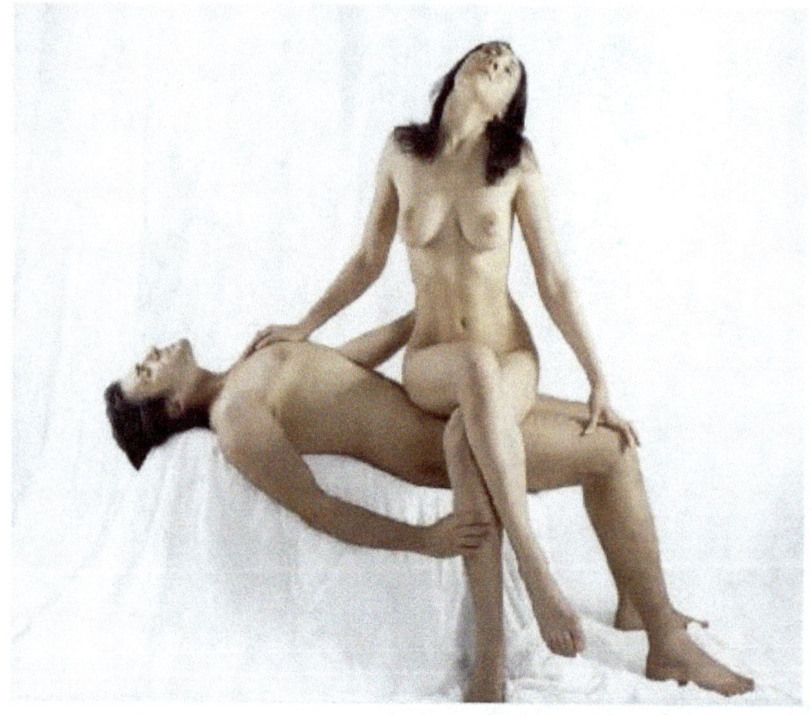

January 4

I love the scent of your hair

This lovers' embrace can do more than serve the greater pleasure of the lovers; if the weather is fine, it affords them the chance to sunbathe.

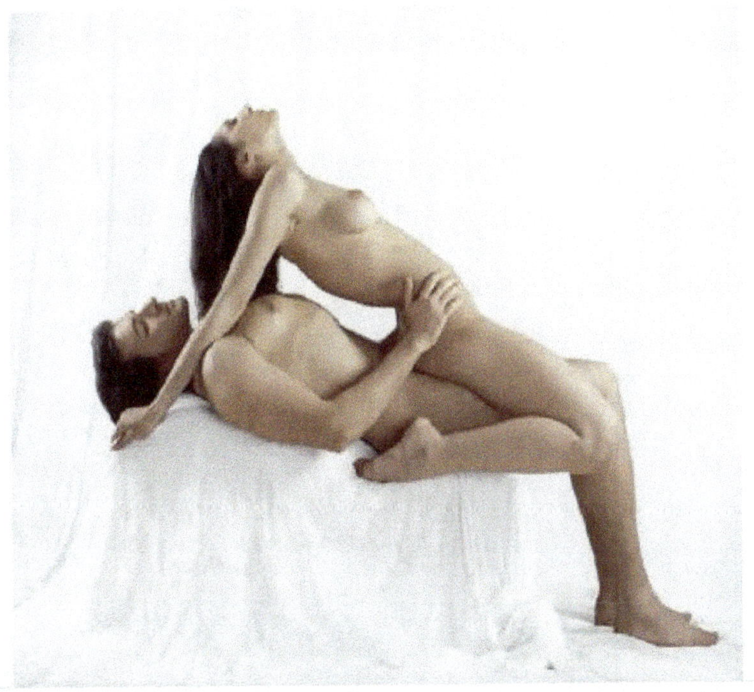

January 5

Absolute

In political terms, an absolute monarchy is a regime in which power is concentrated in the hands of one person who rules unchecked The same is true for absolute love...

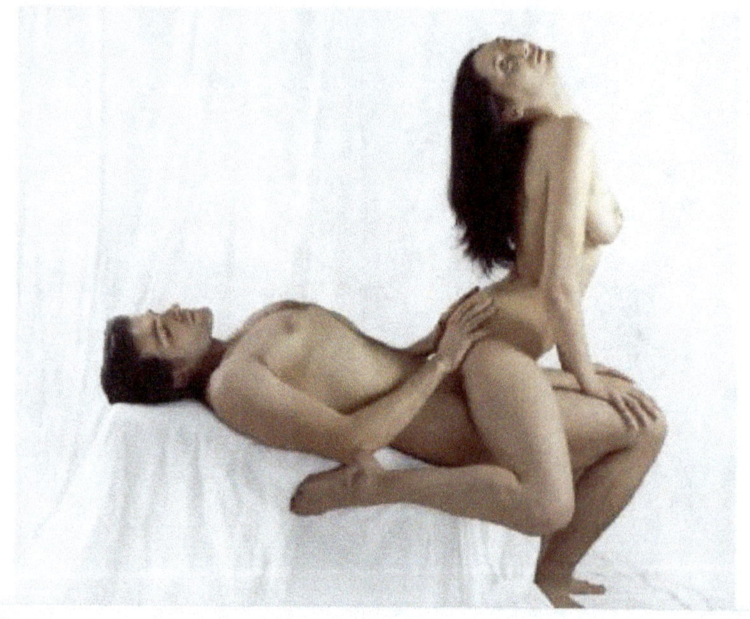

January 6

Paradise Lost

The woman turns her back to her partner and clasps his ankles to perform a dance as exciting as it is sensual. She holds him and she alone is what holds him back…

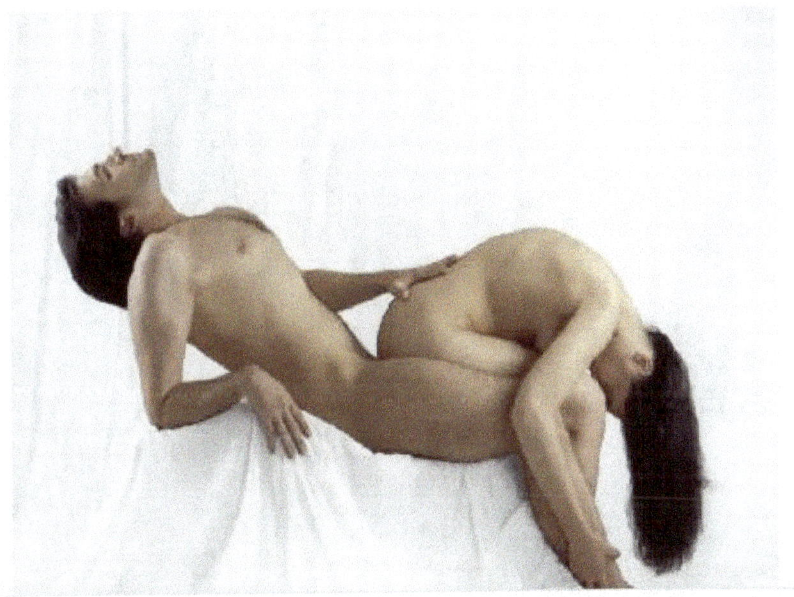

January 7

In the Sunlight

The couple both enjoy themselves and she can take advantage of the rays of sunlight and breezes all over her body. The man is held firmly down to earth by his partner's feet while both take their pleasure.

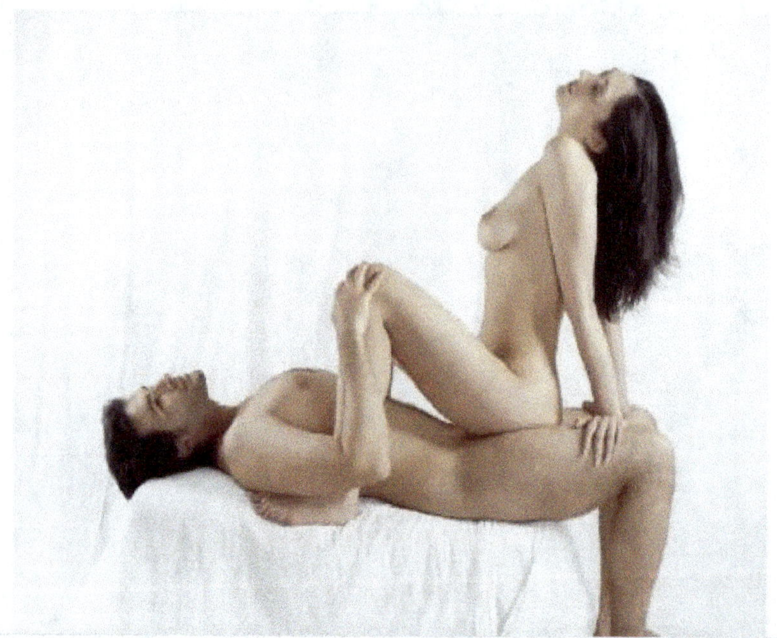

January 8

Excess

Love is synonymous with excess for in search of pleasure it knows no limits. The woman is quite comfortable but has no chance of escape, held tight in her lover's grasp.

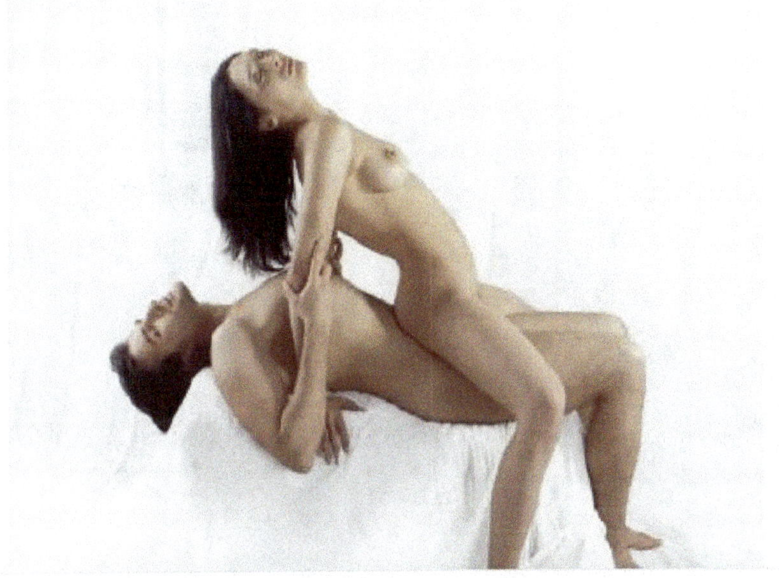

January 9

Budding Rose

A woman may give her lover the gift of a rose. A flower with no thorns, showing off its petals, colours and intricate beauty.

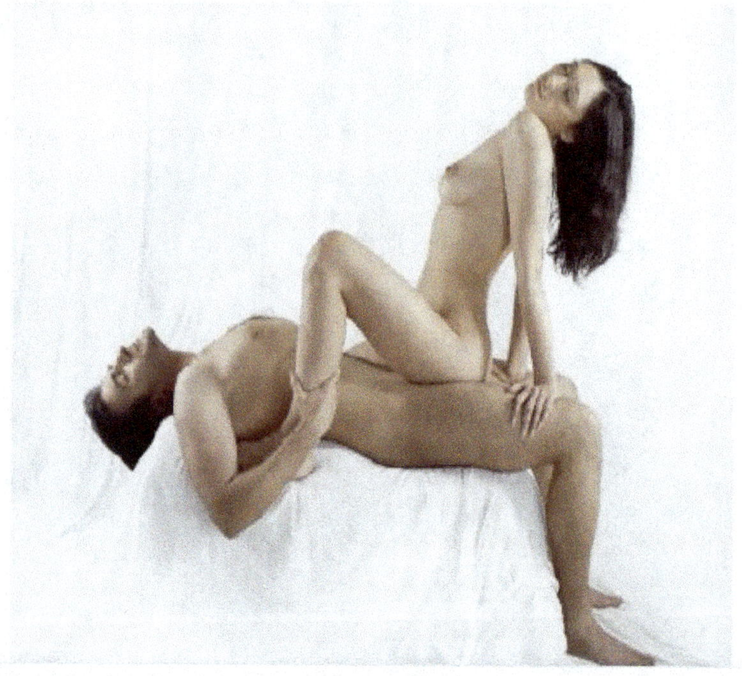

January 10

Busy Hands

There are positions where the man may not have a free hand... but here he can easily caress his partner's whole body. All she has to do is give in then and enjoy his touch.

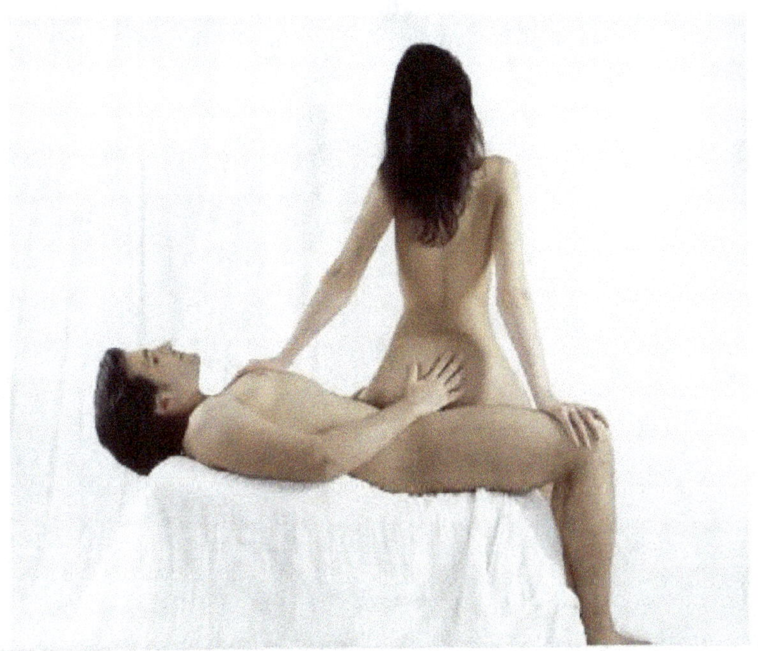

January 11

Sensual Delight

The question of equality of the sexes can be abandoned for the space of a lovemaking session. Shall we say that in this case, the man is a bit more comfortably seated, but any sacrifice is certainly for a good cause.

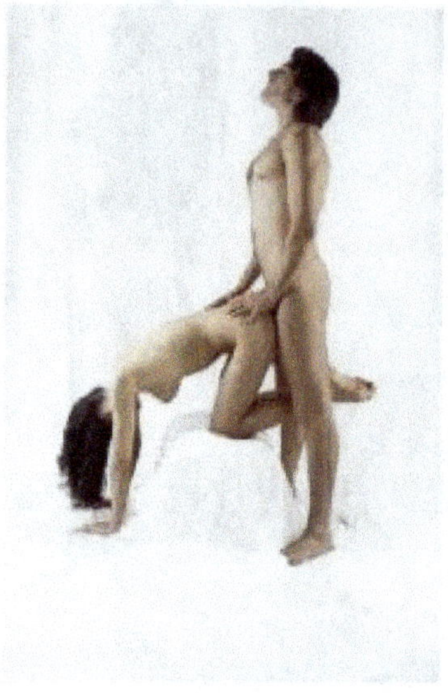

January 12

Intimate Embrace

In the midst of this maze of intertwined legs with the right mixture of caresses and forceful grasps, pleasure always arrives right on time (or a cramp!).

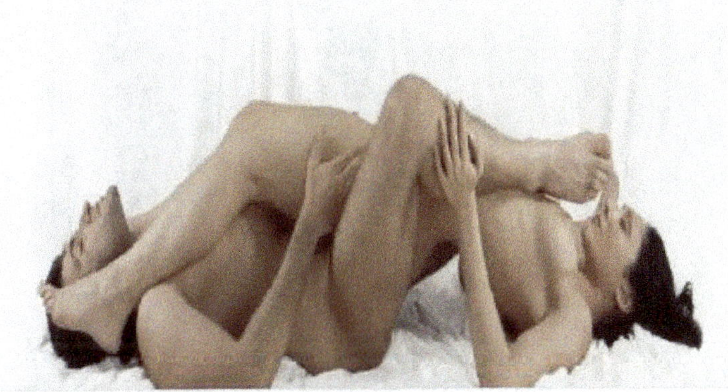

January 13

The Opera Singer

Not unlike intimate relations, singing is rich in emotions. The melody is sweet and caressing and the voice coquettish. Now all you need to do is keep up the rhythm.

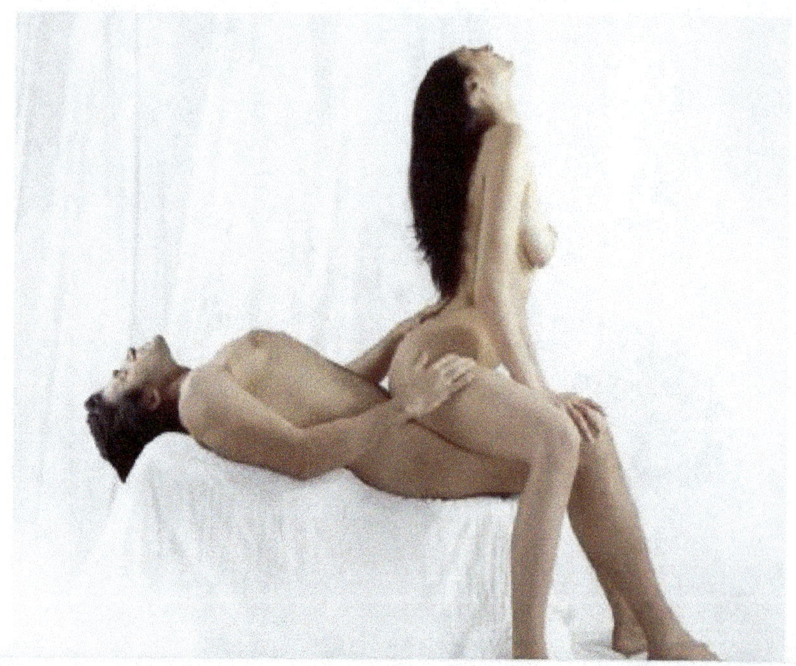

January 14

Lust Upended

With every muscle clinched the lovers begin a powerful embrace. The woman turned upside down by the bold power of her lover must master the acrobatic arts.

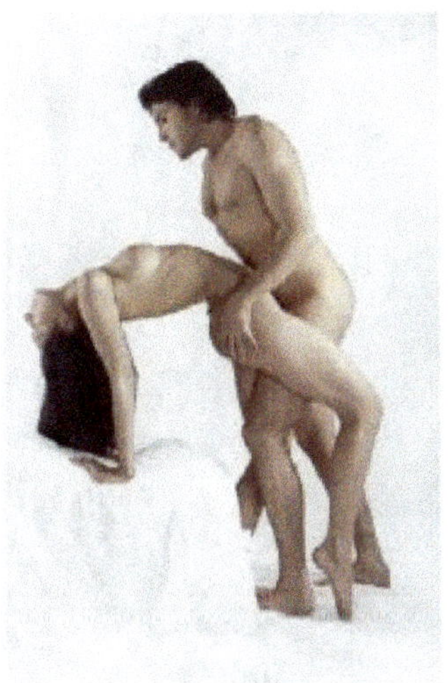

January 15

Ready, steady, go!

Sprinters in top form have the best chances with this type of sensual competition where firmly toned muscles are called for. Long-distance runners will have to wait for next year.

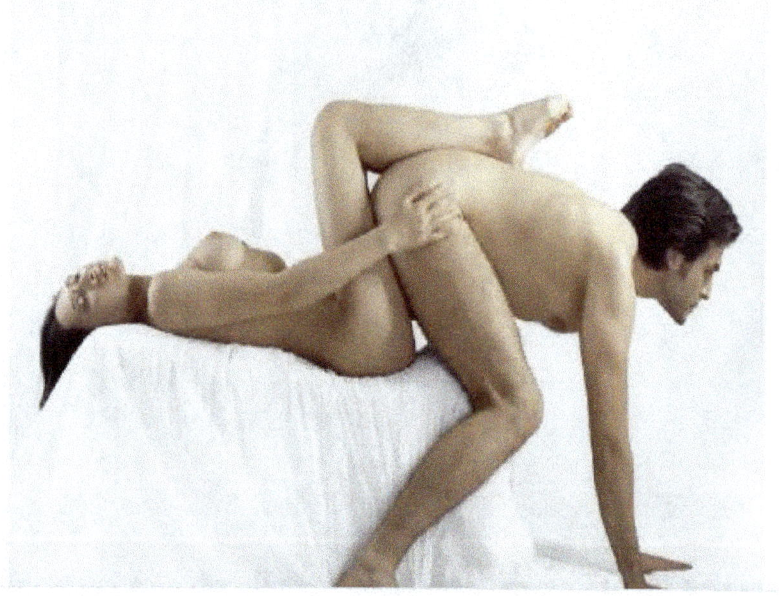

January 16

Risqué Armchair

Comfortably seated, both bodies relax deliciously into one another. The soothed lovers give in to the gentle sway of love.

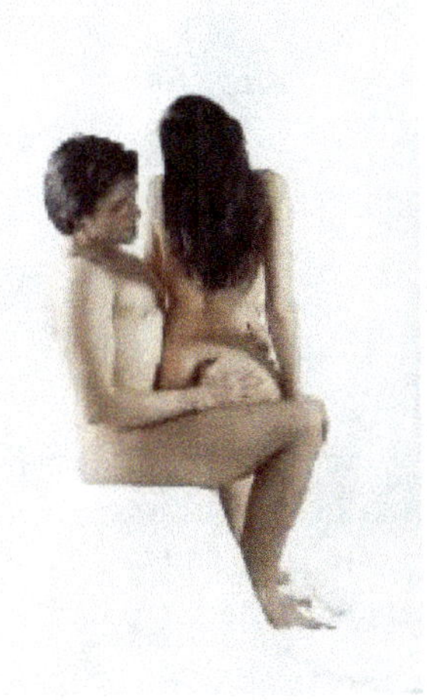

January 17

The Scorpion

In life, there are few occasions to imitate the scorpion. Like this bold creature, it seems as the lovers too can go without food and resist heat or cold.

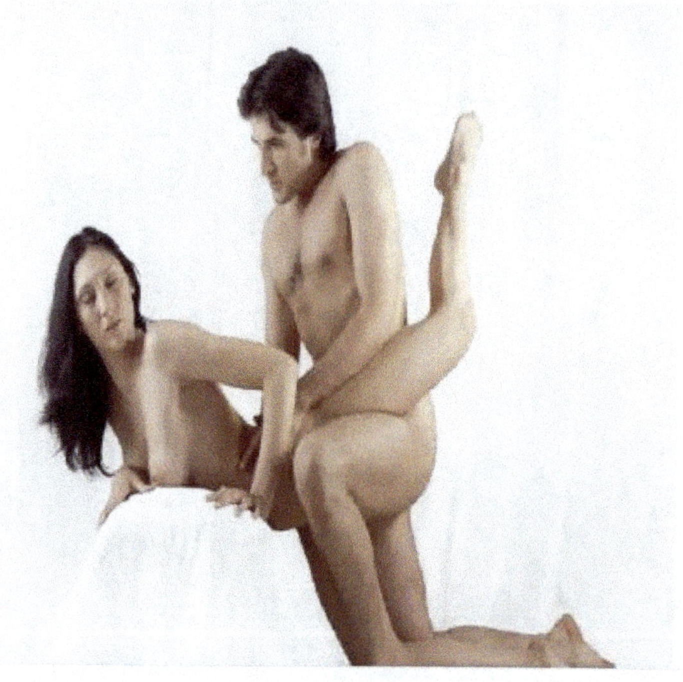

January 18

Swallow Dive

The lover dives in with brio and ardour to join his partner in the swirling waters of passion. The woman shows complete trust and gives in fully to the pleasures of her partner's delicate hands.

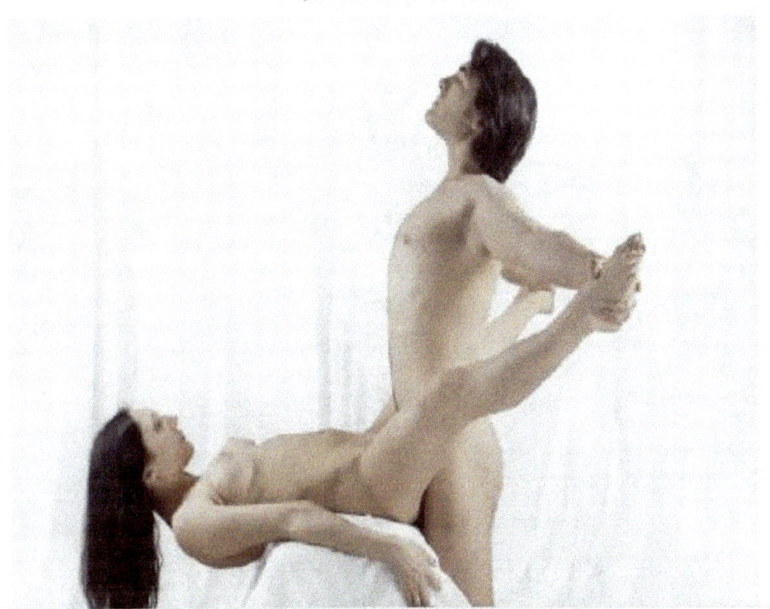

January 19

Harmonic Duet

Lovers use all four hands to play their duet on the world's most beautiful instruments. From half-notes to eighth notes, the tempo accelerates to keep time with passion.

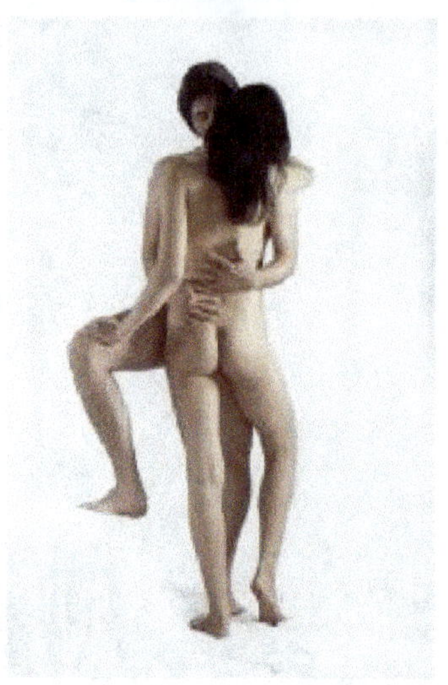

January 20

Birdsong

Birdsong serves to attract a partner to the nest in the season of love. The bird's power of attraction and his direct honesty draws the woman to him so that together they can take flight towards pleasure.

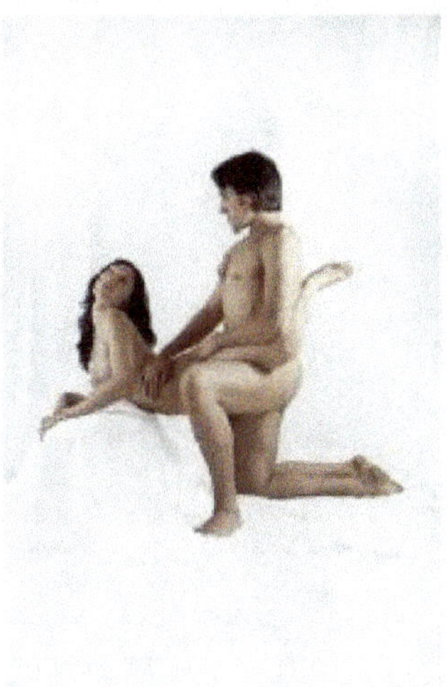

January 21

The Crossbow

To perform this delicious dance, it's best to have a piece of furniture that's the right height and a partner who is both strong and gentle. All the pleasure lies in the suppleness of the bow…

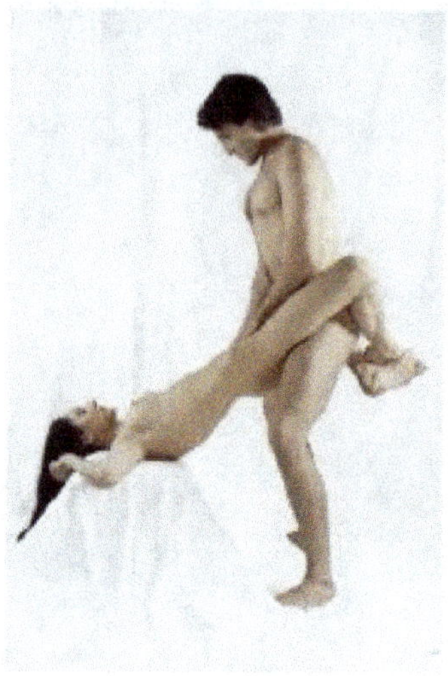

January 22

In the Stairway

This position is easy to perform, unless you're in a 35 storey building (elevators are more likely there) or on the steps up to the Basilica of the Sacré-Cœur (it's full of tourists already).

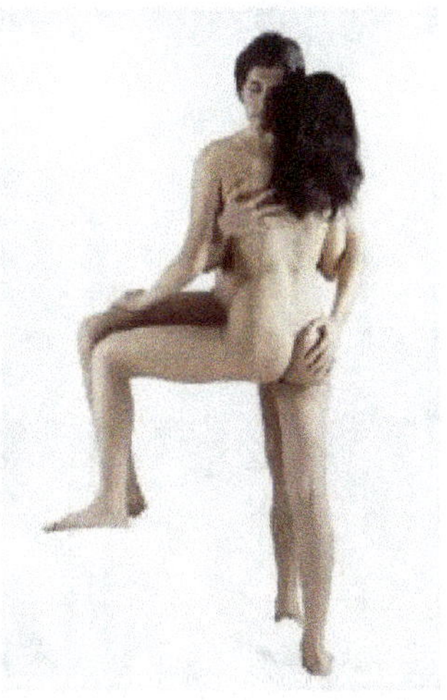

January 23

North-South

This position is surprising to say the least, and the pleasures it provides are every bit as unexpected. Get ready for takeoff; tropical climes await your arrival.

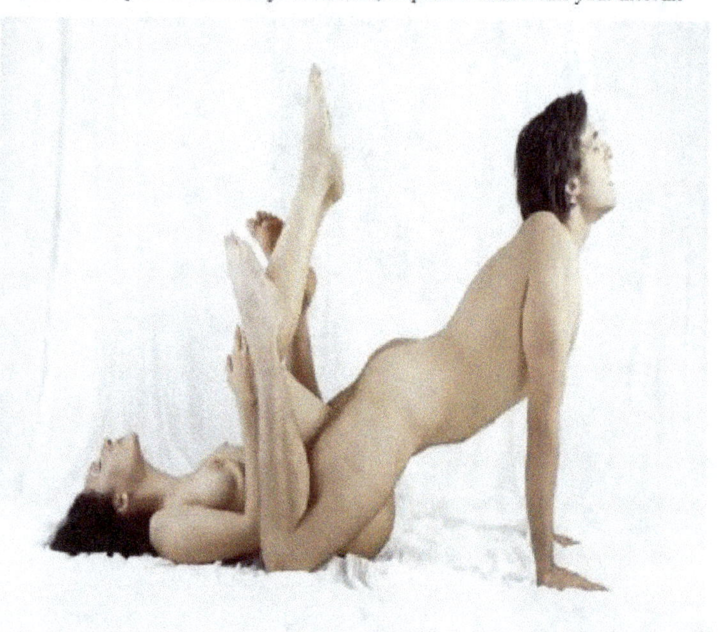

January 24

Upside Down Cake

The recipe is simple: as the woman swings her legs backwards, the man passes his knees under his partner's back. Serve hot, and enjoy...

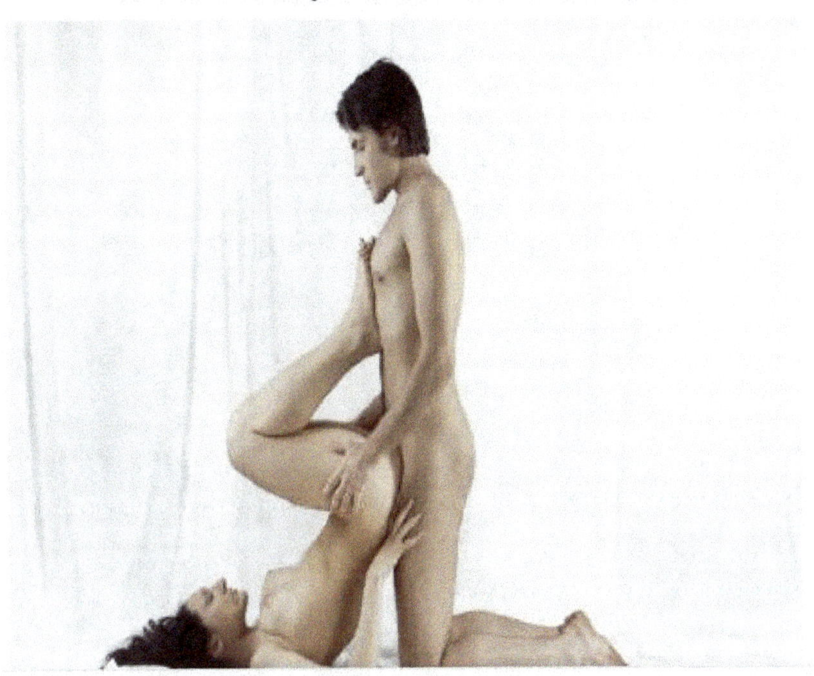

January 25

In the Shower

The air is steamy and hot, the bodies are damp and full of desire. Hidden behind the curtain, the lovers find one another in the torrid heat.

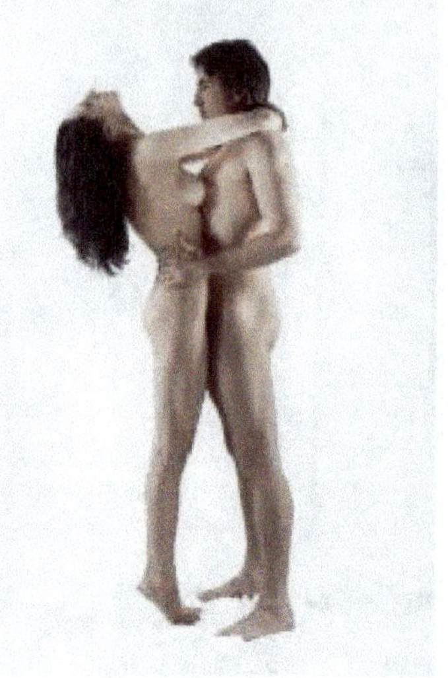

January 26

Delicious Improvisation

Make love standing up, anywhere (in the living room, the office, the great outdoors) and especially… without even seeing each other! A way to be mysterious strangers for each other once again.

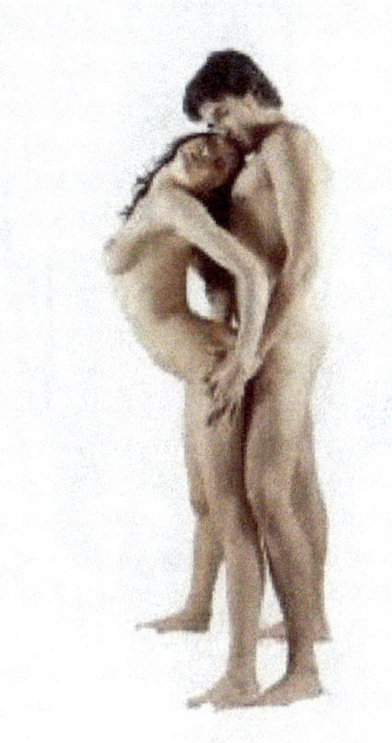

January 27

The Square

Halfway between lying and sitting, a 90° angle makes for more intense pleasures; the man relies on his supported position to find their rhythm and symmetry.

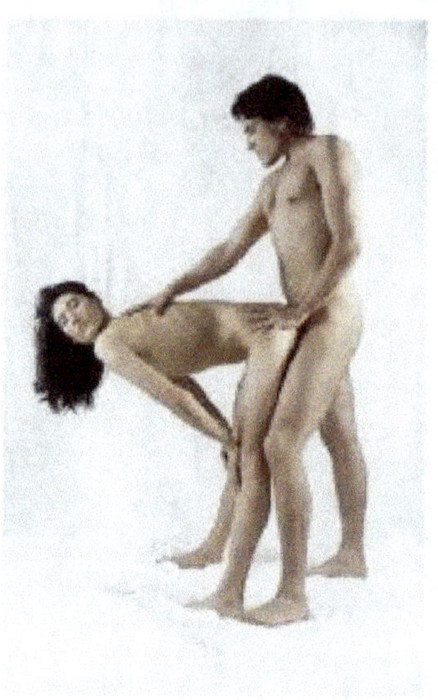

January 28

The Little Bridge

Once she has succeeded in the difficult task of bending over forward far enough to delicately place her hands on the ground, as she wishes, all her partner has to do is pay the proper tribute to the view from this unusual angle.

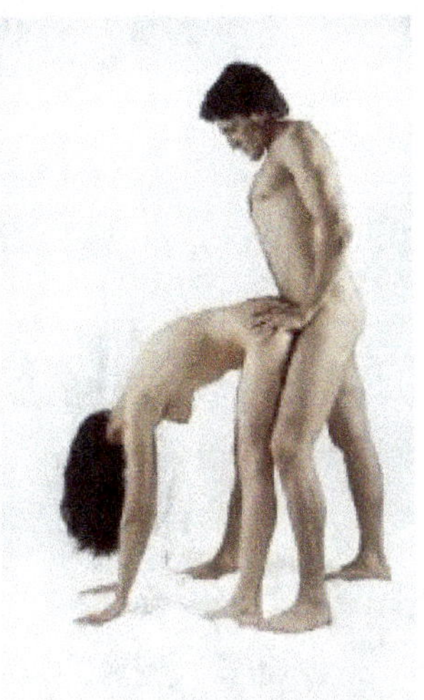

January 29
Gift Wrap

This embrace is just the thing for someone who has dinner on the stove, a load of laundry in the wash or a train to catch at half past 8. This embrace is perfect for someone who needs it to be quick but good… very good.

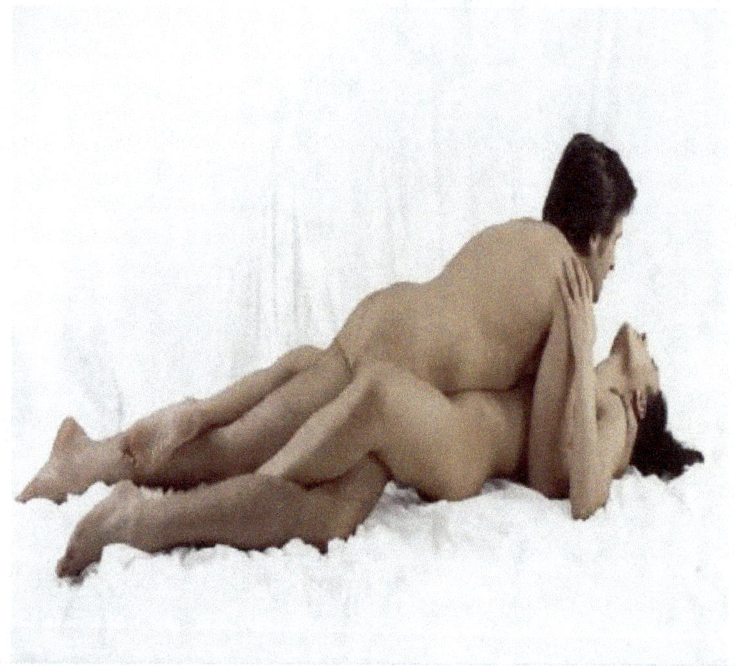

January 30

Nirvana

While the man seems to be seeking the algorithmic to reach Nirvana, the woman appears to have found it instinctively. Getting there requires a lot of love and flexibility.

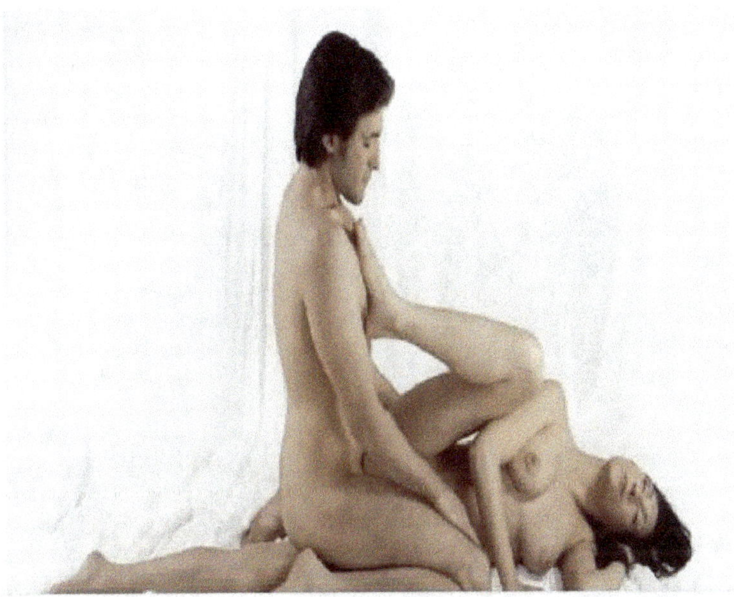

January 31

The Clash of the Titans

Love and hate are sisters, and these emotions are illustrated perfectly in this brave lover's embrace. The fury of love is at its height.

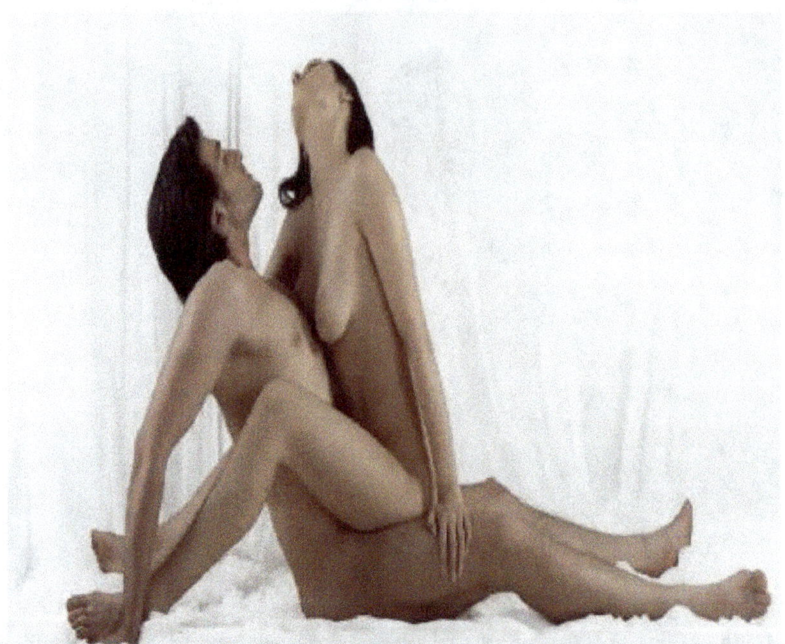

February

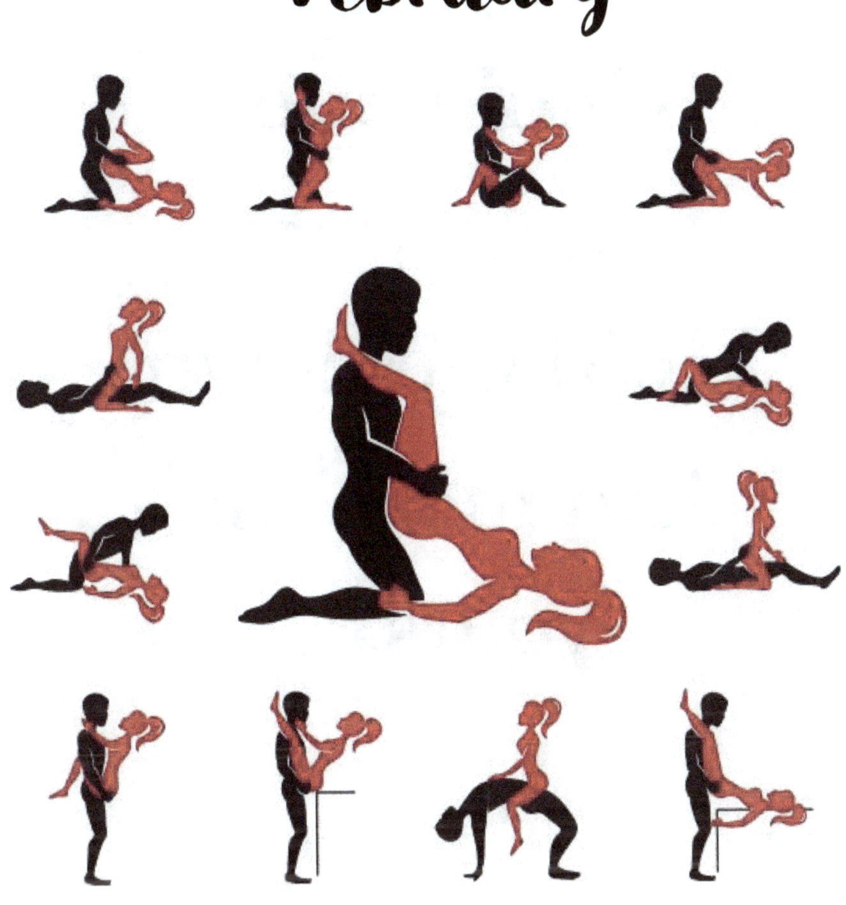

"Pull my hair, Choke me, Slap my ass, Hold me down And make me yours."

The married couples I know who have lasted the longest all have said that, when it comes to foreplay, it's about cultivating an emotional connection, most of all. It's a reminder that building true intimacy isn't just about sex; it's about making sure your partner feels wanted, heard and safe.

February 1
Cross-Legged Cowboy

The intertwined legs of two battle hardened lovers cross like their destinies. As they push the limits of intimacy, this position is intense and unconditional.

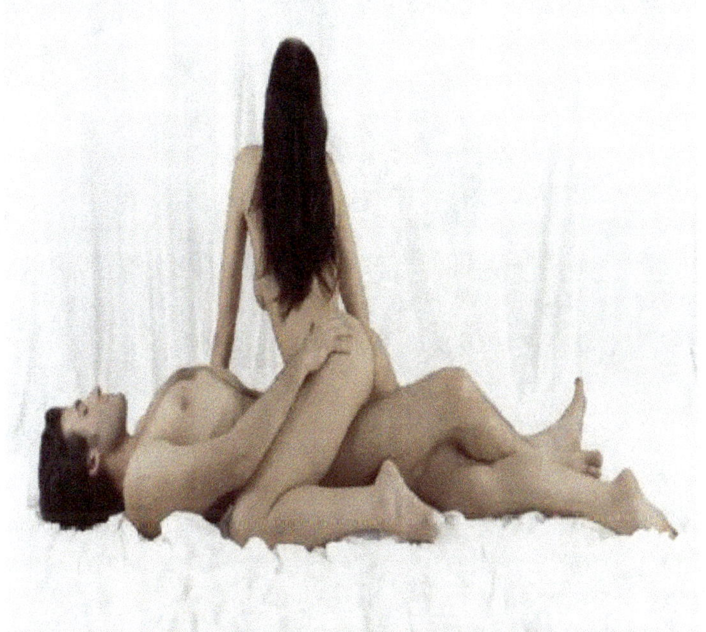

February 2

Yin and Yang

When their dual nature becomes complementary both lovers will reach total ecstasy. They are off in their own perfect world and nothing can stop them.

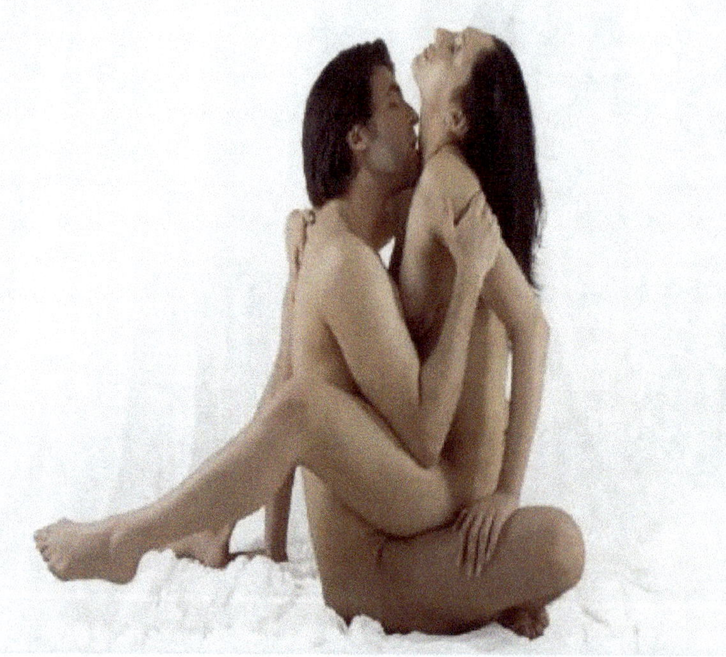

February 3
Hevean's Feel

To reach the heights of this paradise, it's best if you know something about hanging gardens and are keen to work your arm muscles. Now all that's left is to pluck the dangling delights.

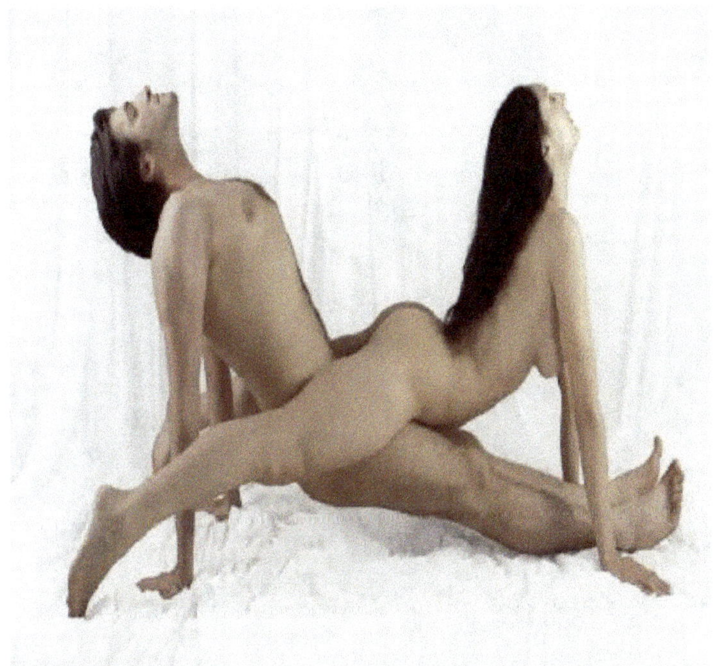

February 4

Coffee, please

Sitting on an improvised bench, the woman savours the pleasure of a chance meeting. From a chance conversation, a more lasting encounter could arise.

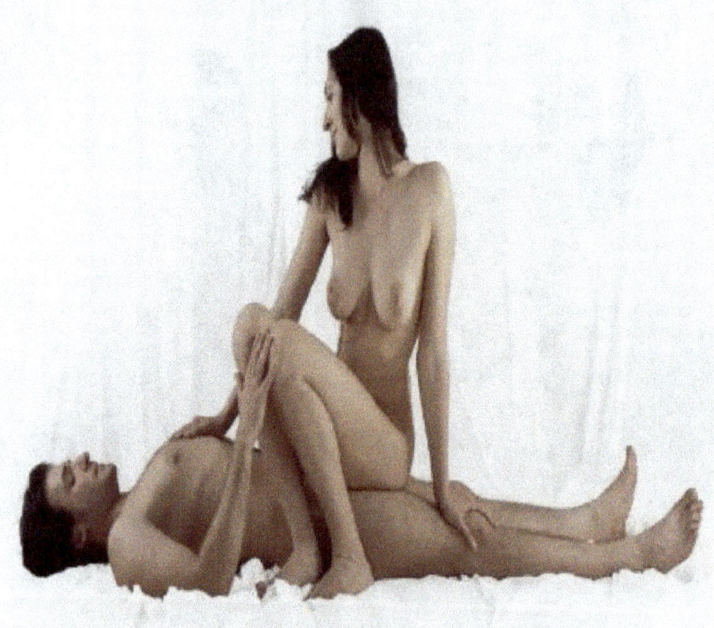

February 5

Back Seat of a Taxi

In this position the woman turns her back to the man and straddles him, the best position to control the dance and the rhythm. From that angle, no matter where you are you'll enjoy the city more than you would in the back of a taxi.

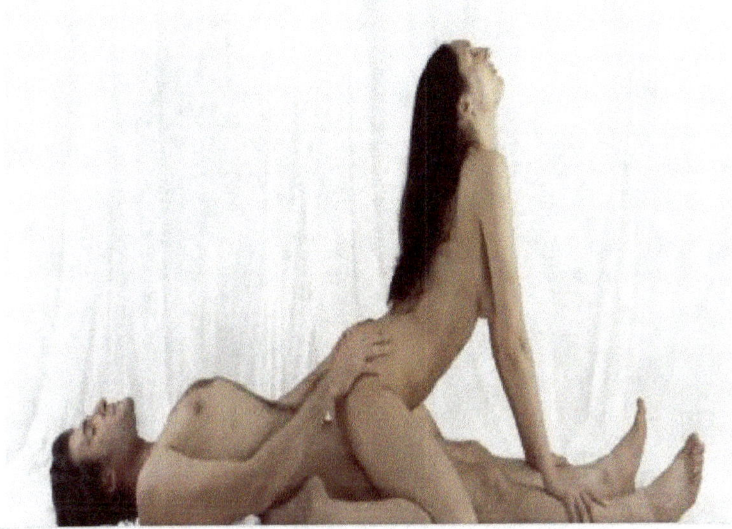

February 6

Waves of Pleasure

On stormy days, the wildest waves make for turbulent waters and undercurrents, making even the most seaworthy sailors close both their eyes.

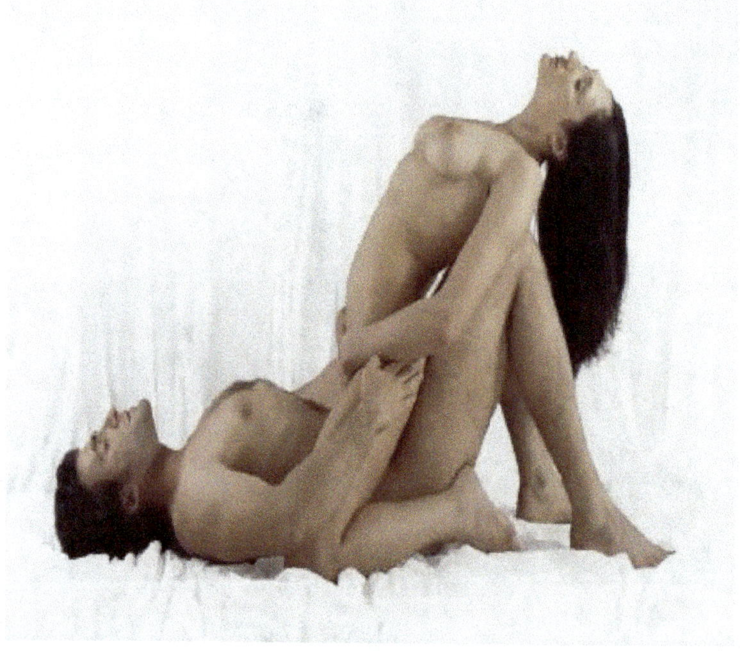

February 7

The Promise of Dawn

Clutching tightly, the man holding his partners buttocks and the woman holding her own ankles, the lovers are looking to the same horizon, faces turned toward the promise of the dawn.

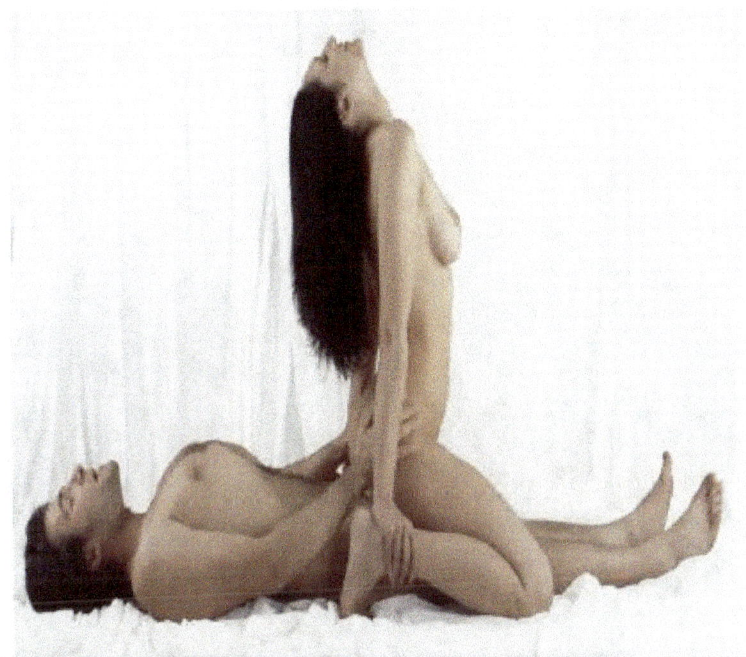

February 8

Down the Road to Joy

In love, your partner's happiness is essential if both bodies are to unite in total harmony. Travel together down the road littered with sensuous ideas.

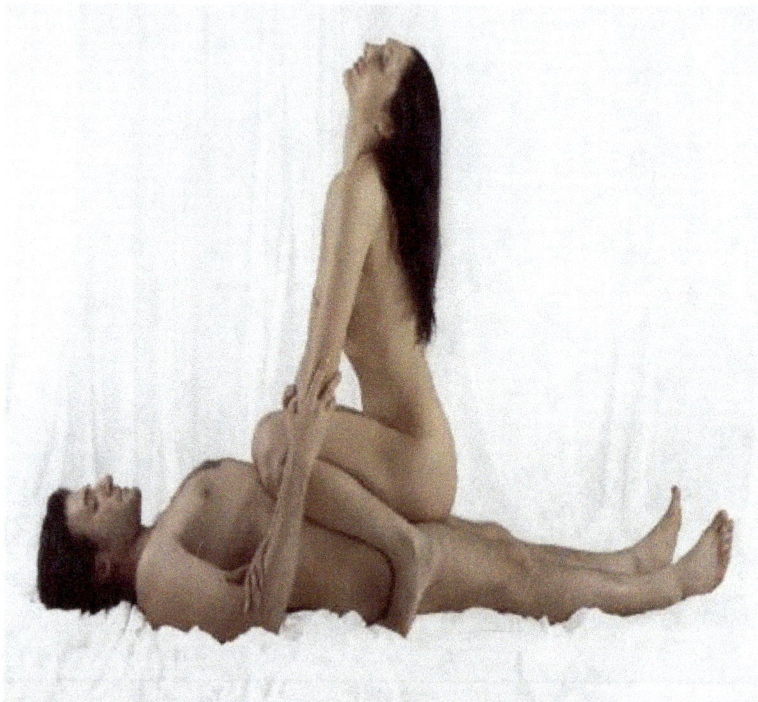

February 9

Hercules and Goliath

The clash of two heroes is always a formidable affair and a meeting such as this is one for the history books. Every sense is piqued and this moment will be an unforgettable one.

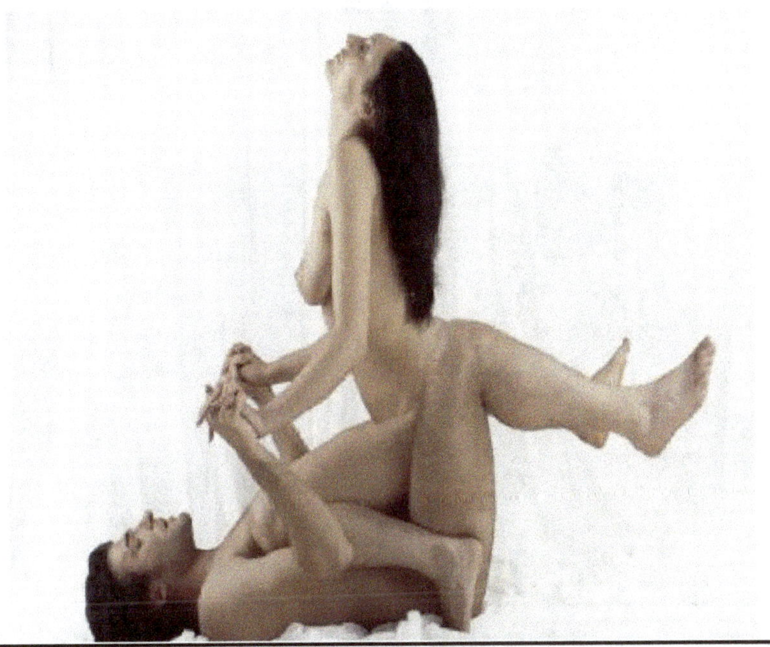

February 10

Extreme Supreme

To climb to the mountain peak, you'll have to do a little back and forth; you must not be afraid of touch the extreme, reach out for the tip - extreme satisfaction. It's not unlike an ice cream cone.

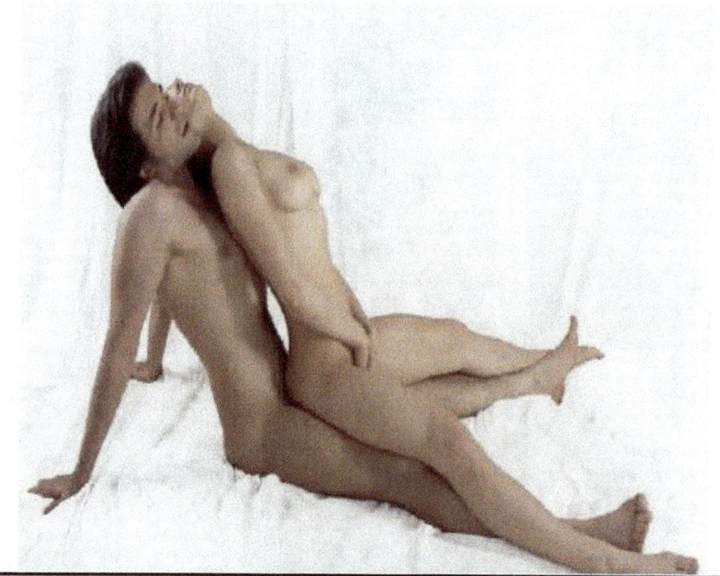

February 11

Dominatrix

A woman can be an angel of domination whenever she wants; all she has to do is use her wiles to make her partner fall under her spell. It's pure magnetism!

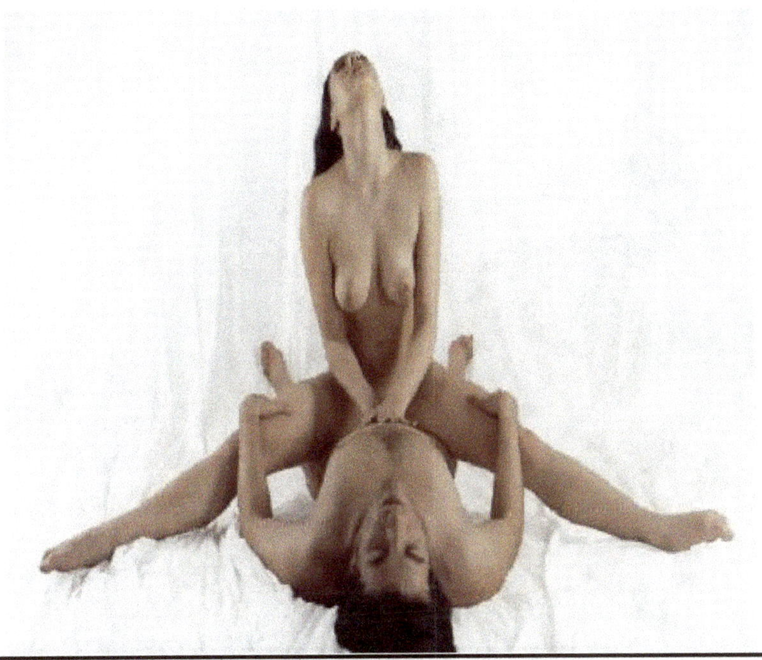

February 12

Takeoff

If the friction and the caresses are well placed and well timed, both lovers will be ready for launch in five, four, three, two, one, blast-off!

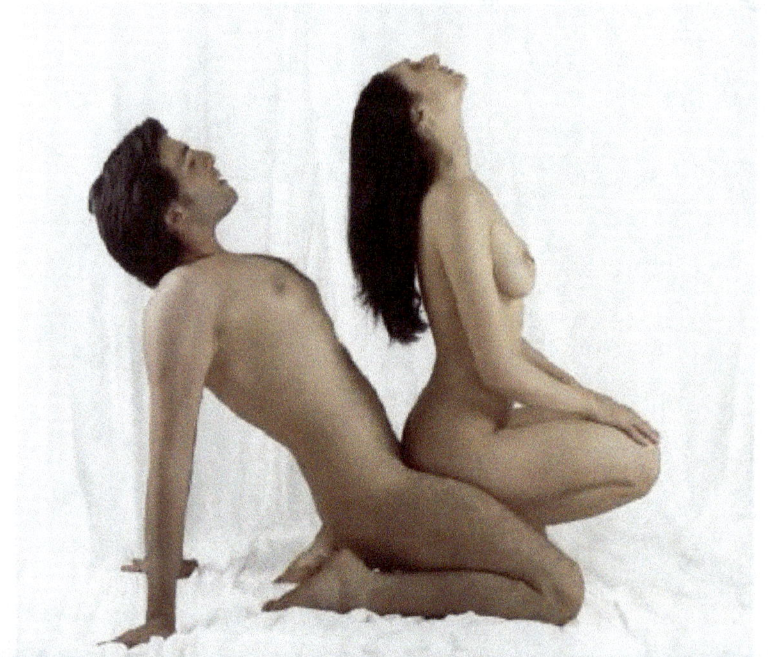

February 13
Secret Garden

There are hidden entrances, tucked away from prying eyes that give access to secret gardens. With the lover's feet placed on the man's chest, there is no finer stage door entrance!

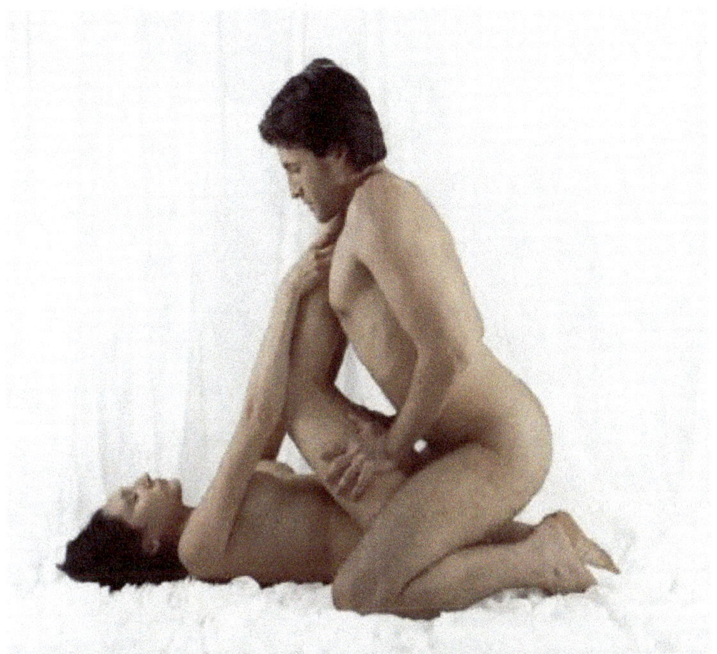

February 14

All Yours

This position ends in two bodies closely intertwined, a favourite with Argentine tango lovers. Just don't forget to take off the dress and suit!

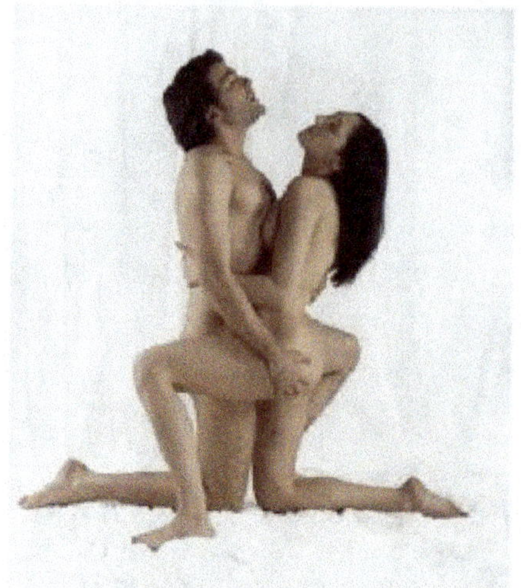

February 15

$1 + 1 = 69$

Mathematics has proven that if two perfect strangers total their love quotient, the sum is equal to or greater than the proportionally perfect geometric figure they create…

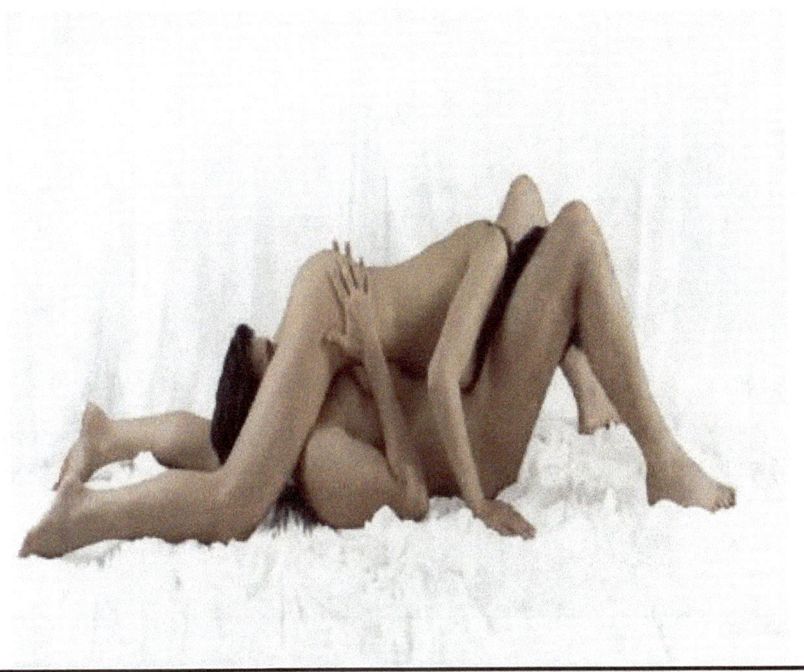

February 16

Equation with Two Unknowns

Science and love might not make good bedfellows - pleasure is the result of spontaneous generation and the explosion that results can't be defined by any natural law. Passion is anything but rational!

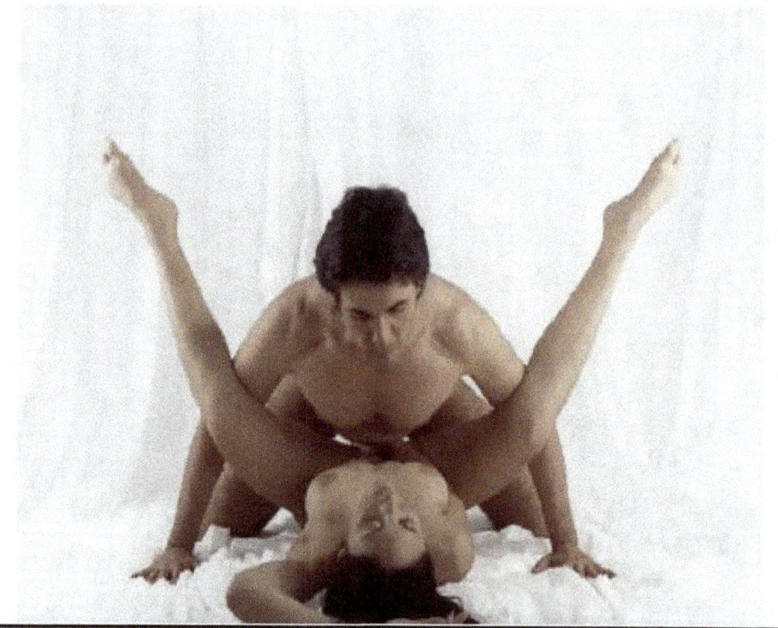

February 17

Look at Me

It's important to look at one another no matter what the position is. In a moment of pure passion, the man can take a moment to glance at his dear one and make sure that she is enjoying the moment as much as he is.

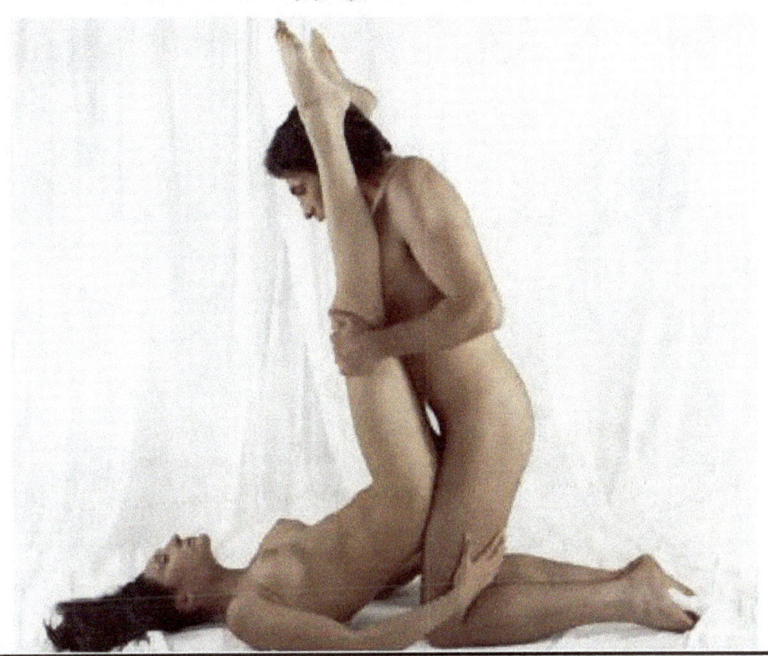

February 18

A Man and a Woman

The balance found between lovers is upset when they stretch out on a bed and conform to the shape of the other. Positions and power can be reversed - to each his own pleasure dome!

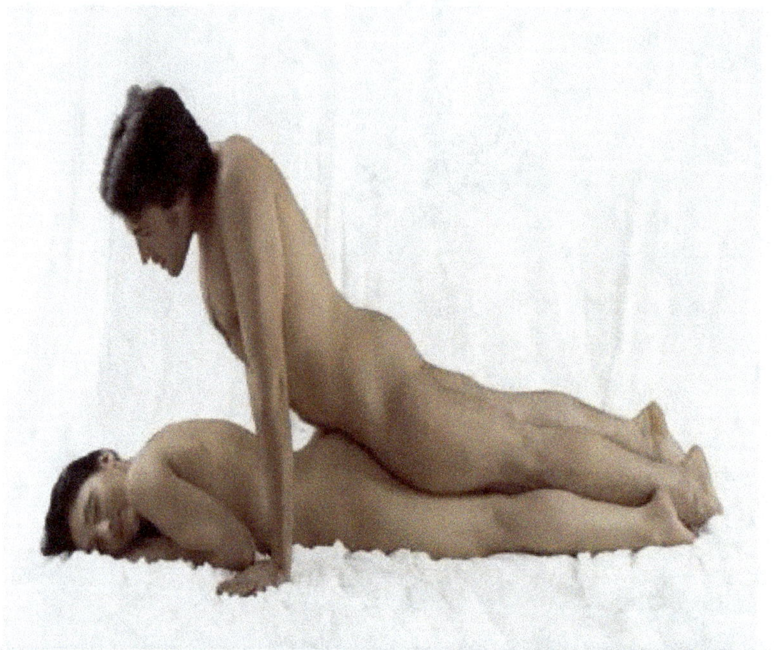

February 19

In My House

It seems almost as if this position was discovered by two lovers who fell together on the last stair step, and they are only too happy to have landed where they did!

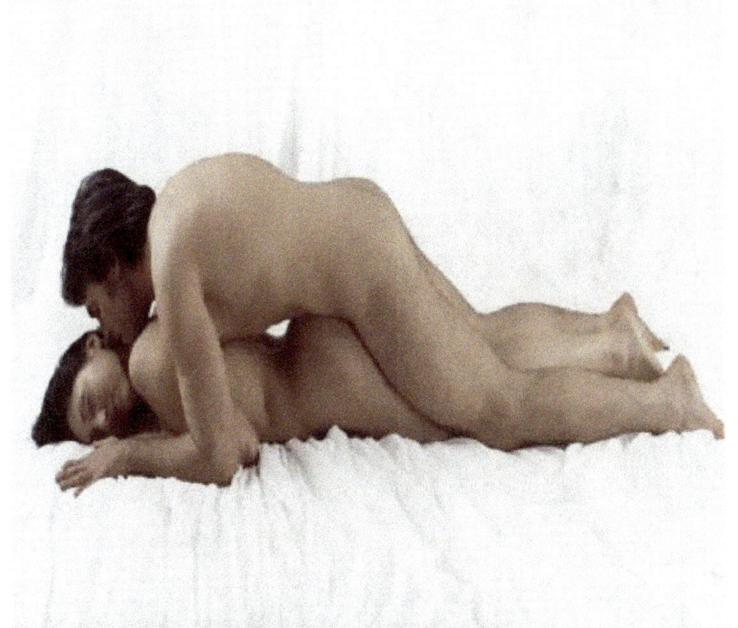

February 20

Torrid Moment

Pressed against each other, both can drink in the sight of their beloved in this position. Self-assured gentleness or boldly brave passion can both work to make this a night to be remembered.

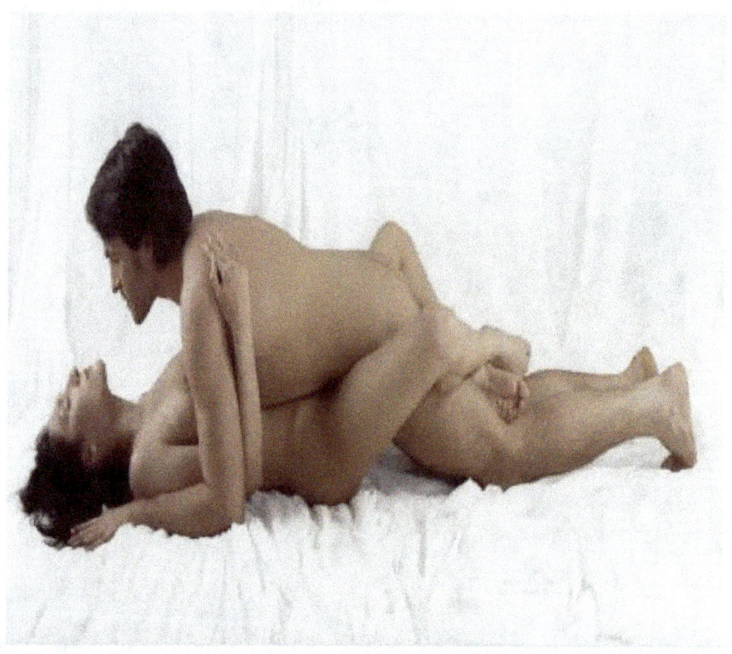

February 21

Again and Again

Pleasure is at a fever-pitch and the woman just keeps asking for more to reach nirvana. Inch by inch her body will rise up and claim what is hers by right.

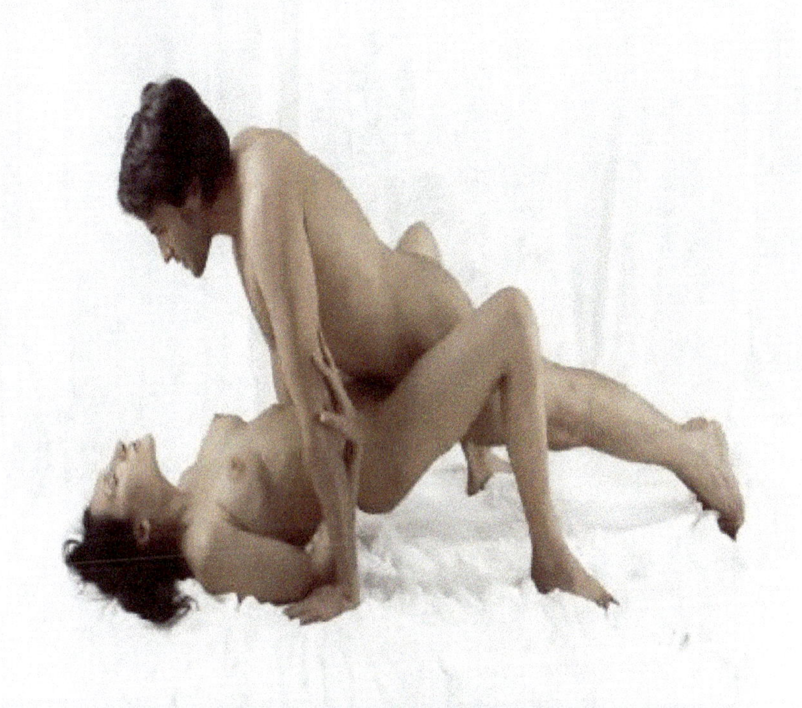

February 22

I'll take you there

Placed perpendicularly, bodies attract and repel each other at the same time. The connecting point is crucial for holding together two unlike beings.

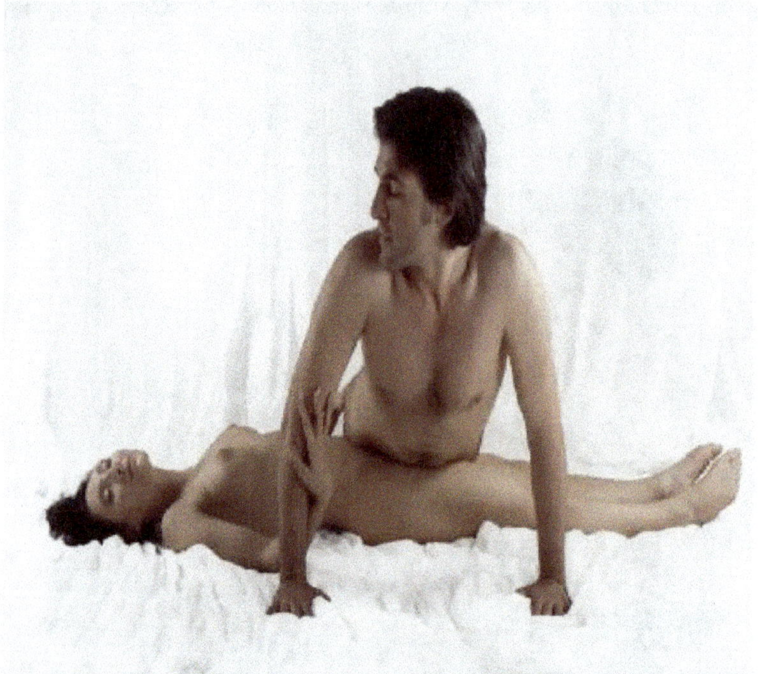

February 23

Discovery

The discovery of the attraction of bodies will always be more interesting than any discovery in sea life or underwater travel; it has the advantage of being practiced naked and with a partner.

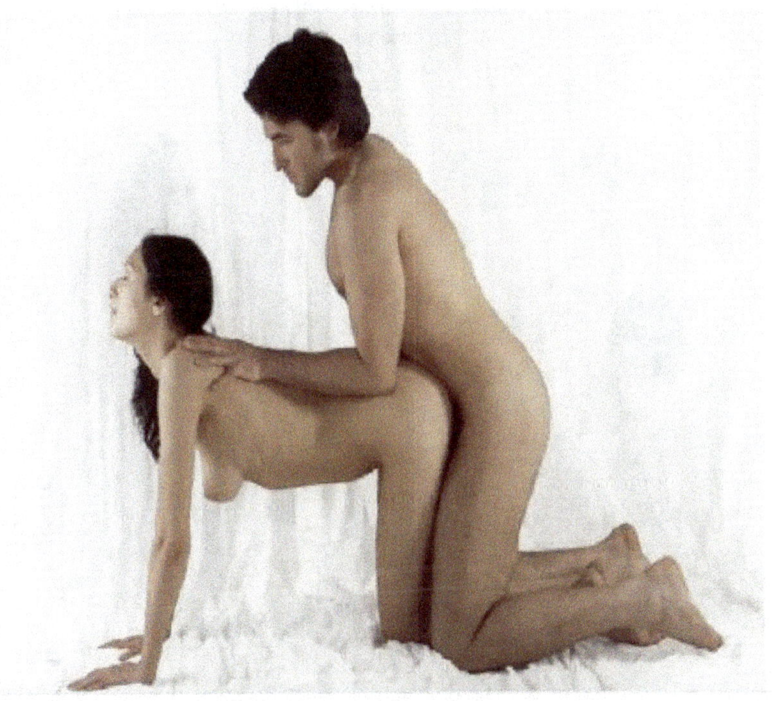

February 24

February 25

Dagger and Sheath

Legs spread and feet forward, man and woman fit together perfectly. The stars of their bodies together makes a new constellation, the most fleeting and most beautiful.

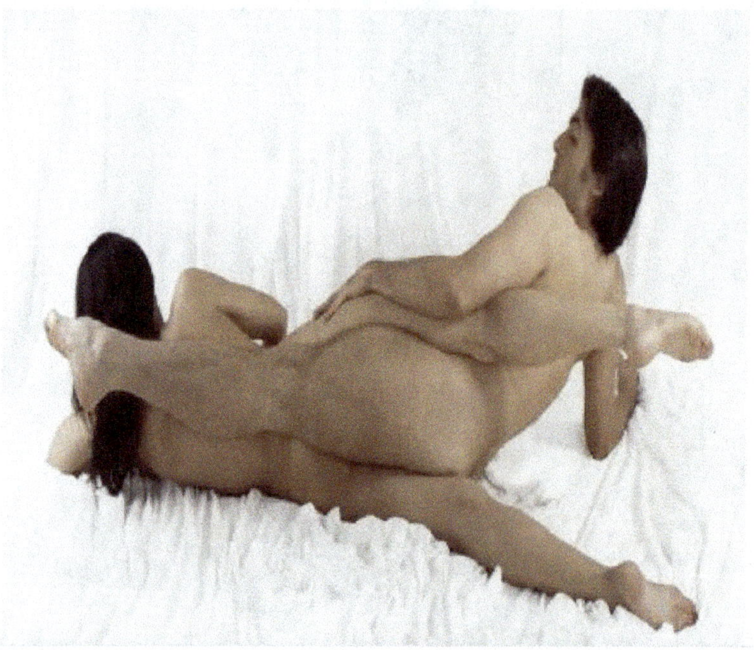

February 26

The Rite of Love

Kneeling at the feet of her king, the woman gives sacred caresses. With the warmth of her mouth are born new royal desires, to kneel in turn at the feet of his queen.

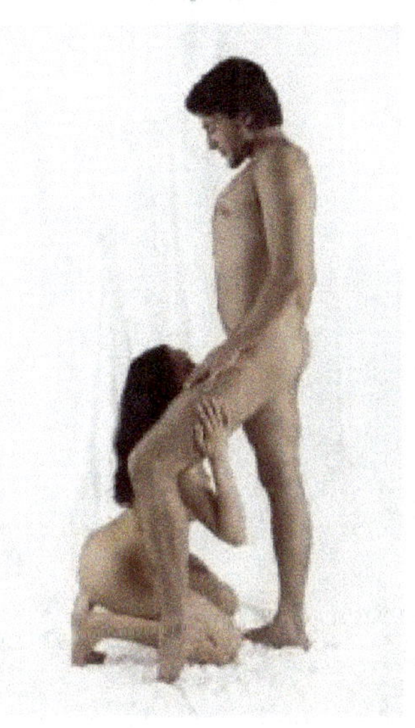

February 27

In the Shade of the Trees

Beneath the branches of hundred year old trees, the welcoming shadows call for a nap and a cuddle. The lovers stretch out to enjoy the torpor of a fine afternoon.

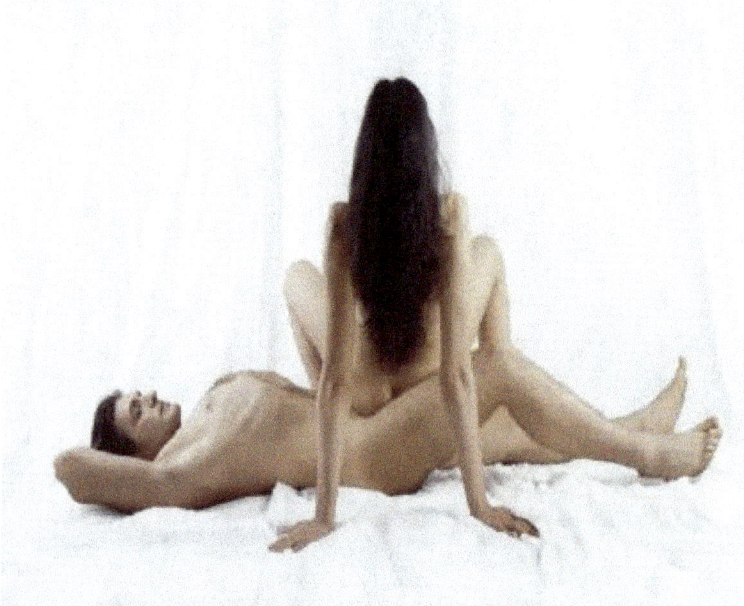

February 28

Ambushed

Hidden in a blind, the huntress may await her prey for many long hours. When the man is finally captured, she will eat her catch alive.

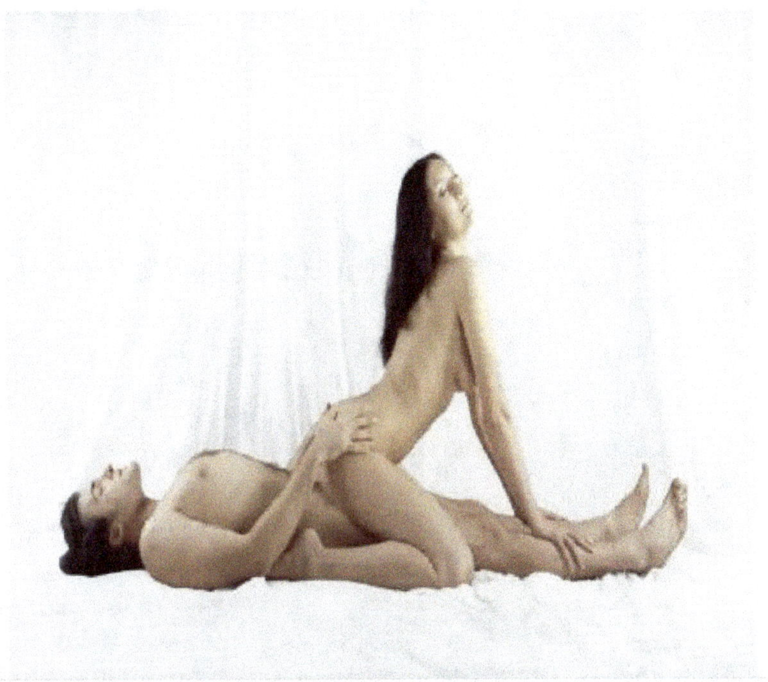

March

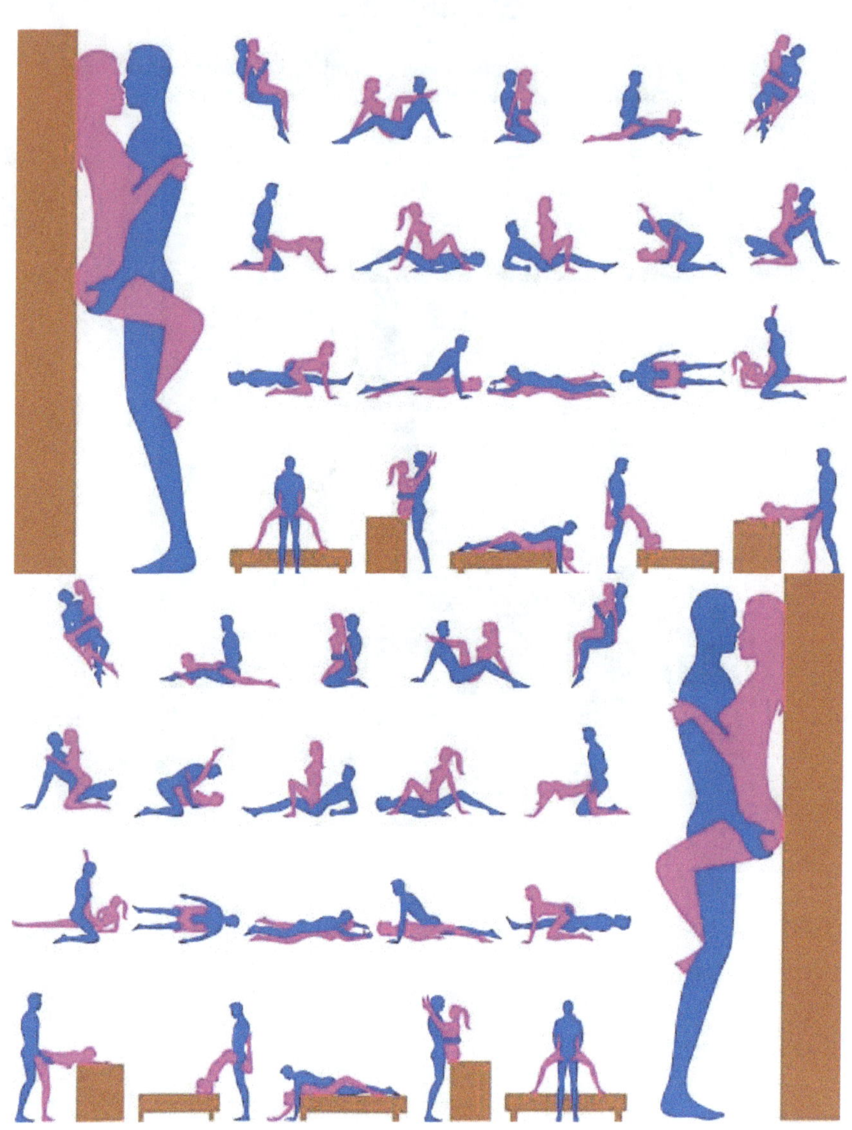

"God, you drive me
absolutely wild."

"I lose my mind
when I'm with you"

"You make me
so horny."

"I need you.
I need all of you."

Foreplay is all about building anticipation. Even if money is a little tight right now, that doesn't mean that the two of you can't dream.

March 1

The Call of Passion

The man is howling at the moon like a wolf when suddenly, overtaken by a sensual frenzy, he pays tribute to his beloved. A pleasant surprise!

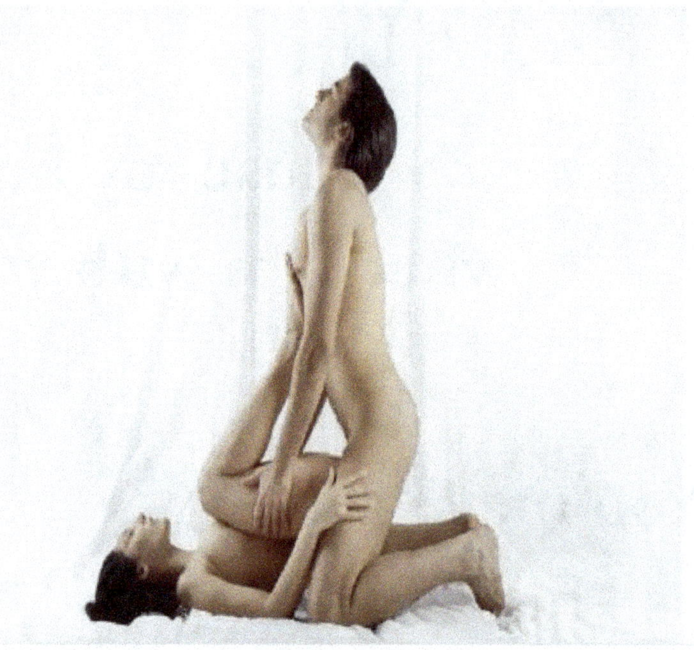

March 2

Don't Go

Holding back a free woman in a vice-like grip, far from easy. Only love can control a wild spirit.

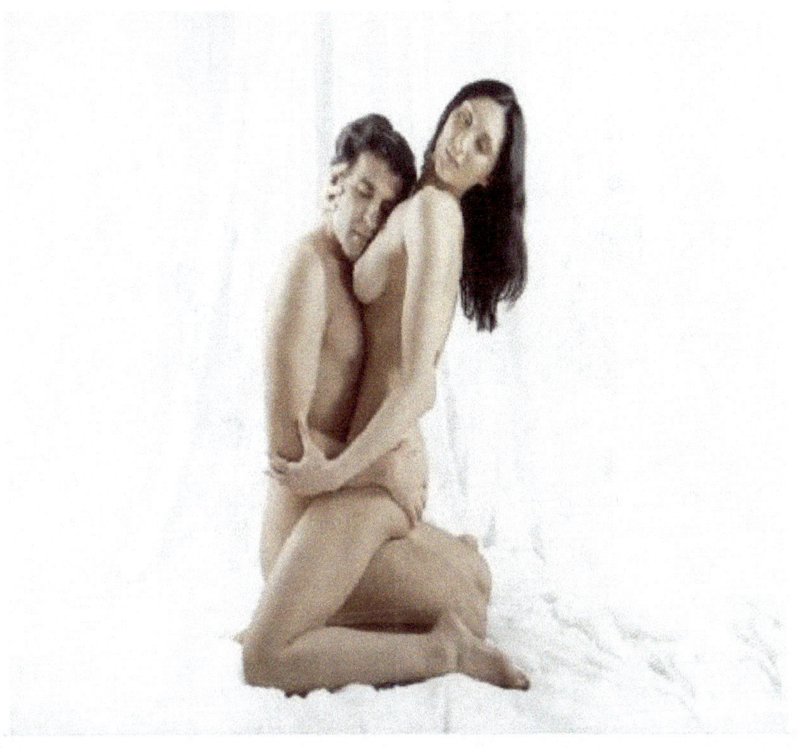

March 3

The Renaissance

Like two butterflies emerging from their cocoon, the two lovers watch their pleasure reborn in this sensual Renaissance period.

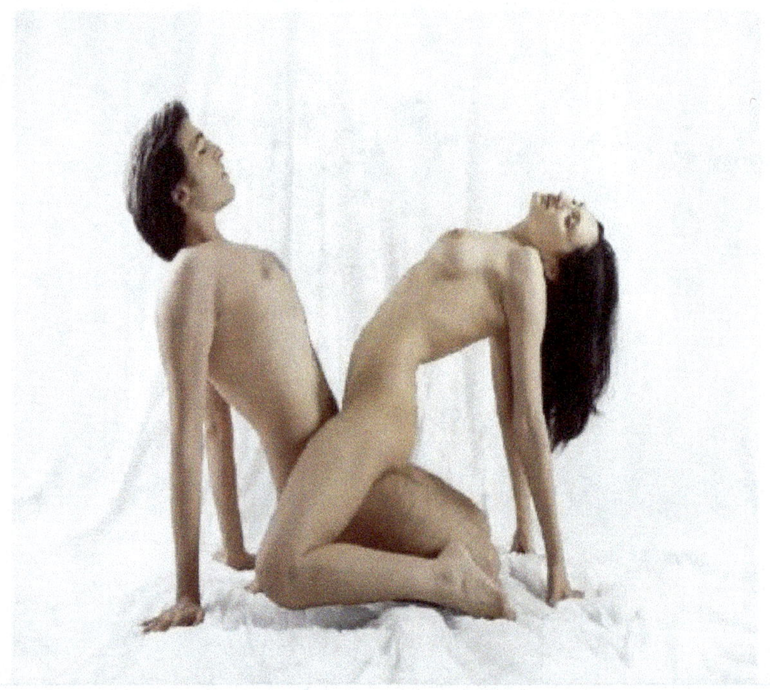

March 4

Now you see me

Tucked into the hollow behind his lover's knees, it is up to the gentleman to control the motion. If the woman wants to play an active role, she'll need firm abs.

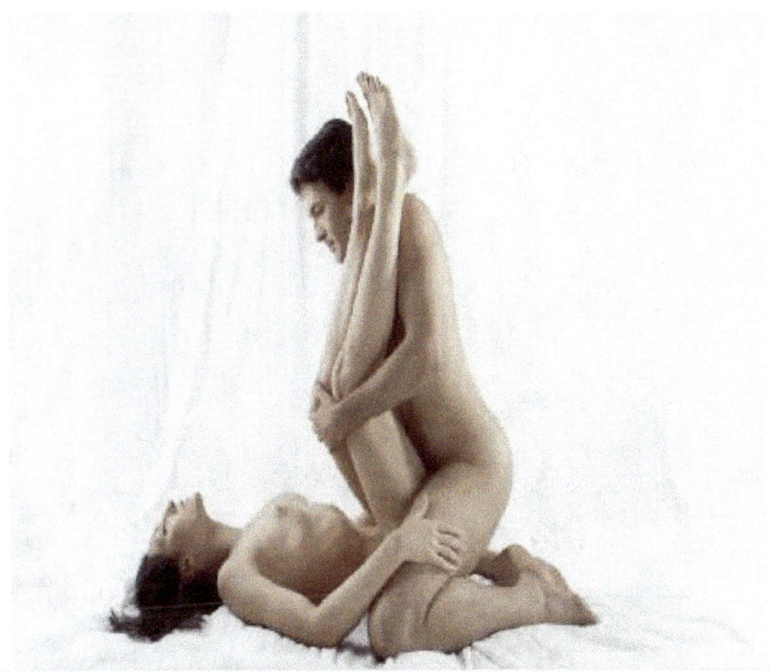

March 5

A Merry-Go-Round

Love will make you lose your head, everybody knows that, and it can also make you lose all sense of backward and forward, left and right, up and down. Love will turn you inside out!

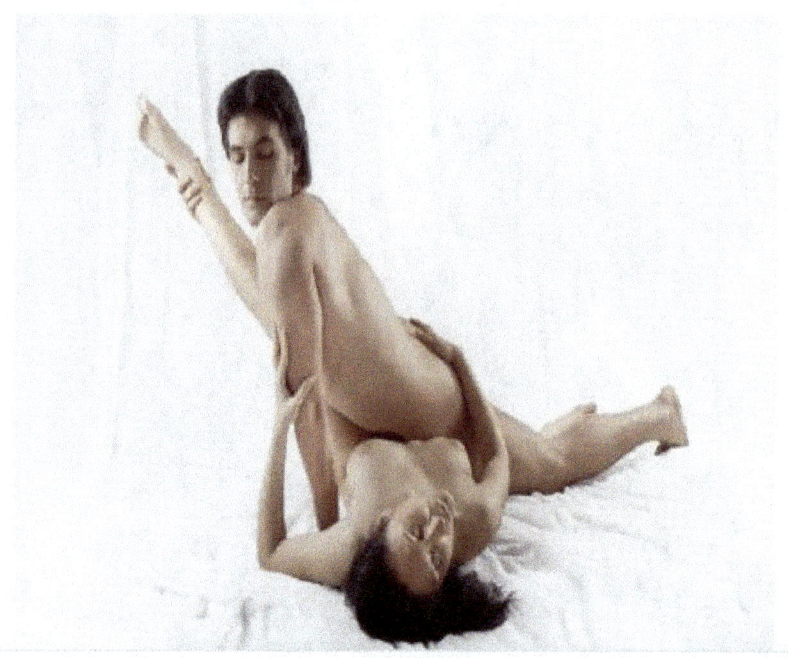

March 6

Look me in the eyes

Contemplating the flash of pleasure in your partner's eyes isn't always possible. Enjoy this position to admire the curves of their face and the expression of delight.

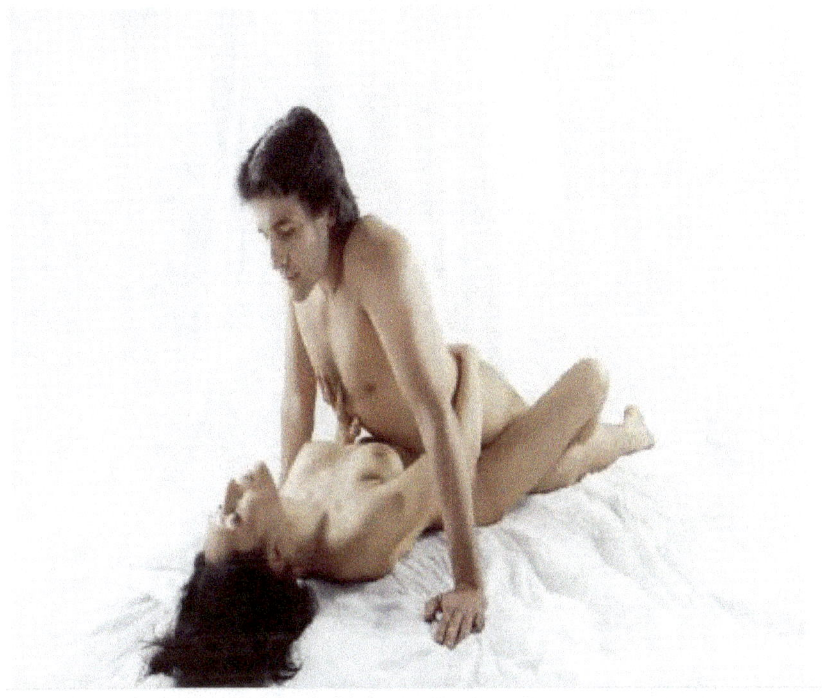

March 7

The Keystone

Forming a couple is like constructing a building. The man is the load-bearing wall and the woman the keystone. A creation to last a thousand years!

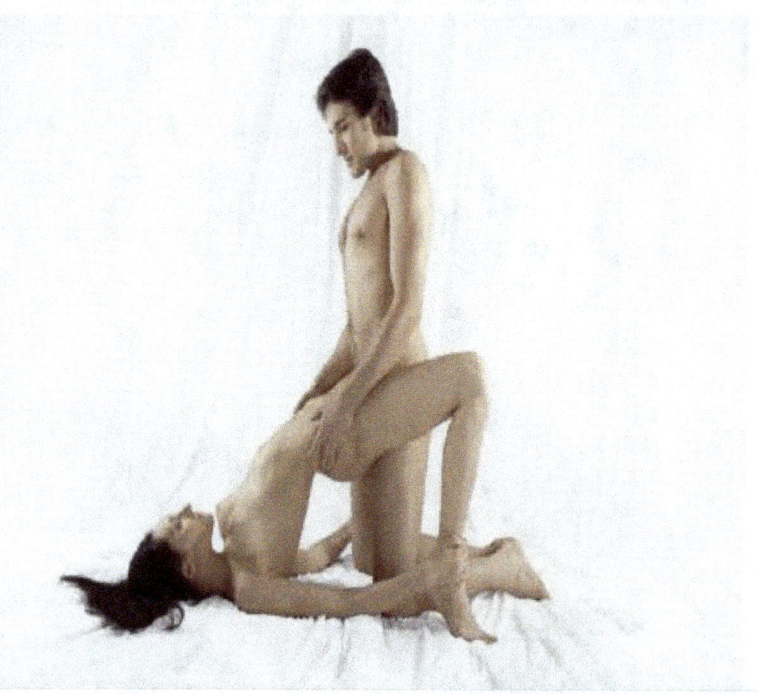

March 8

The Candle

With bodies at right angles, one lying down, the other kneeling, the lovers rise like the flame of a candle to reach new heights.

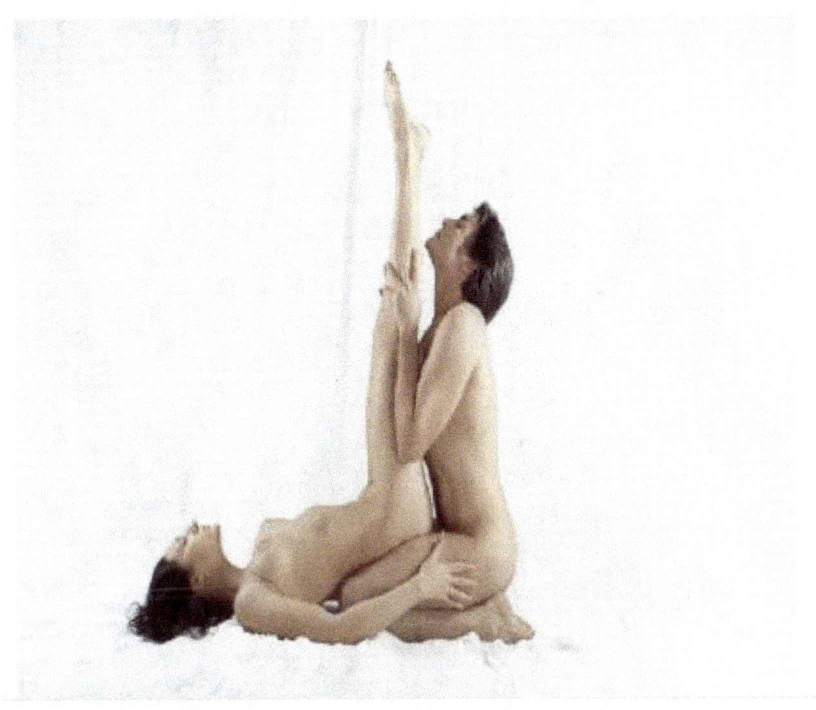

March 9

The Other Profile

Take advantage of this spot with a side view of her feminine curves. It's not everyday that you find yourself on the side so let this be an opportunity for innovation.

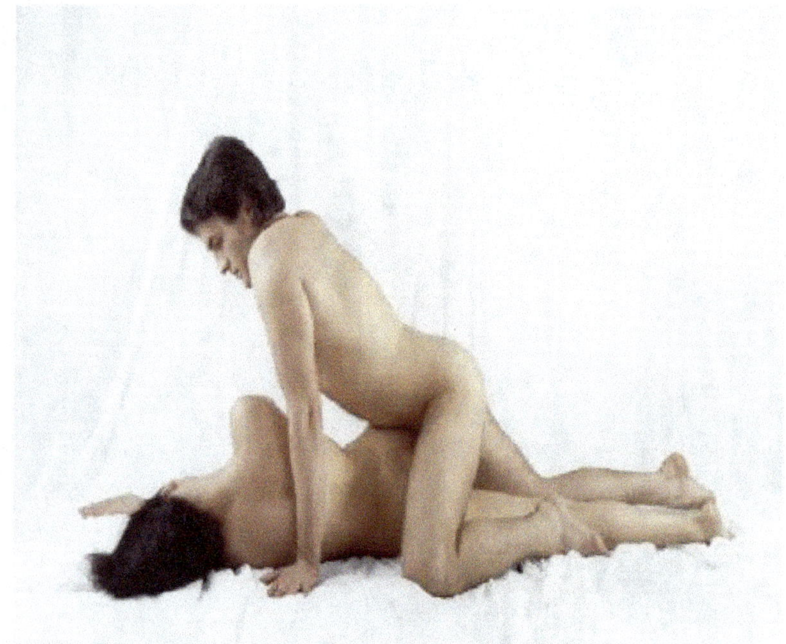

March 10

Indiscrete Little Nook

Wrapped in the warmth of the sheets, the couple takes no more precautions for their privacy. She gently guides her lover's motions so that their caresses are harmonious, matched to the same rhythm.

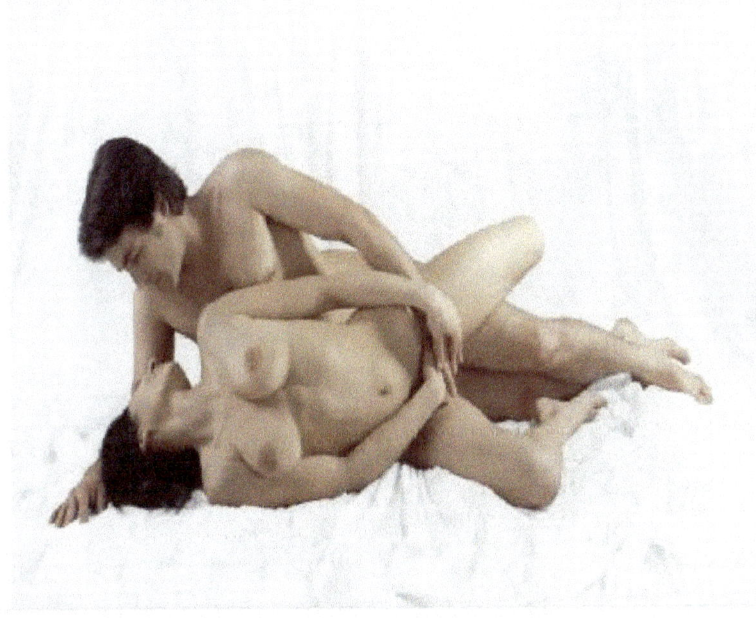

March 11

I'm all yours

Flexibility is a primary quality of good lovers. Extended limbs brush by one another, interlace, intertwine in the most satisfying waltz for the senses.

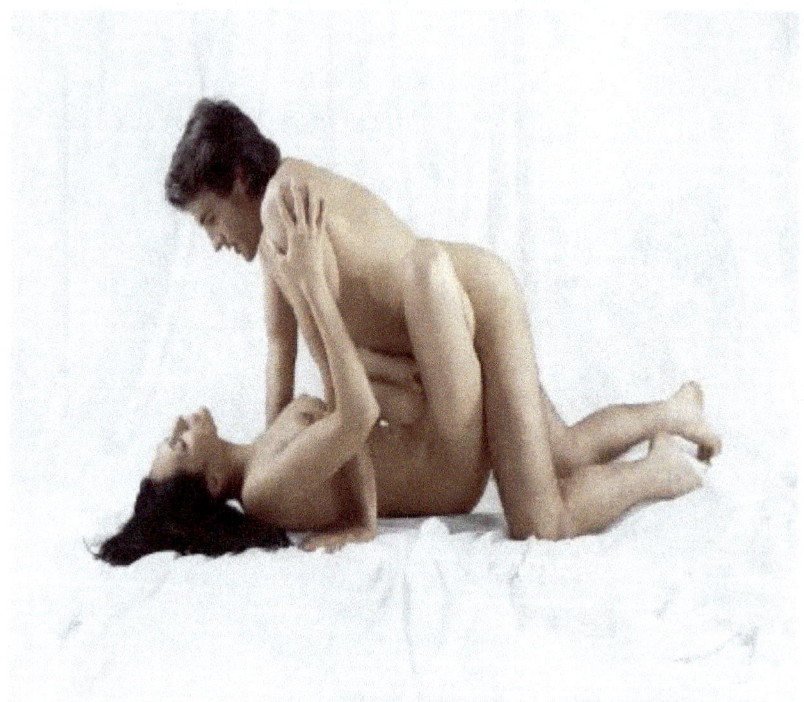

March 12

Masterful Release

Each partner's role is rather distinct, according to their position. The woman may look like she is in a less dominant position but she is the one holding her lover tightly between her legs. You just have to figure out who sets things in motion.

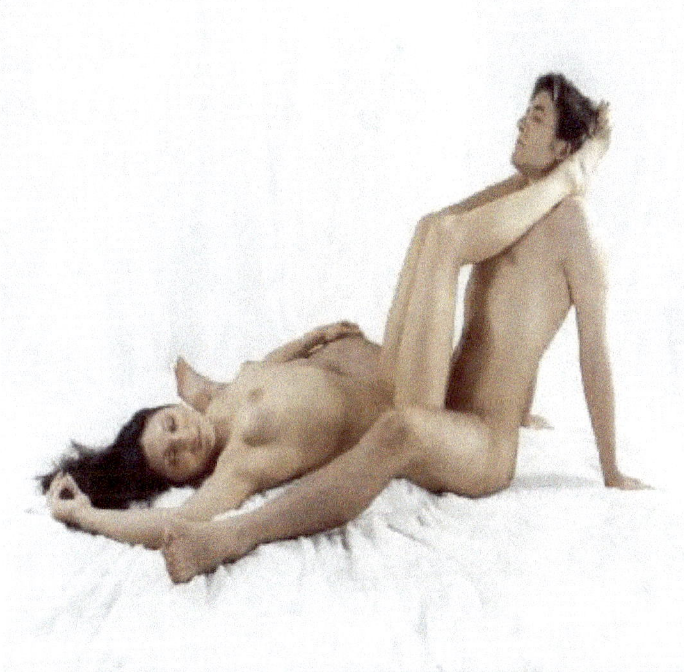

March 13

The Prisoner

With her ankles linked around her lover's neck, the lady has to give in to his masterful thrusts. The libidinous beauty can however draw him towards her or push him away with just the power of her legs.

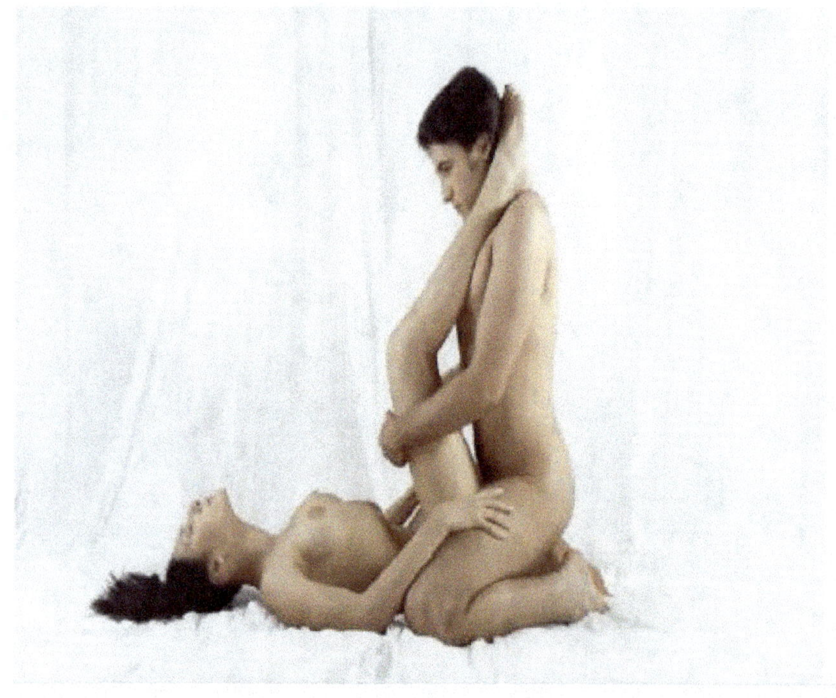

March 14

B as in beautiful

The alphabet can give us quite a few postures, much to the delight of lovers everywhere. This position requires some self-control, but with a little savoir-faire what a beauty!

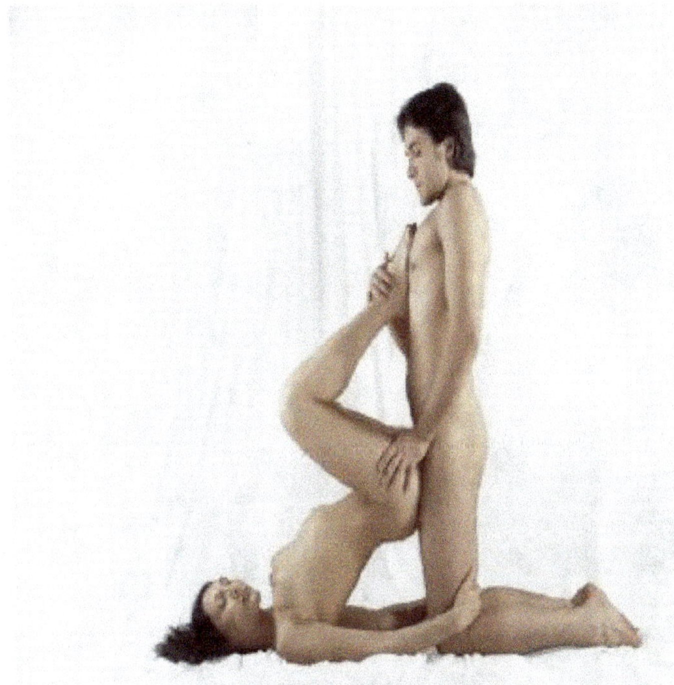

March 15

Savage Lift-off

As hips rise off the ground to meet their partner, they reveal their impatience and pure desire. It is a savage lift-off, a sensual being's gesture that hides nothing of its intentions.

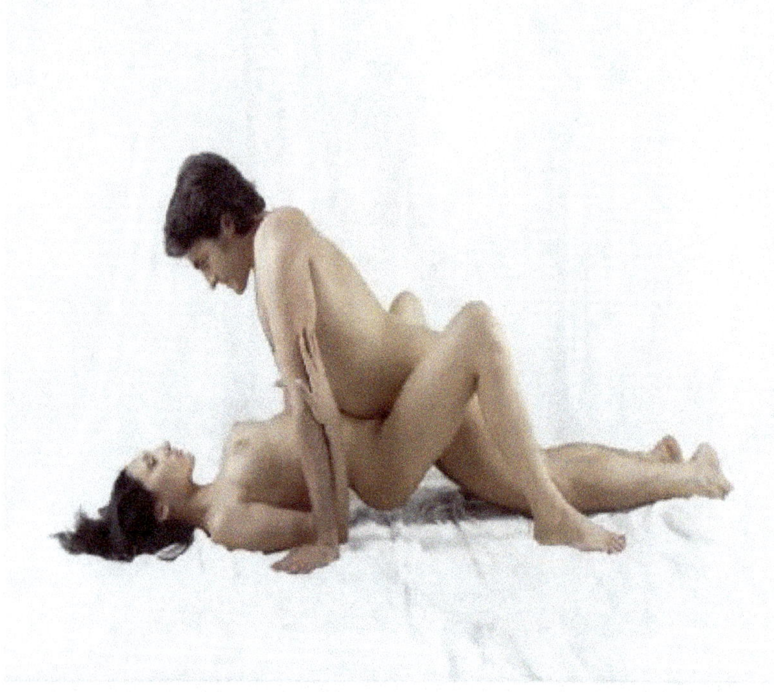

March 16

Tell Me

Sharing one's feelings is a most delicate operation. You have to find just the right moment to move her heart and win her over. A declaration in bed seems right, when she is susceptible.

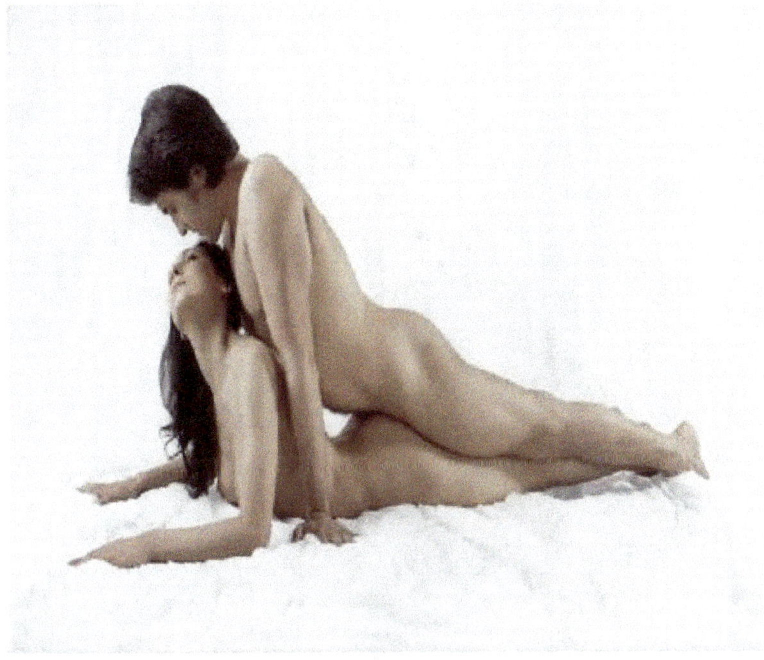

March 17

My Slave

Passion reduces men and women to slaves. Here the man dominates the woman with his imposing frame and she bows before him.

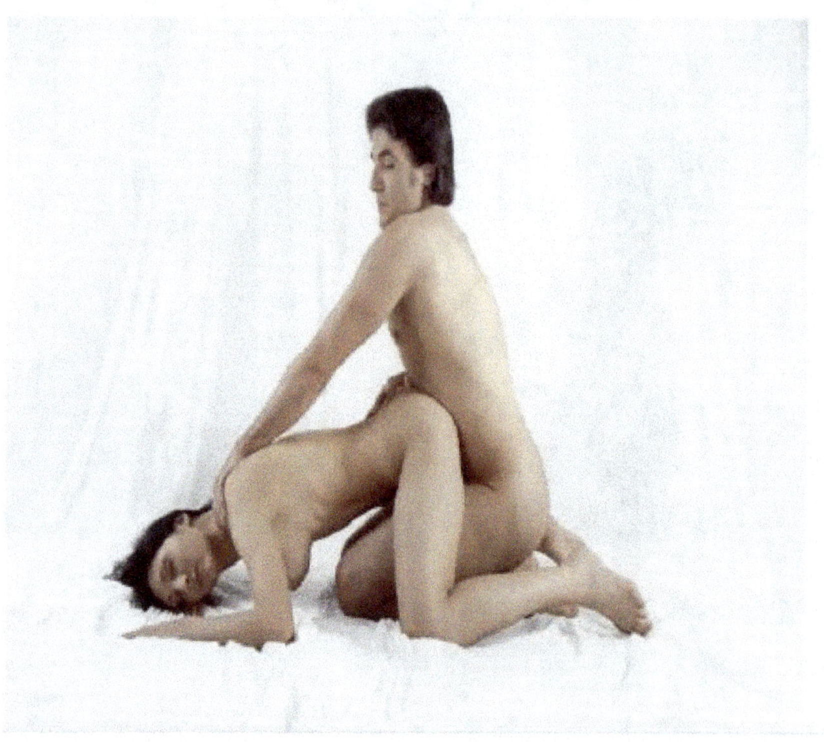

March 18

By Surprise

It's a surprise because the woman can't see who is behind her. She knows perfectly well, but sensations may be heightened when she gives herself free rein to fantasize.

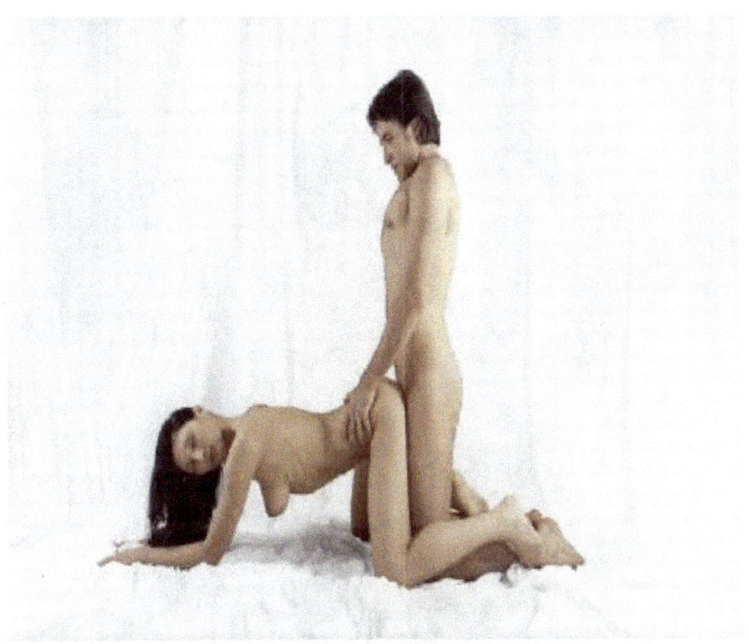

March 19

Height of Delicacy

This pose seems so discrete to the eyes of anyone else; sitting demurely on her partner's lap, what could be simpler? And therein lies the pleasure of this exercise.

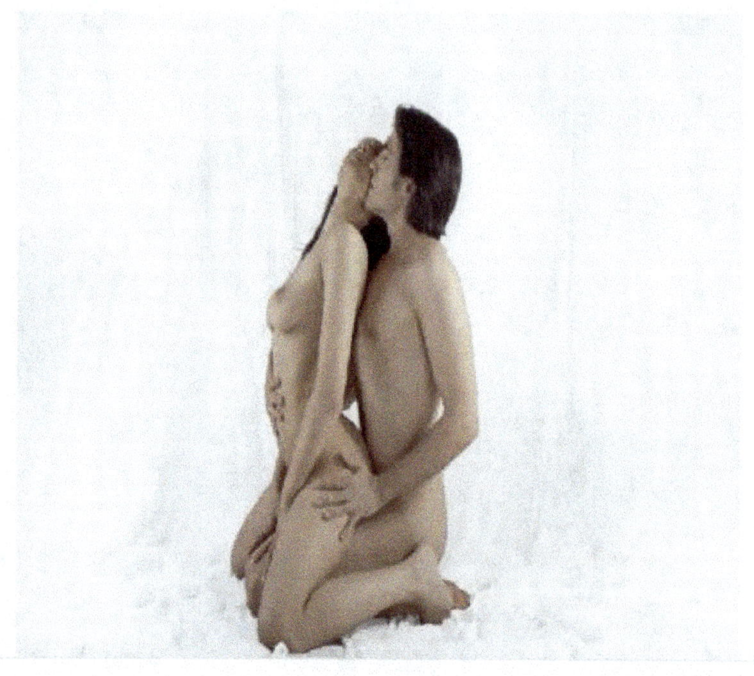

March 20

Cattily Sweet

When a woman acts sweet and cuddly as a kitten, she rounds her back, stretches, arches and rubs against her partner. With a little purr of contentment the metamorphosis is complete.

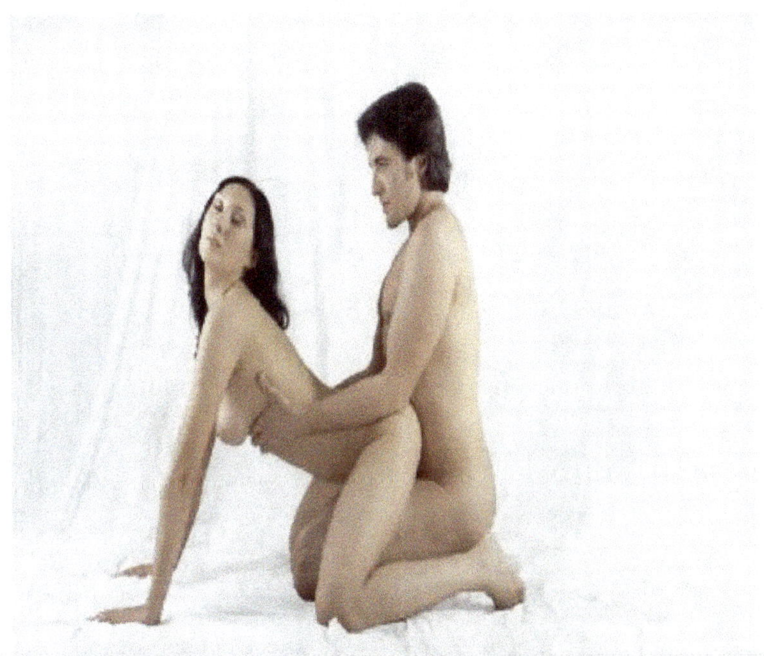

March 21

The Cavern

Held fast by his partner's legs wrapped around his waist, the man discovers the ecstasy behind a few simple truths. This knowledge is a forbidden fruit with a wild flavour!

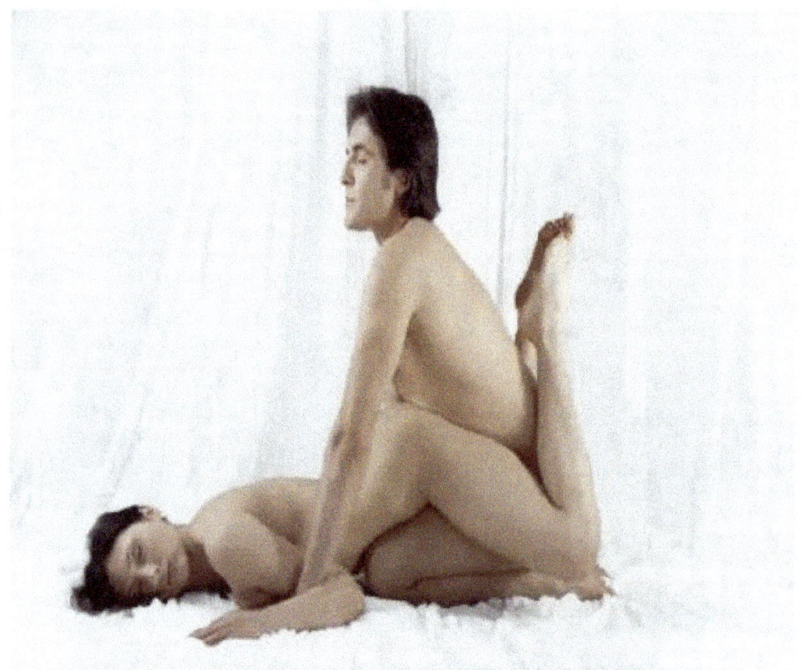

March 22

The Sofa

Giving in to their delights, the couple floats away on an imaginary sofa savouring this magical moment. Their cheeks pressed together thrill with their hot breath, mingling and mixing in a shared rhythm.

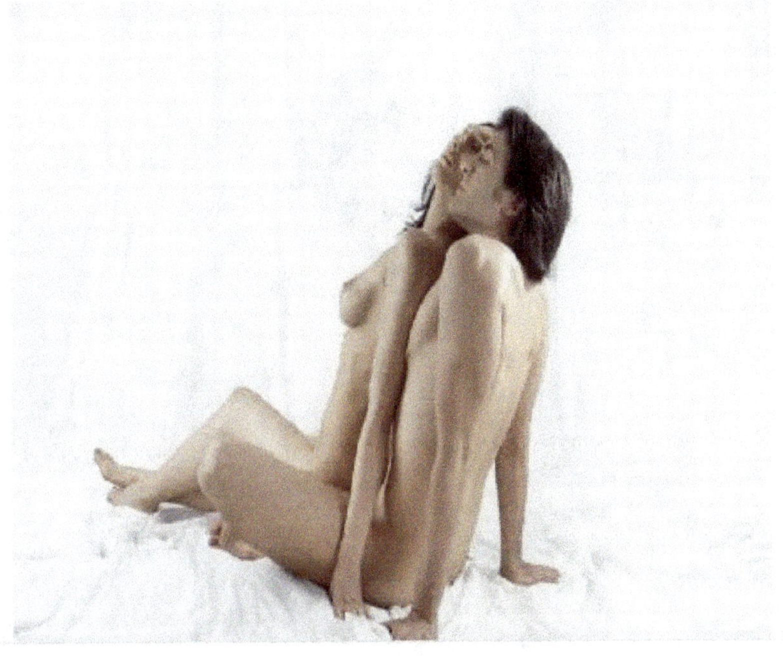

March 23

Comfortable Seating

With her partner's hands locked around her waist the woman can concentrate all her energy on a particular axis, multiplying sensations and vibrations. The soft seat balances out the heat at the core.

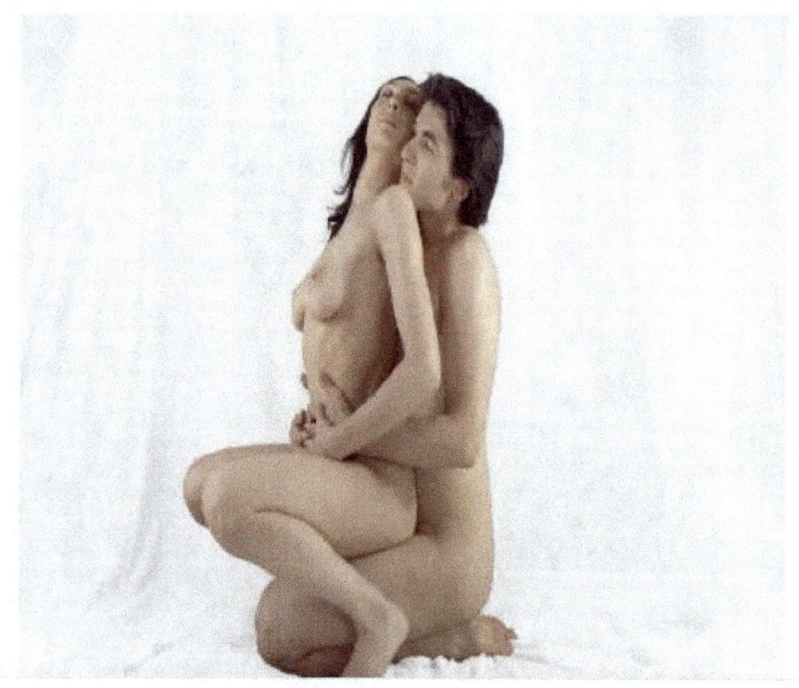

March 24

The Sphinx

Forearms and knees on the ground, the sphinx nonchalantly dominates the ages. His graceful, eternal face, just made to be worshiped, reminds mere mortals how fleeting is their own beauty.

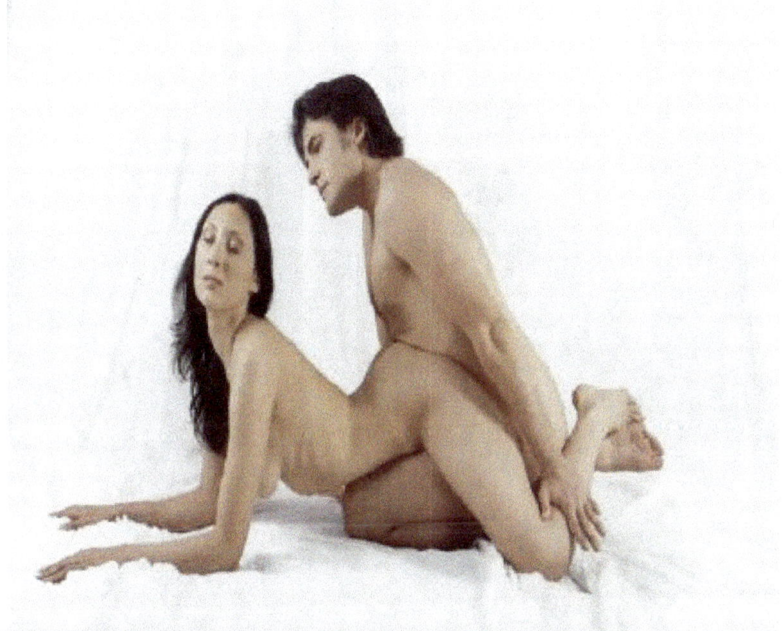

March 25

The Duel

Armed to the teeth, highway robbers never hesitate when it comes to taking advantage of someone weaker. But his victim has a trick or two in her bag as well and so a duel it is. This is just the beginning of close combat.

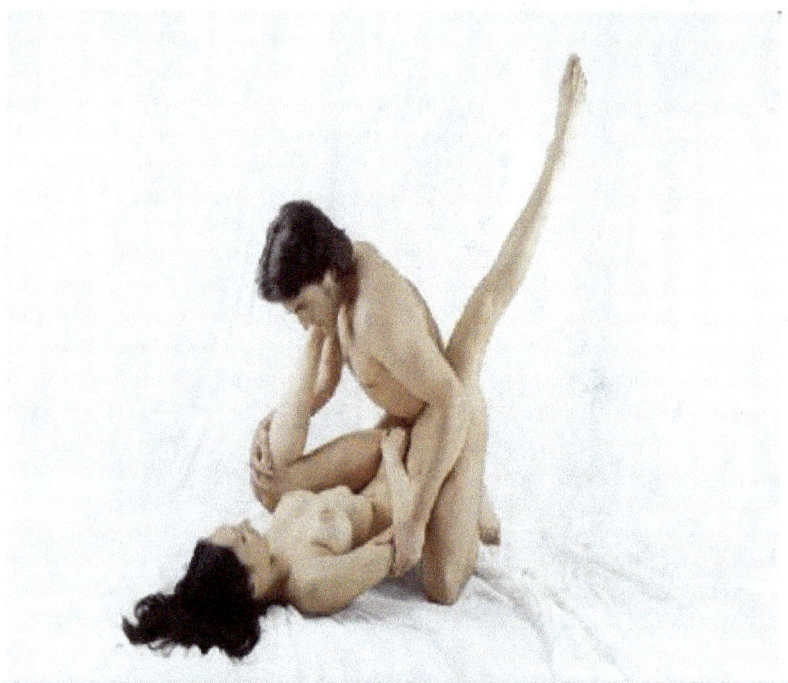

March 26

Sensuous Stroll

Seated on her partner, the woman can perfectly control the back and forth motion of her hips. By leaning slightly forward or backward she can find just the right angle for dizzying, sensational effects.

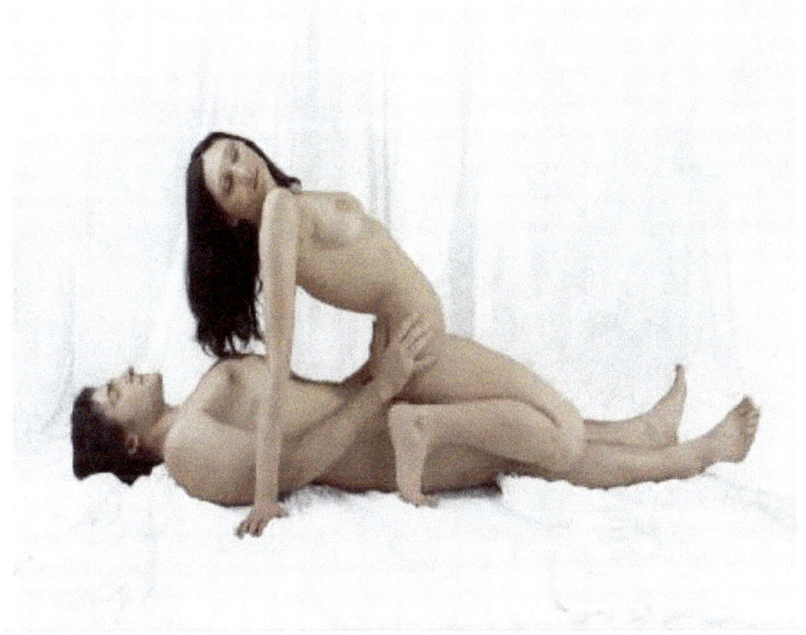

March 27

Fusion

Linked together and on their side, the lovers meeting here is one of the deepest. Staring into each others eyes and with their bodies intertwined, they are brought home riding the same wave of pleasure.

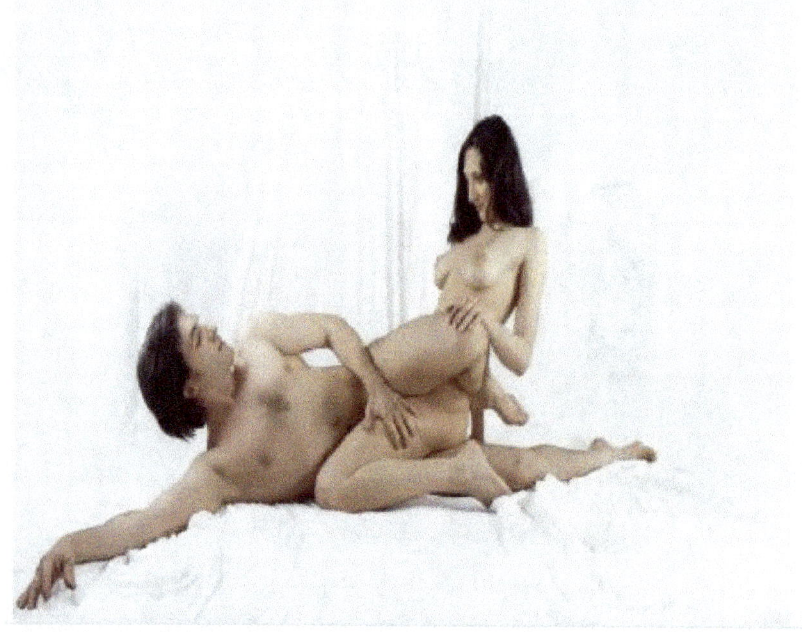

March 28

Tell me who you are

Tell me who you are and I'll tell you who I am. This isn't an interrogation but it's true that during intimate moments you learn the most about someone, so enjoy!

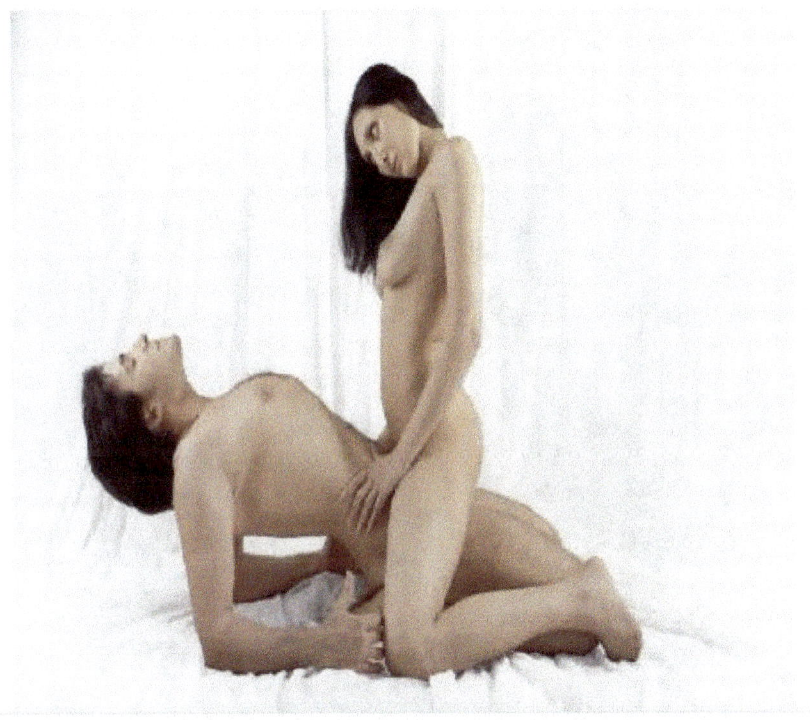

March 29

Guilty as charged

The woman feels the need to take matters into her own hands and call the shots for a while. The man doesn't really have much choice here, but what he doesn't mention is that he loves it this way...

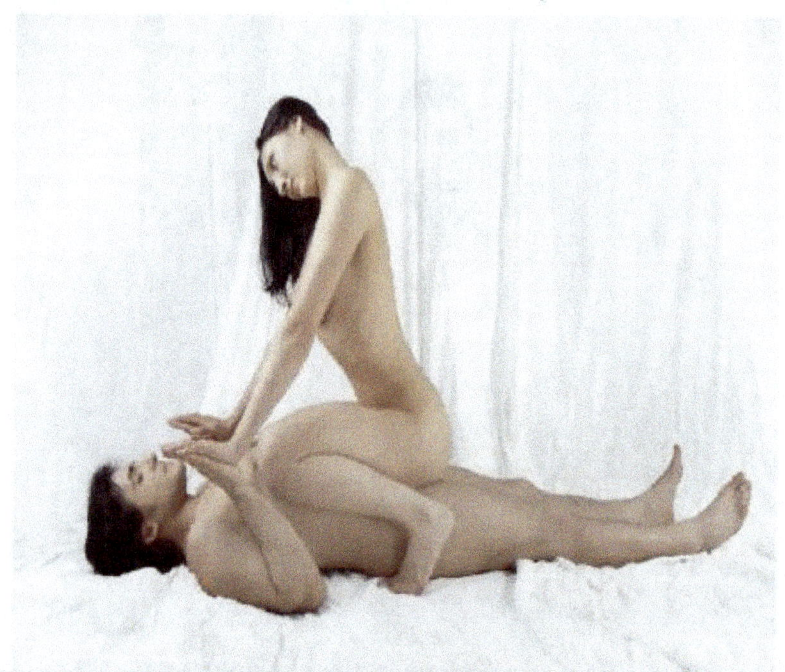

March 30

The Conquering Heroine

In this position, the woman can take control and make the decisions - especially the rhythm and depth of their relations. The man is caught in her trap and must submit to the desires of his beloved.

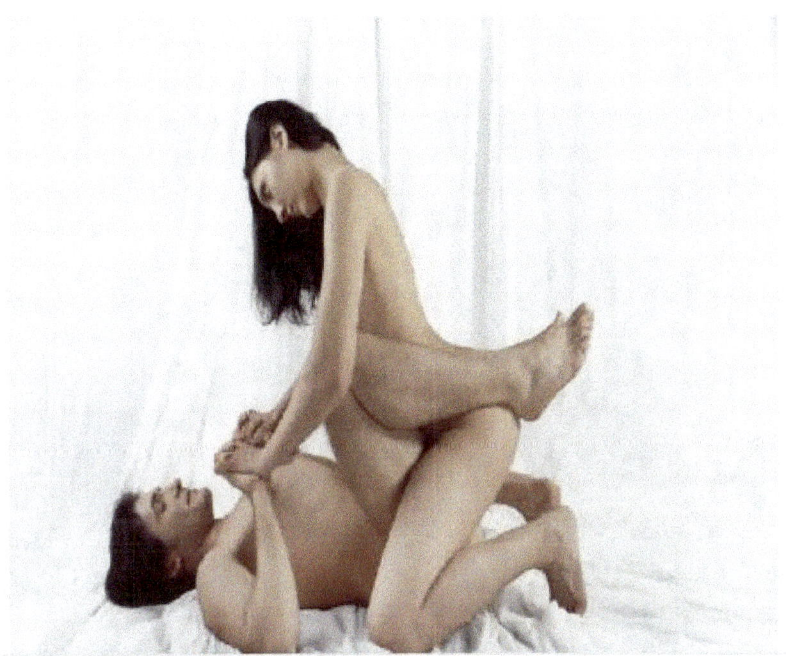

March 31

Caught in a Trap

The man is caught in a trap and completely at his partner's mercy. She takes advantage of the moment and immobilises his feet to avoid any uncontrolled movement. We can tell who's in charge here.

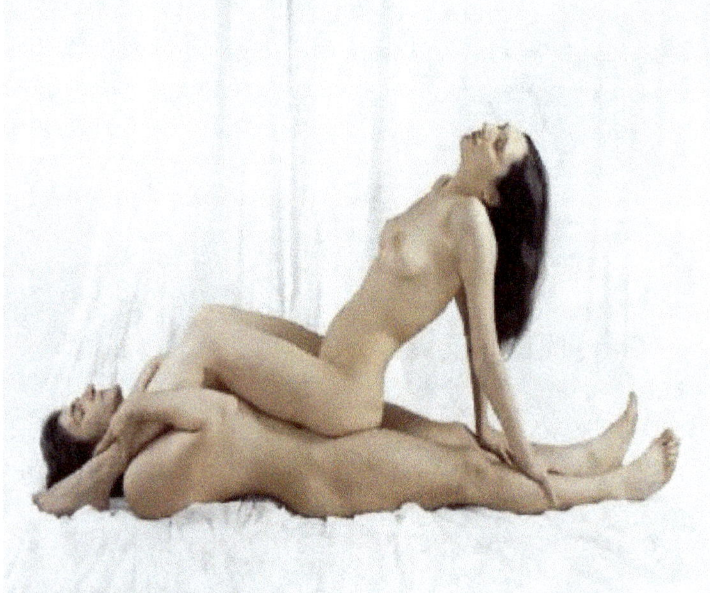

April

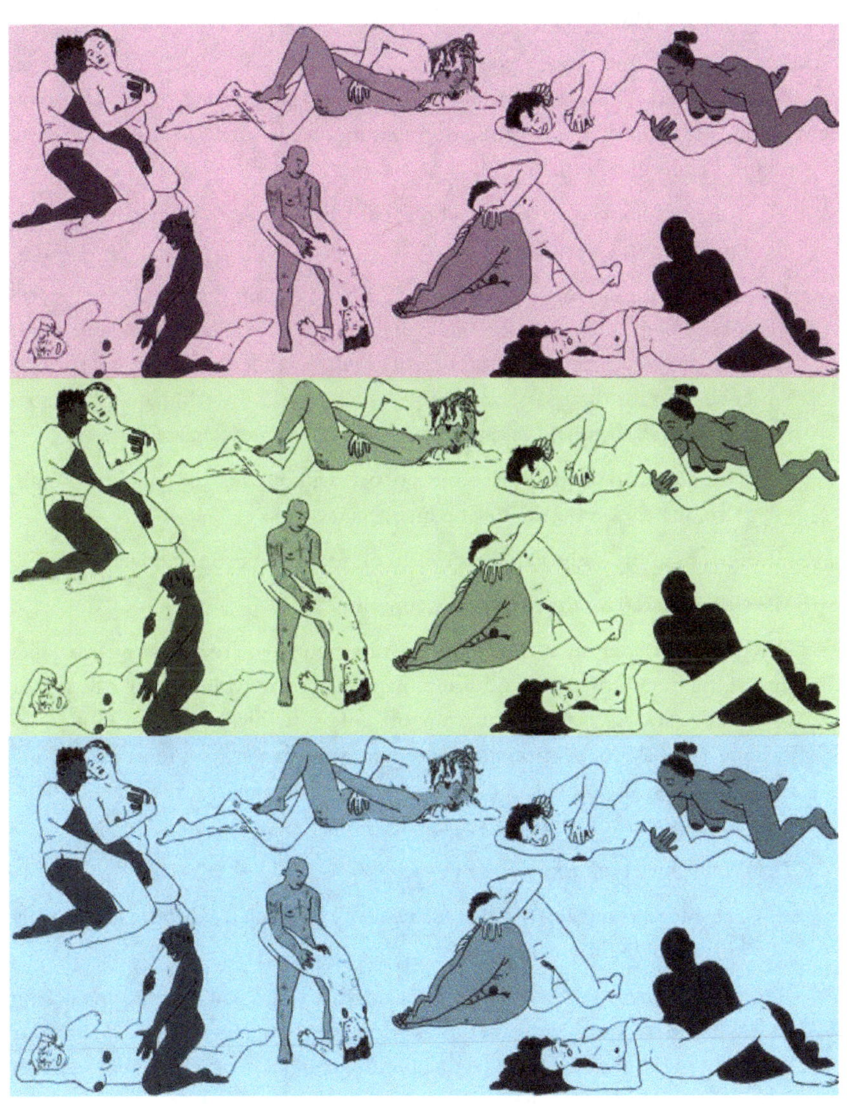

Ally's Dirty Talk Hall of Fame

➢ The guy who wouldn't let me cum unless I begged him for it. Orgasms are just so much more enjoyable when you earn them.

ME: "I'm going to cum!"

HIM: "Don't you dare! Don't you fucking dare cum yet! I did NOT give you permission to cum. Do you hear me? You CANNOT cum until daddy gives you permission, so if you want my permission to cum, you're going to have to fucking beg me for it like a good little slut."

➢ The guy I hooked up with at a hotel bar who seemed to have a very specific fantasy… Still, **very** hot.

"I'm going to throw you down on the bed, rip off all your fucking clothes, ravish your naked body, then fuck the everloving shit out of you until I get your squirt on every single surface in the hotel. Better hydrate while you can, baby, because I'm going to turn that pussy into motherfucking Big Foot Rapid. And grab a fucking snorkel, sugar tits, because there **WILL** be water damage."

➢ The guy who wouldn't let me go pee without his dick in my mouth. Also, the reason buying toilet paper gets me wet.

HIM: (kicks in the bathroom door) "The fuck you think you're doing in here?"

ME (sitting naked on the toilet) "Uh… peeing?"

HIM: "Not without my fucking cock in your mouth, you're not. Now open that slutty little mouth of yours and listen. Anytime you're with me, my rule is that you're not allowed to take your pants off unless my dick is in your mouth. So anytime you have to go pee and every time you shower, you must be sucking daddy's cock at all times. And if I ever catch you breaking my rules, there will be punishments and you will be disciplined."

Thankfully, he let me take a shit in peace.

➢ The guy who screamed this at me while I was riding his dick was apparently a blackbelt in dirty talk:

"I'm going to cum inside of you so fucking hard that you're going to fucking taste it in the back of your throat for weeks! Then I'm going to cum down your throat for good measure, and keep cumming until all my fucking cum replaces your brains that I fucked all the way out of your fucking skull and you have cum dripping down your fucking ears, and I'm not going to fucking stop until you're positively drenched in my cum, from the inside out, so when you go to do a DNA test it'll say you're 99.9% made up of cum!"

April 1

The Butterfly

The lovers' legs make the shape of a butterfly. The woman leads the dance and is able to alter the thrusting of her hips as she wishes.

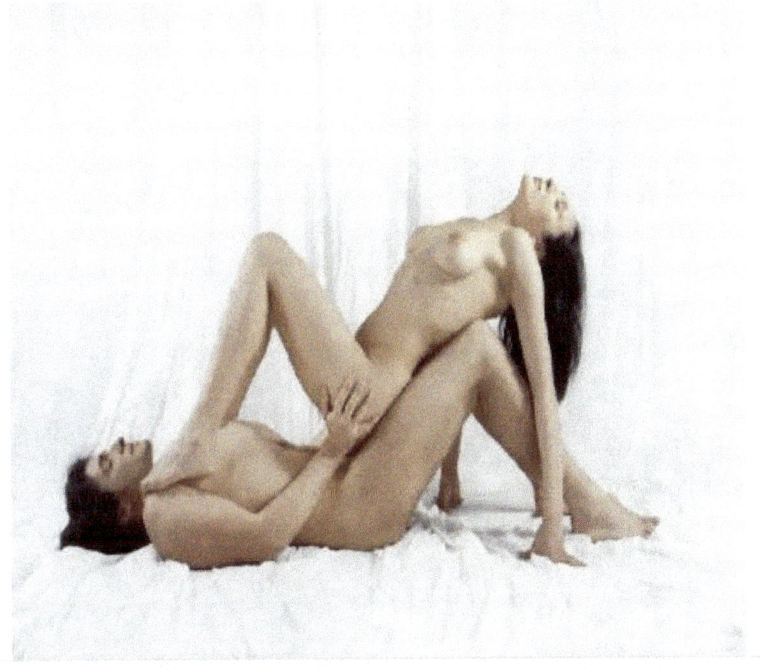

April 2

Andromeda

Skin against skin, this position leaves the woman free to lead the lovers' dance to new heights of ecstasy. The man can increase her pleasure by running his hands over her back.

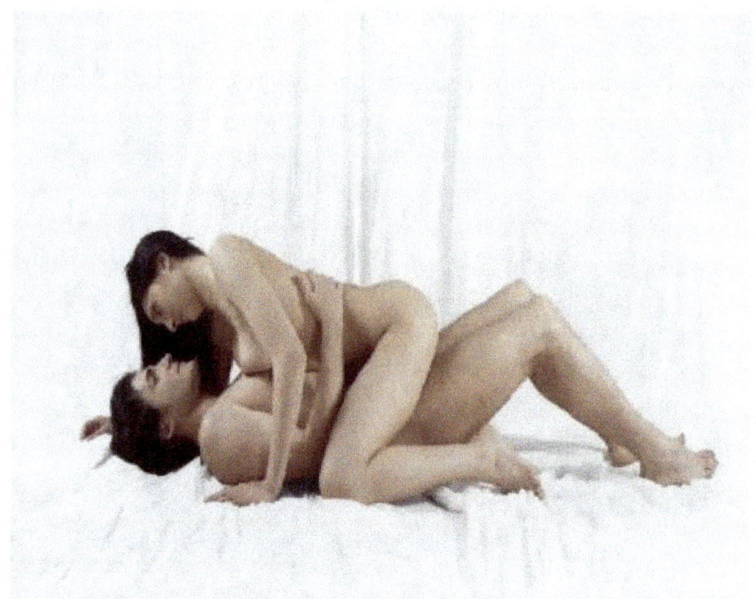

April 3

From a Different Angle

Sitting on her partner's stomach, the woman can watch his reactions to the motion of her hips. He can hold her and help her find the most attractive angle.

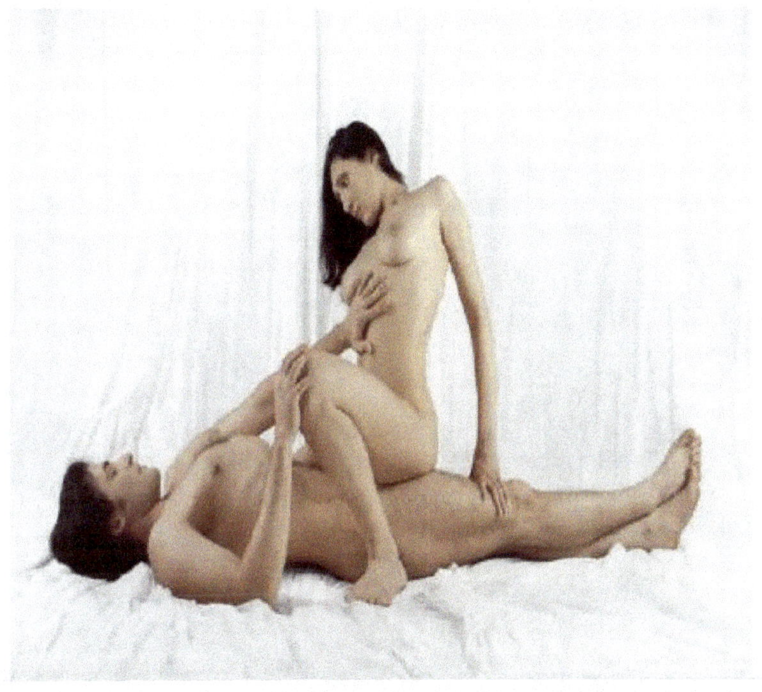

April 4

With Emotion

In addition to the unbelievable sensations that this position provides, the angle allows the lover to admire his partner's fantastic shapes and the curves of waist, hips and buttocks.

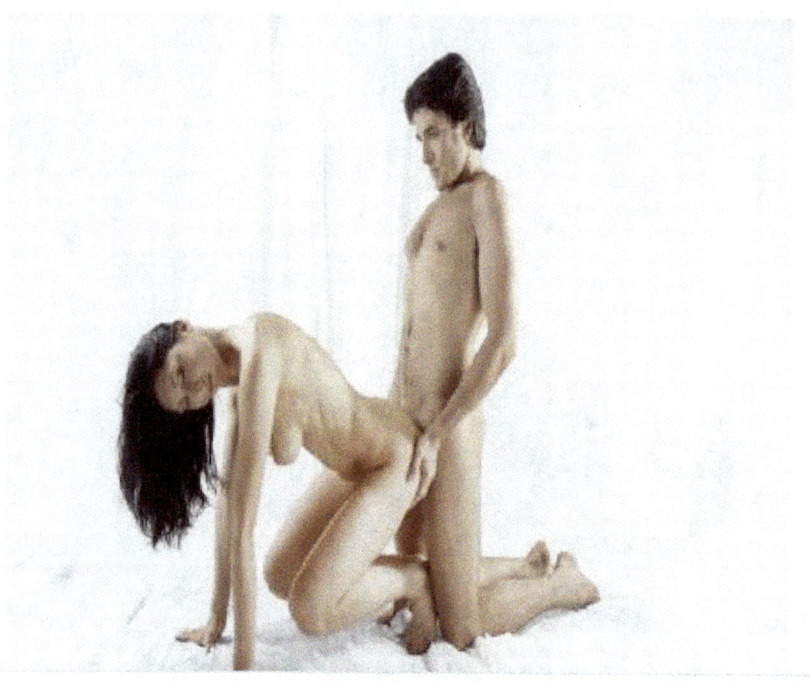

April 5

Perfect Union

This position requires flexibility and an ability to let go on the woman's part but allows a very deep union between the couple. Their coming together is perfect, their looks lascivious.

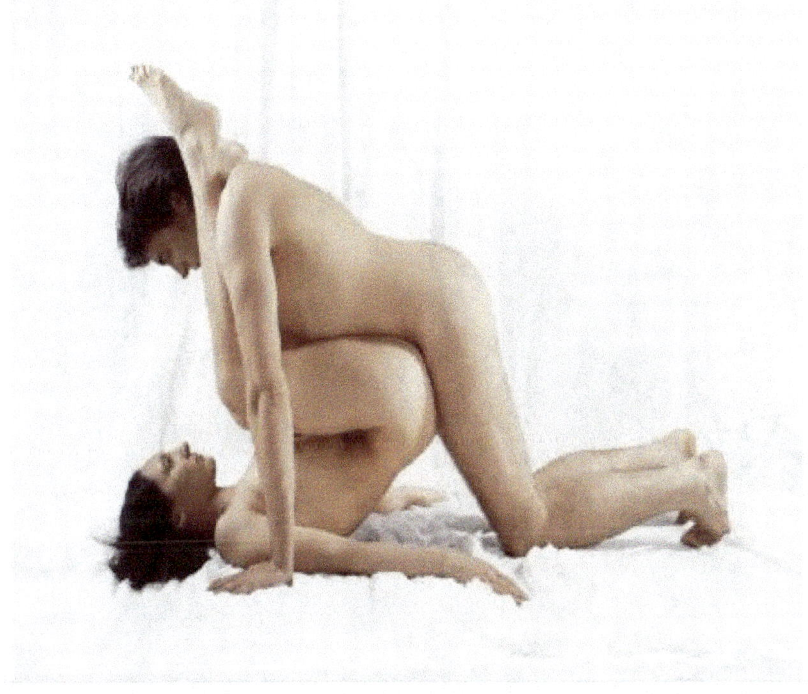

April 6

So Supple

This might look uncomfortable but that's not necessarily the case if you go about it right. The man will need to make use of his hips to reach the desired results.

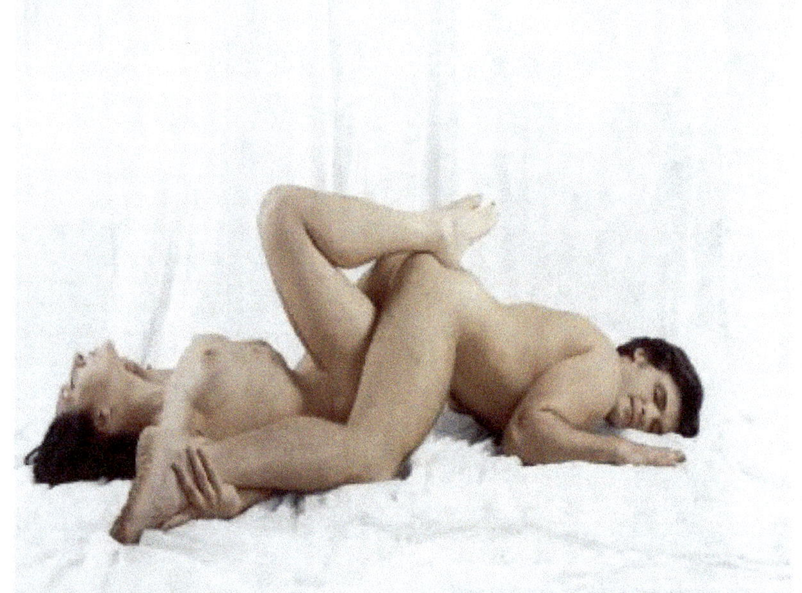

April 7

Upside Down

The symmetry of the position means both lovers can devote their full attention to a single thing - the movements of their hips which will lead them to ecstasy.

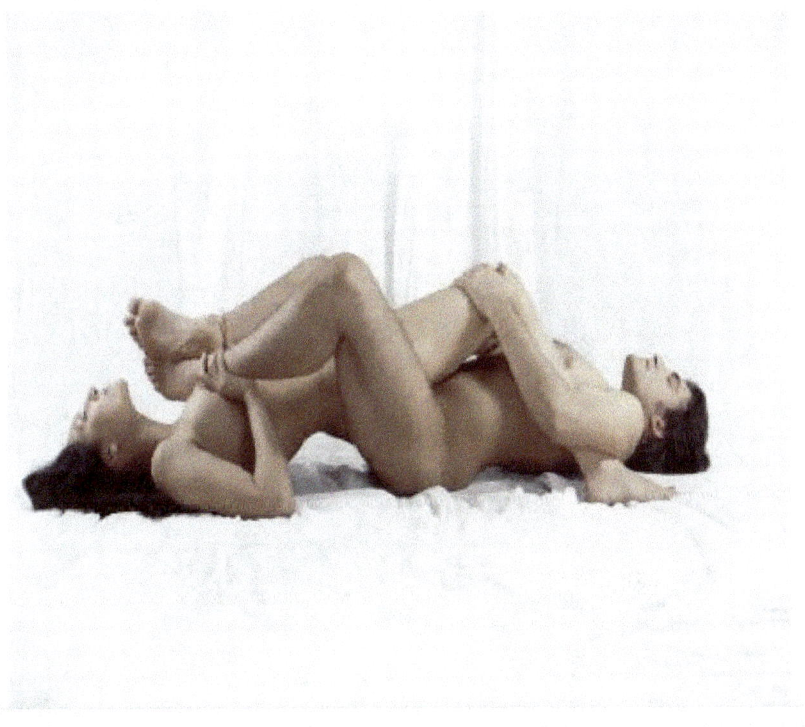

April 8

The Swing

With her back to her partner, the woman directs the sensual rhythm of these games. Meanwhile, her lover's unoccupied hands can travel freely across her swinging body.

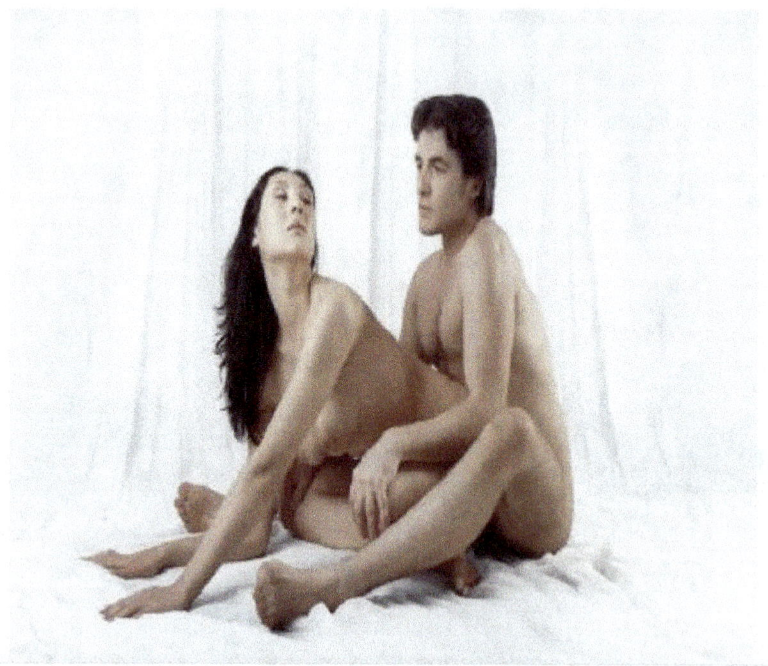

April 9

Flying Trapeze

As if weightless, the woman's body stretches as she gives in completely to her partner's desire. Here, a quick break gives flight to their desire.

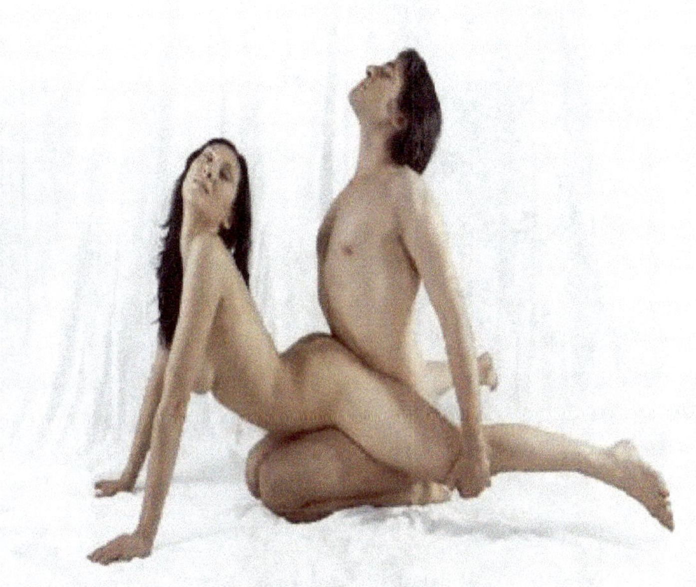

April 10

With Relish

The man kneels to accommodate his flexible partner on his stomach. The beautiful man-eater holds the hottest prey in her grasp. It's going to be a good meal.

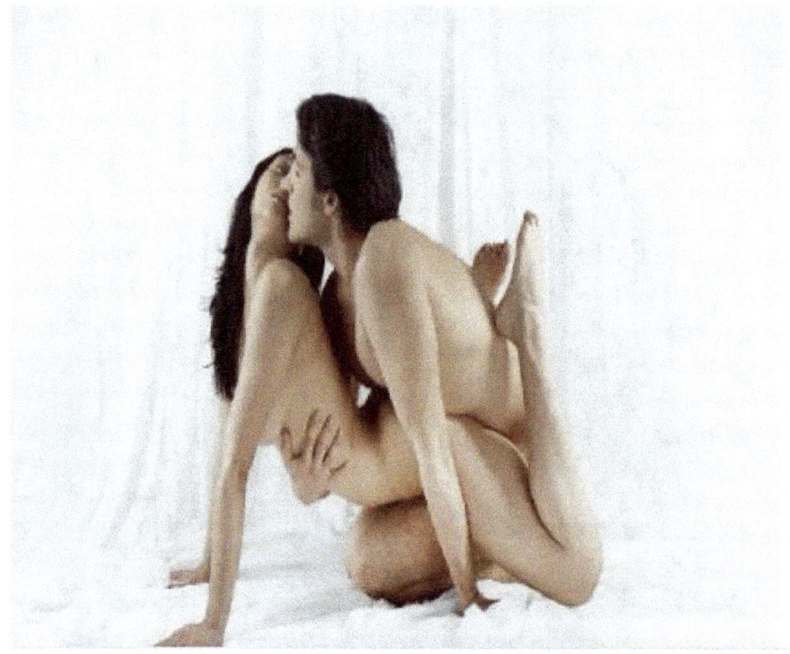

April 11

Hot Seat

The woman takes her pleasure on the most comfortable of divans. A soft seat for her, an audacious angle for him, and both partners will rise to new heights.

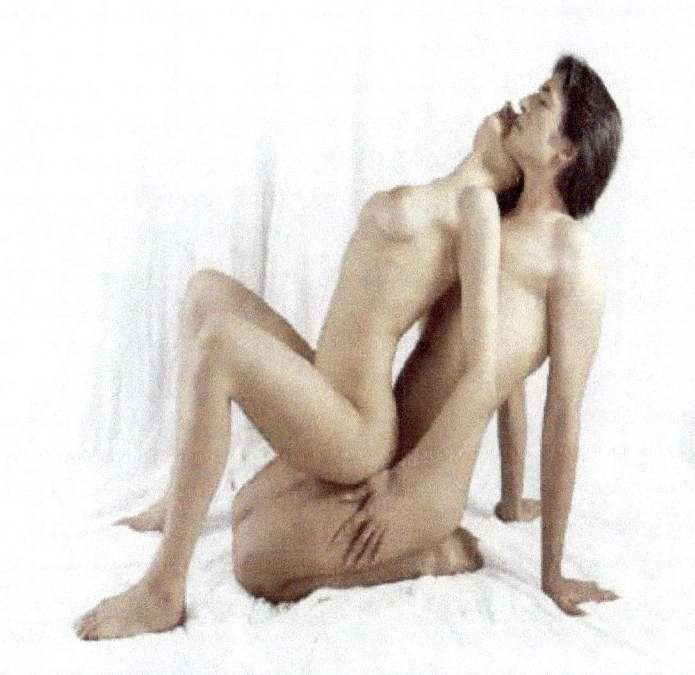

April 12

Devilish Massage

This position looks like it's for an innocent massage while it is anything but that. The partners use touch to increase the pleasure of this intense moment.

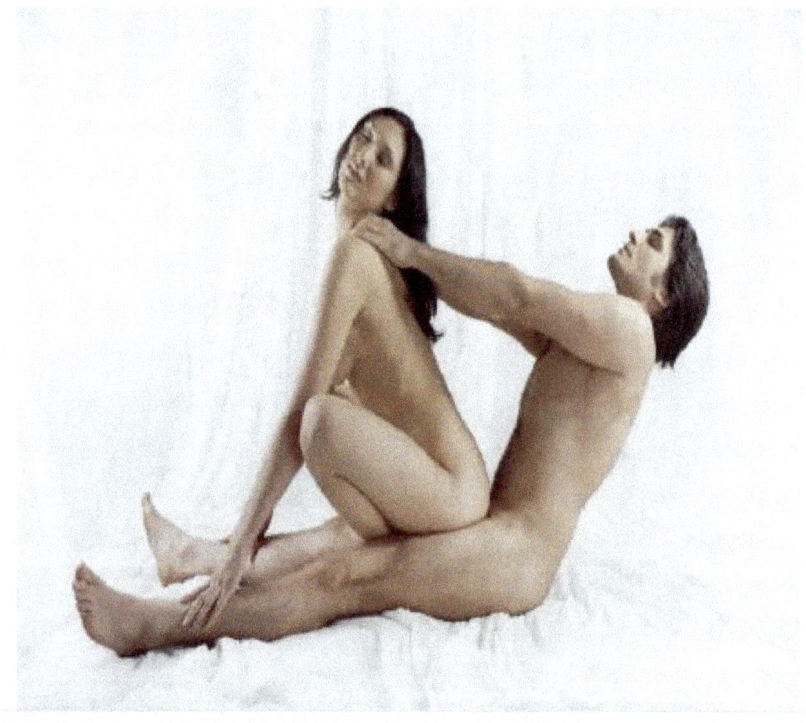

April 13

Sweet Tooth

The lovers are seated facing each other in the most intimate pose. This posture means the man can explore with lips and tongue every inch of his partner's sweet skin.

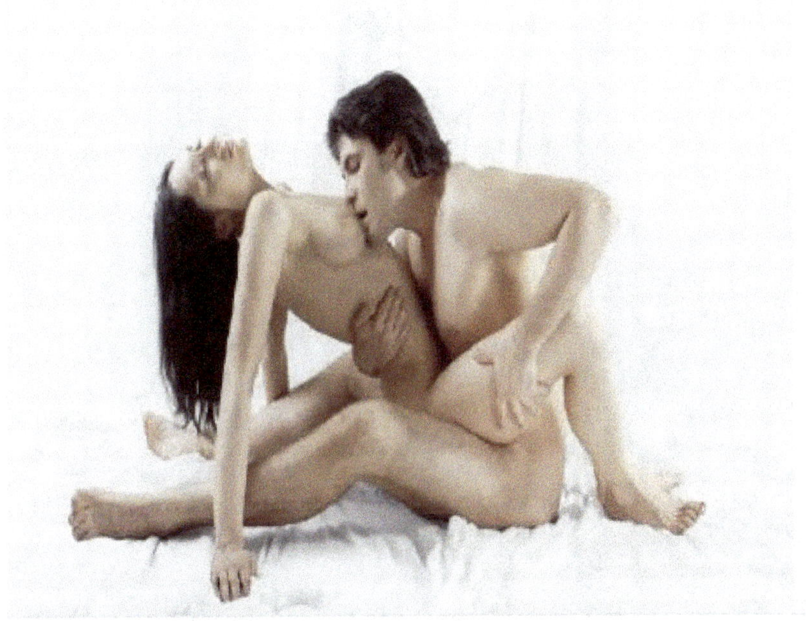

April 14

The Gardener

With support from his beloved's hips, the man can start gathering the forbidden fruits of pleasure early. Admiring the curve of her back he can hope for a good harvest of spicy delights, euphoria and joy.

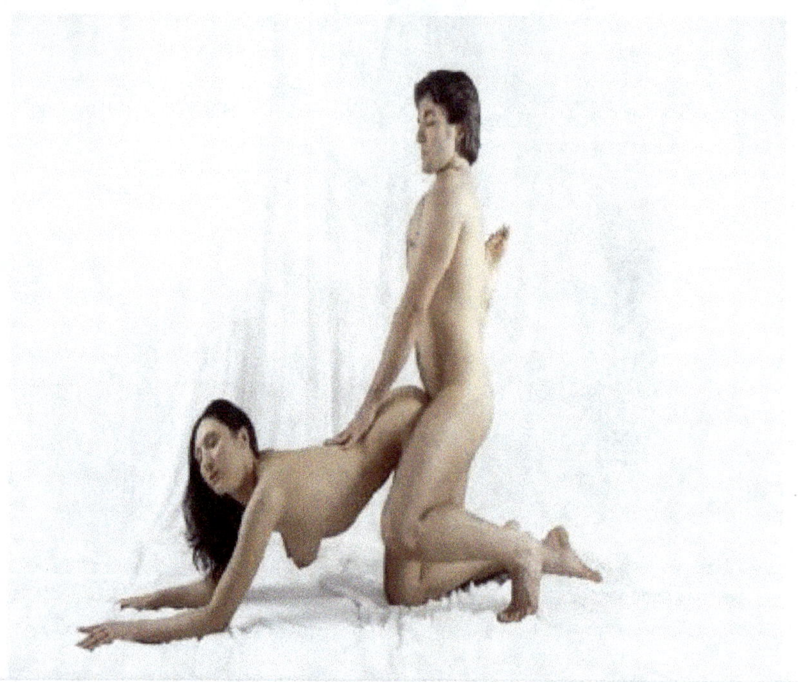

April 15

Over the Waves

In this position, the man is the boat and his companion the prow head. They will sail together over the seas of pleasure where every wave takes them closer to ecstasy.

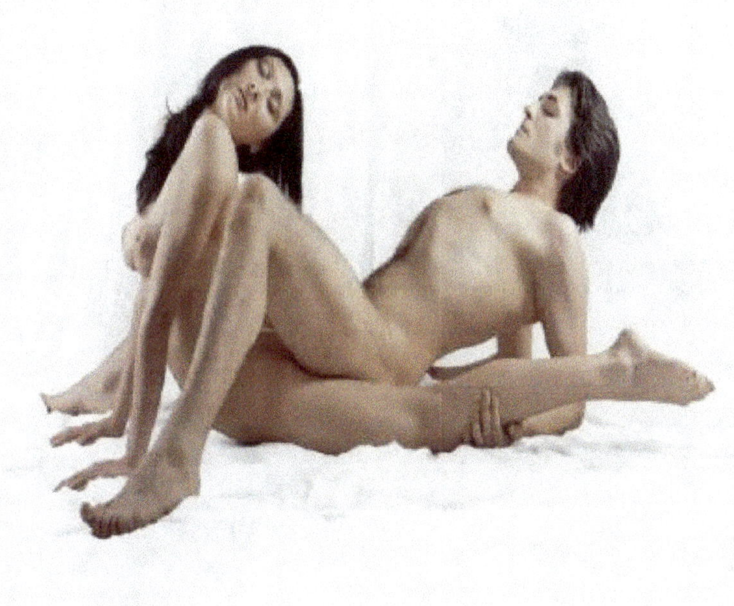

April 16

Abandonment

Horizontal love is by far the most relaxing, but you mustn't think you can let go completely. Every embrace demands the most attentive commitment.

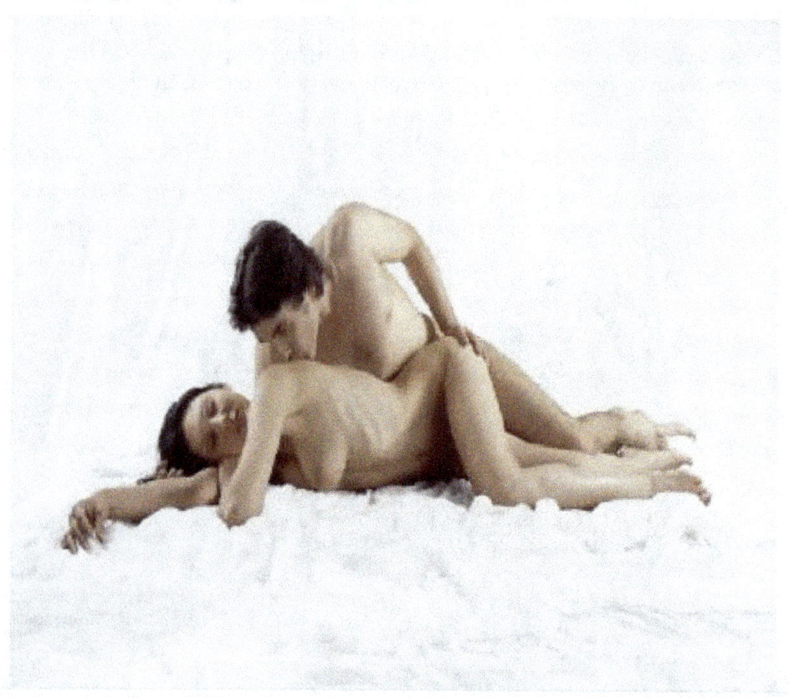

April 17

Letting Go

The woman let's it all go in her lover's arms. Head back, with hands between her legs, she enjoys completely the pleasure he gives her. The man will be perfectly satisfied with this too.

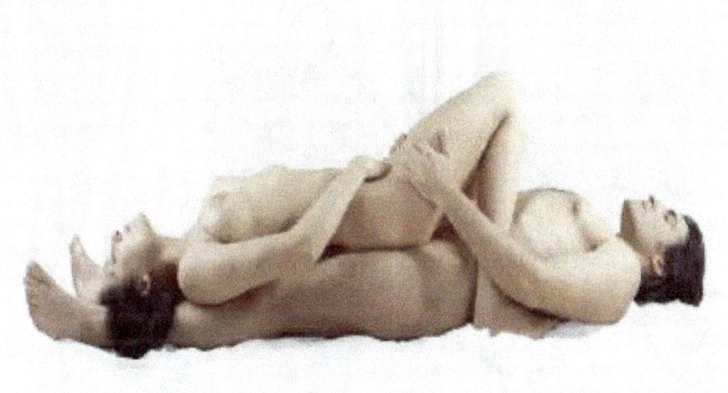

April 18

The Hostage

With both hands held firmly, the man has no choice but to give in to the hot agony devised for him by his lascivious captor. And he hopes it's going to be a long night.

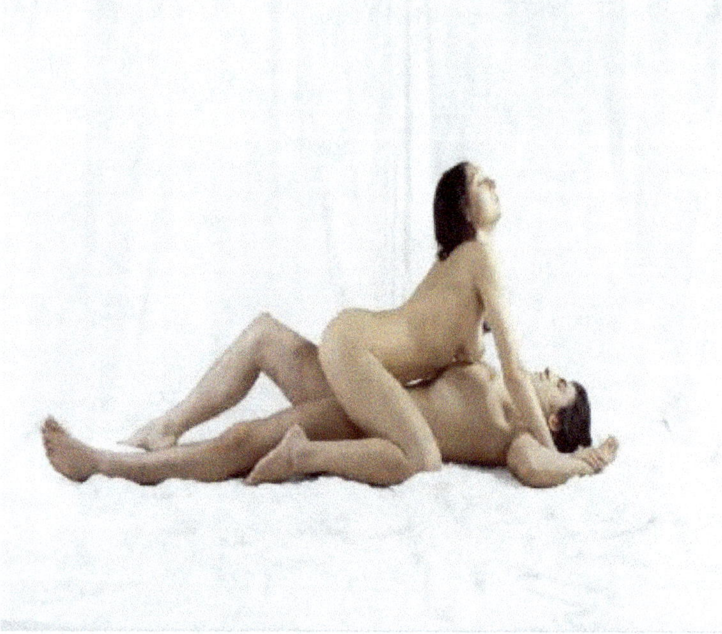

April 19

The Windmill

Artful and passionate, the woman is on her side in order to make the rotational motions that will quickly make her lovers head spin with delight.

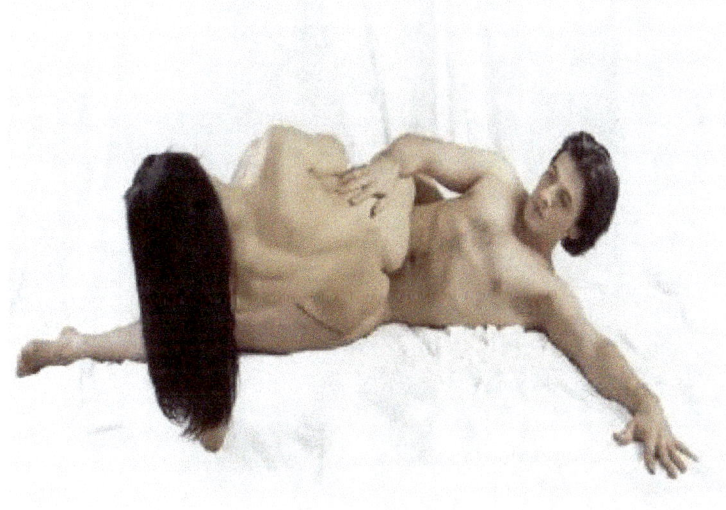

April 20

Rocker

The woman straddles her partner and rests her back on his bare chest. With the precision action of her legs she sets in motion a delicious back-and-forth.

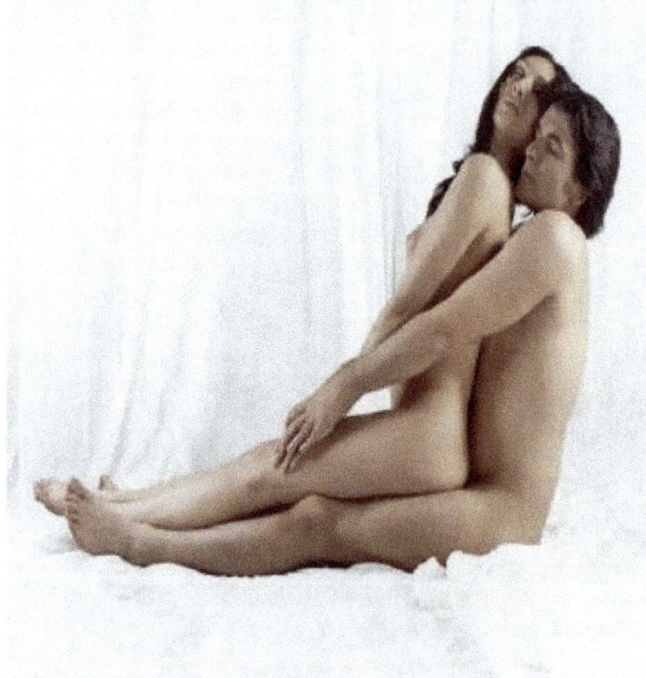

April 21

The Reed

Like the famous reed, the woman bends but doesn't break. In this position with the handsome arch of her back she can welcome her partner's full manliness and take him to undreamt of heights.

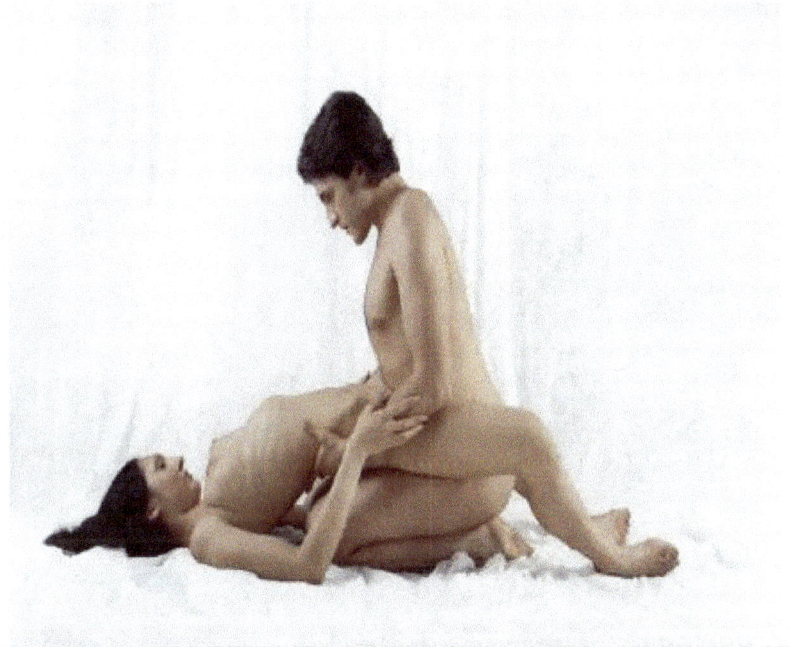

April 22
Roulette

In this position, the woman turns her back on her partner and kneels with her legs on either side of his hips. With the self-assured confidence of a winner, you can bet on fun!

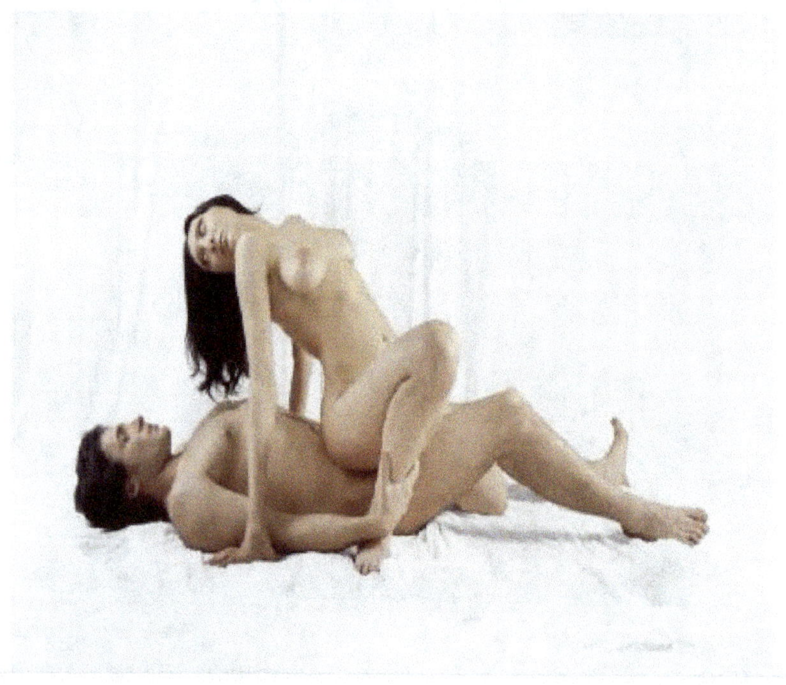

April 23

Waltz

By leaning farther forward or backwards, the woman leads this dance. With her partner's hands on the nape of her neck, she is both leader and led, brusque and tender.

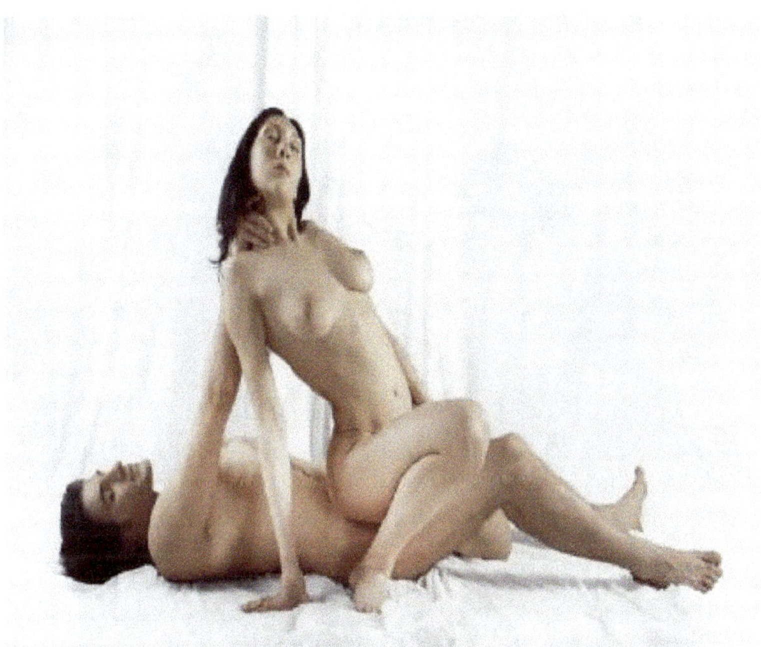

April 24

The Grasp

With her knees drawn to her chest and her legs playfully bound the woman becomes the object of her partner's carnal domination. This combat will end in nirvana.

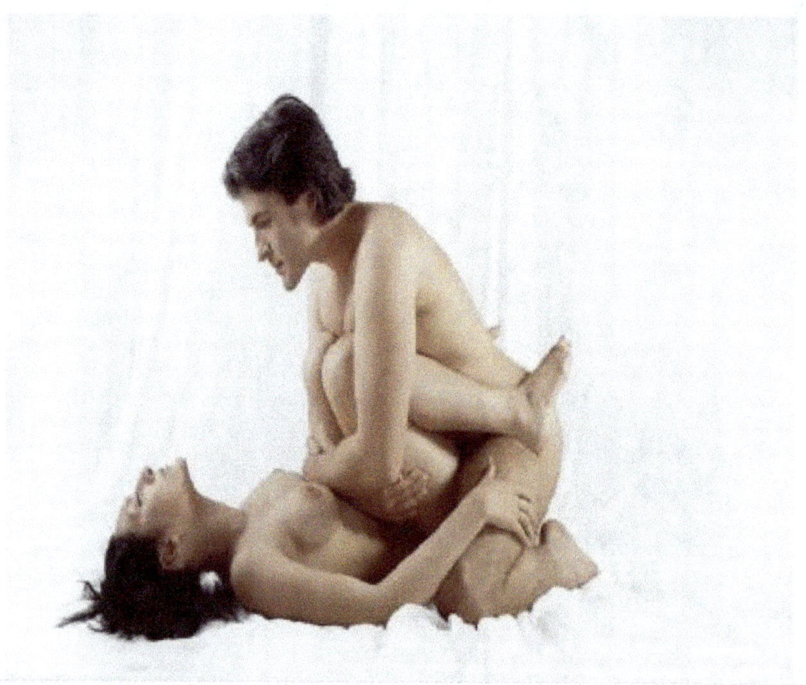

April 25

Prince Charming

Stretched out on his sleeping beauty, the prince wakes her gently. He does his utmost to slip between her legs, conform to her back, lightly, gently.

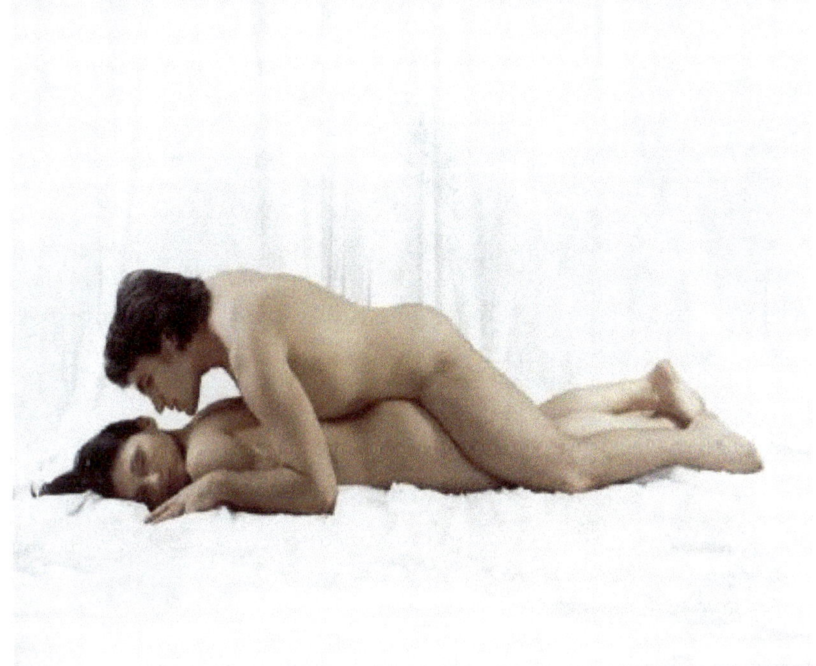

April 26

Sensual Ascension

In this position, the man's immobility is matched by the woman's sensuous aspirations. They are both looking in the same direction, to the heights of pleasure.

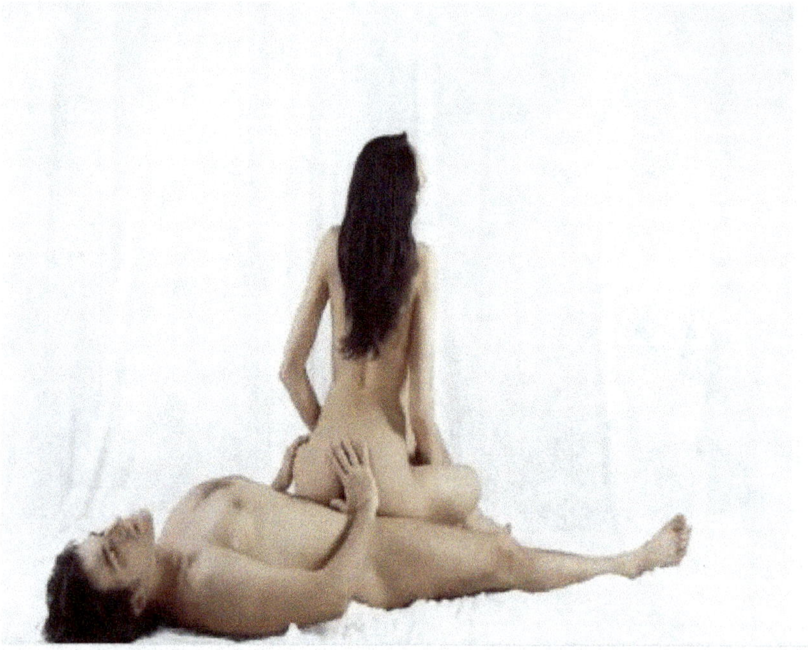

April 27

Love Trance

Stunned by love, these two partners are inseparable and just want to melt into one another. Tightly held, body on body, they don't miss a second of the show before them.

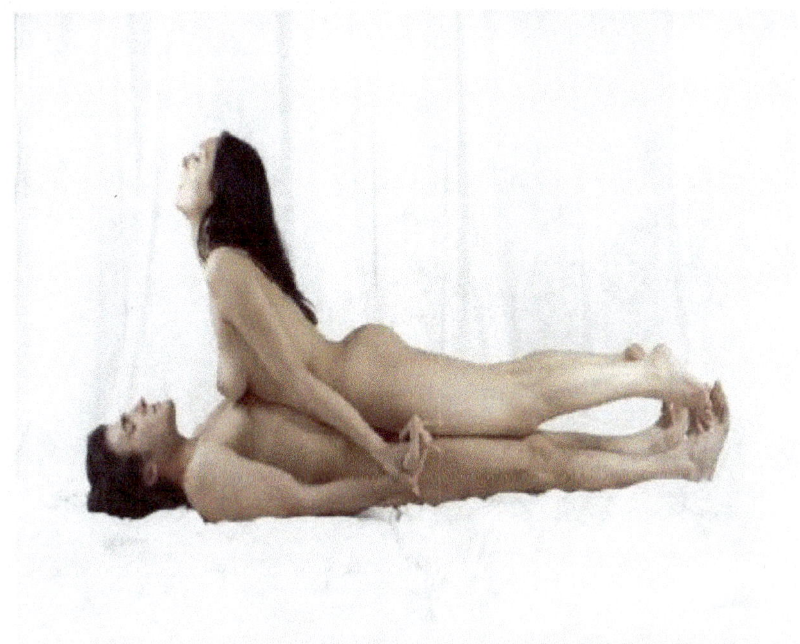

April 28

The Conquest

Legs intertwined with their growing desire, the man stands like a conqueror before his obedient but flirtatious partner. He has come to rescue her from crushing lust.

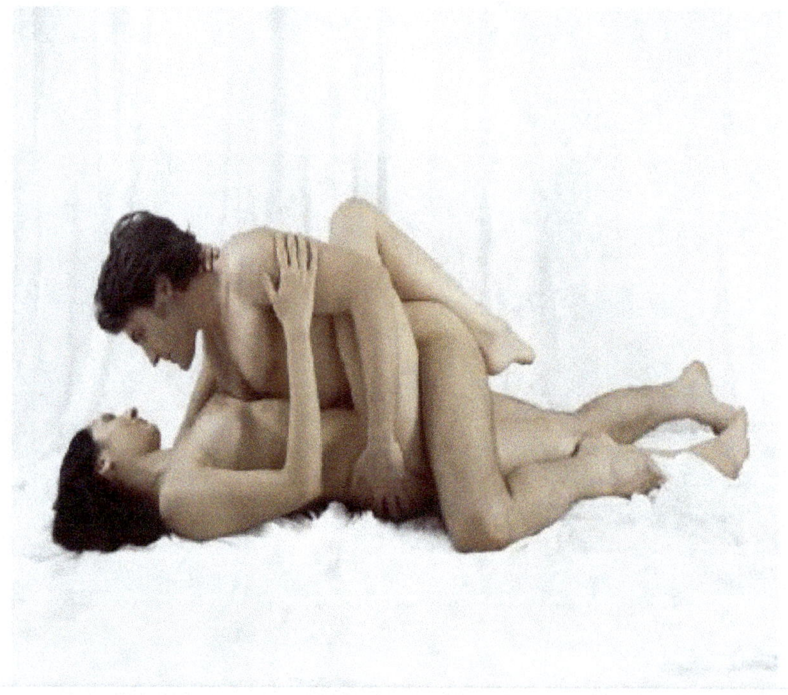

April 29

Cross-legged

In this position, the woman holds the key to both partner's pleasure in her hips. She arches her lower back, rocks her hips to the limit and brings them both to Nirvana.

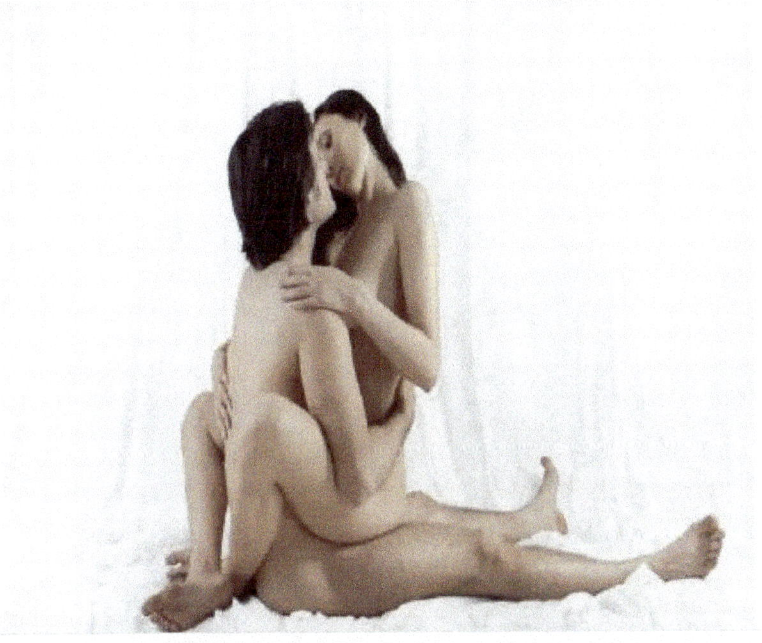

April 30

The Long Ride

Rocking back and forth, forward and back, the woman takes a risqué ride on her partner who lies stretched out on his back. He is a docile mount and will take them both the summit of desire.

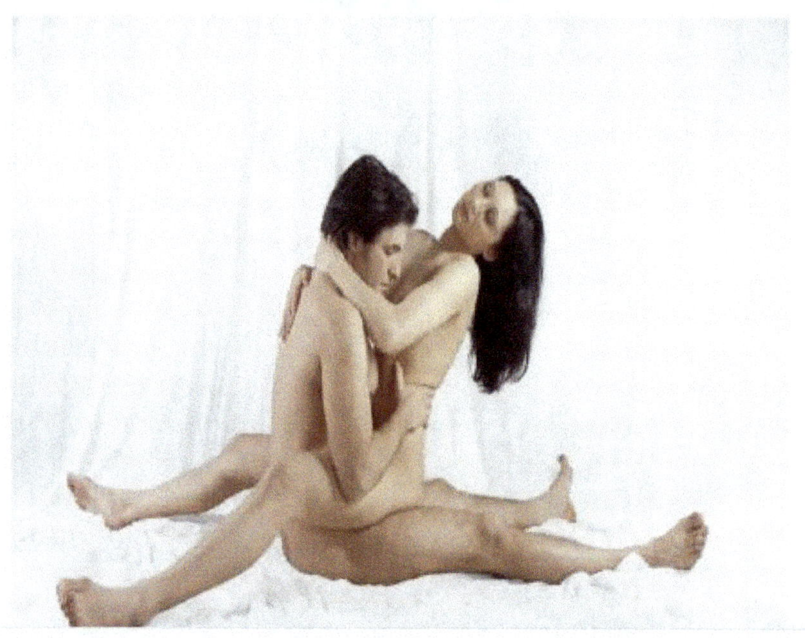

May

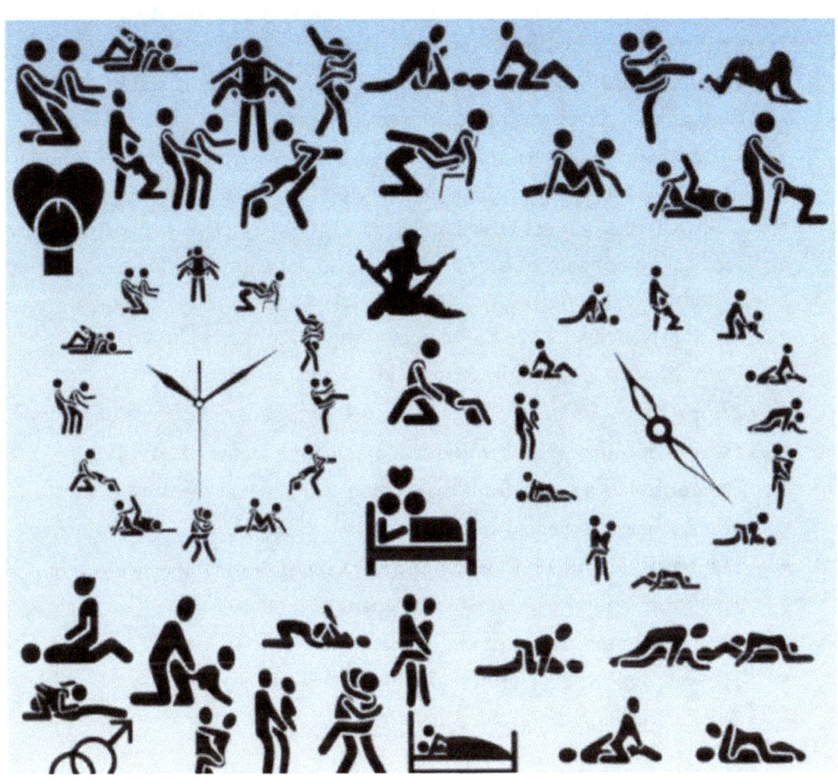

Role-Play Scenarios

- **Age play** - a form of roleplay between adults in which both parties act in different ages, e.g. infantilism, Daddy/daughter play.
- **Aliens** - a fantasy about having sex with aliens which often happens in an abduction or forced scenario.
- **Impregnation** - sexually turned on by the possibility of getting pregnant during unprotected vaginal intercourse for both parties.
- **Infantilism** - a form of roleplay in which one participant acts like an infant or baby, the other one plays a parental role.
- **Medical Play** - a medical-themed roleplay in which sexual partners use medical equipment and wear uniforms to take on relevant roles in that scenario.
- **Pet Play** - a kink in which one person dresses and acts like a pet.
- **Pony Play** - a kink for dressing up and acting like a pony.
- **Puppy Play** - a type of roleplay in which one takes on the role of a puppy.
- **Harpaxophilia** - sexual arousal from being the victim of a robbery.
- **Phygephilia** - a sexual thrill from being a fugitive on the run.
- The teacher and the bad student
- The frisky construction worker and the lonely housewife
- The horny landlord and the broke tenant
- The peeping tom and the exhibitionist
- The jock and the cheerleader
- The doctor / nurse and the patient
- The dominatrix and the submissive slave
- The safari hunter and the wild animal
- The talent agent and the aspiring starlet
- The vampire and the vampire hunter/huntress

You can get all your role-play costumes directly from Festival Drip here.

Use promo code **CSET10** for $10 off all costumes at FestivalDripOfficial.com

May 1

The Vine

In this position, the woman is like a creeping vine around a tree, and this position has a serious advantage, it can be practiced anywhere, for a quick, sensuous escape, always exciting.

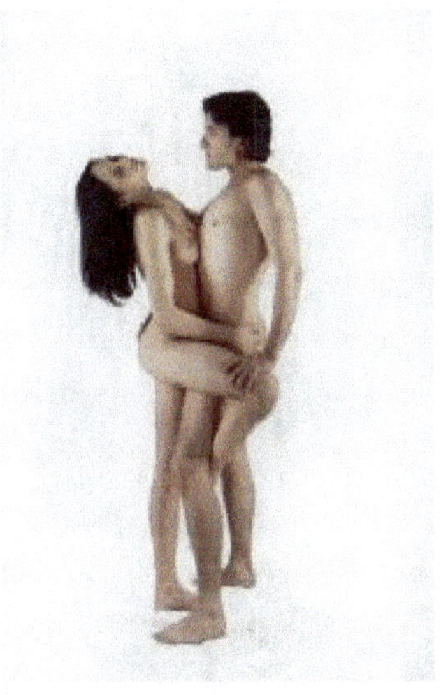

May 2

The Other Side of the Moon

This is an extremely acrobatic posture! When done vertically, it is heads and shoulders above the simple 69. The lovers look as if they were overcome by desire and simply couldn't wait to find a more appropriate bed.

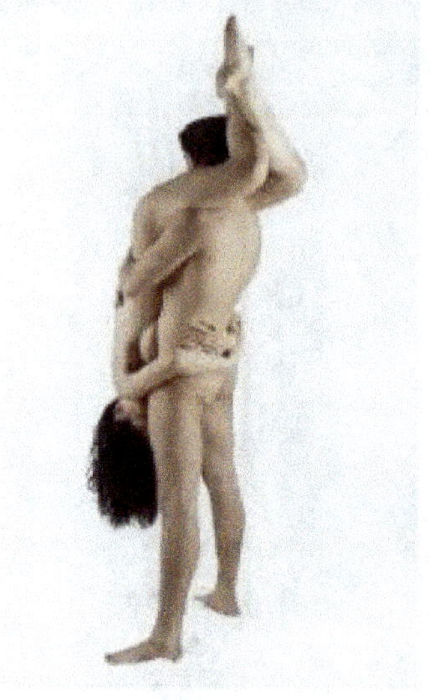

May 3

Suspended

The woman, with her legs around her partner's waist, gives in completely to his charms. The man here has only one responsibility - supporting his love and her delight.

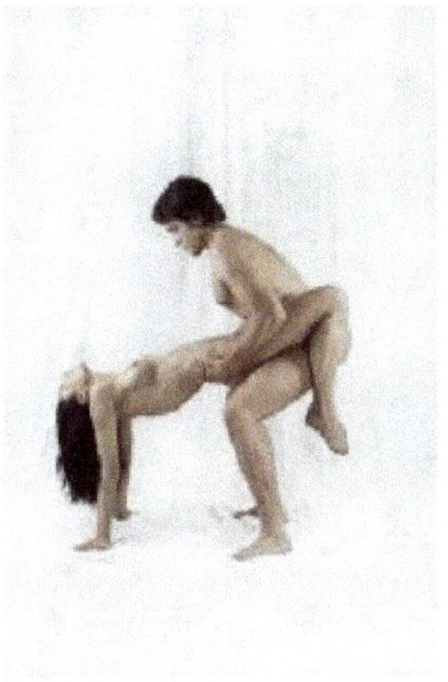

May 4

The Dance

In this position, she is standing, facing away from her partner. By arching her back slightly, she can make the dance more subtle, more natural, more exciting.

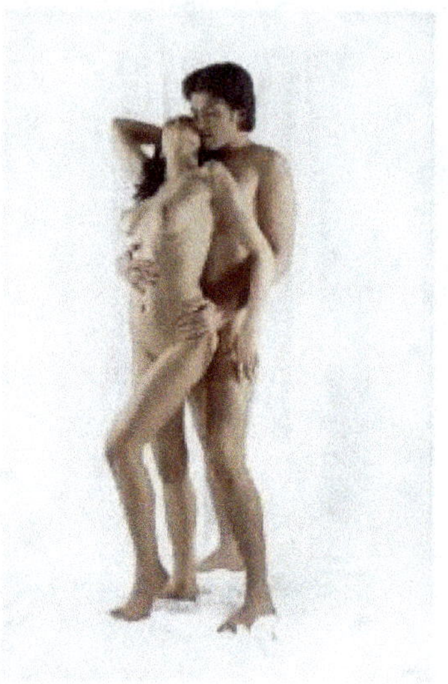

May 5

At the Crossroads

This is perfect symmetry of lovers - chest to chest, staring into each others eyes, their locked knees support the lover's tent that they make together.

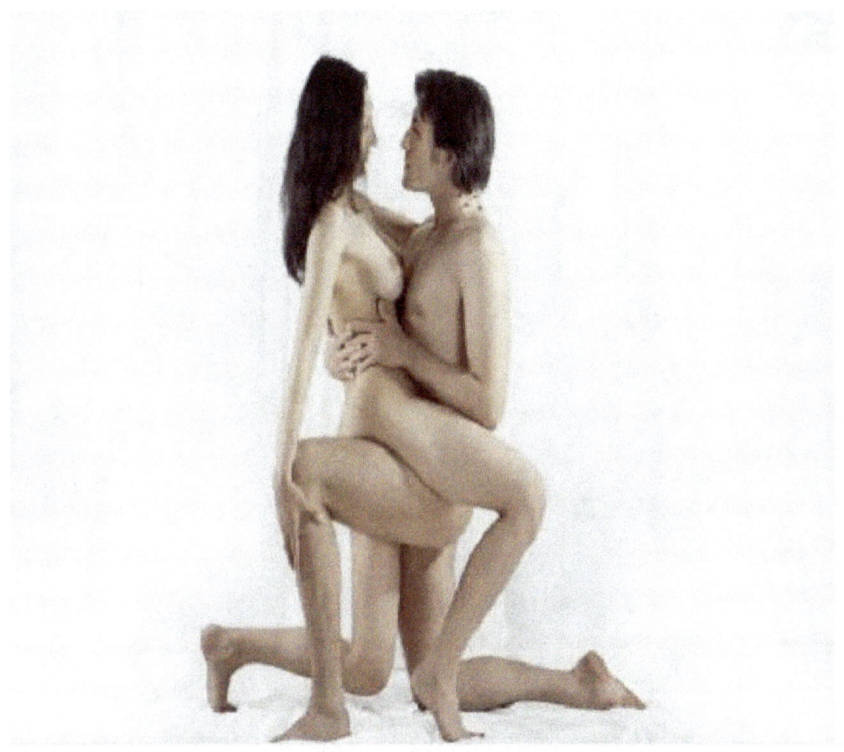

May 6

Spirit standing

Small things can be important and here the small of her back is what guarantees the success of this position. With head and hips thrust backwards, her support shapes the lovers' silhouette.

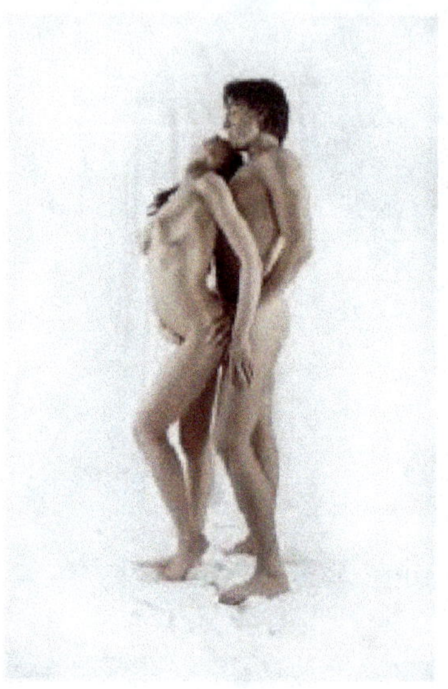

May 7

Pirouette

Pleasure seeking and the search for excitement are key in a physical relationship. Here flexibility and balance are essential!

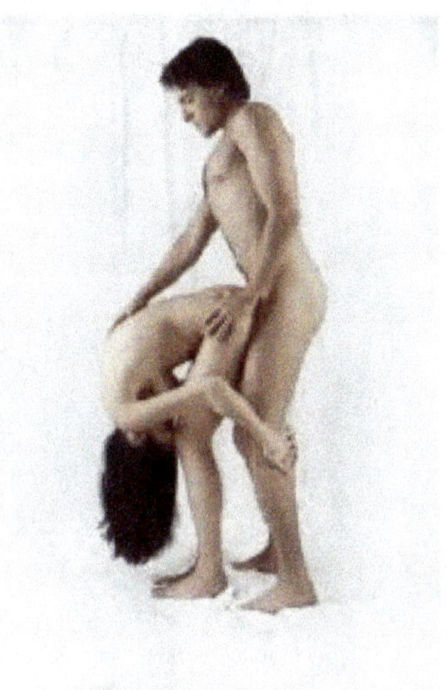

May 8

Flamingo

Standing on one foot, the flamingo preens his feathers, puffing out his breast and showing off. With all his finery in place, he begins the nuptial dance, the prelude to a night of passion where he will be the king of lovers.

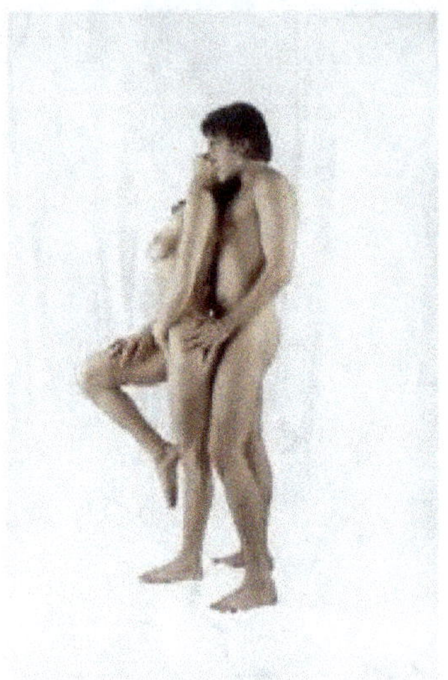

May 9

On Bended knee

Kneeling before each other, the lovers declare their love with promises and stolen kisses. No need to hold back because love just can't wait!

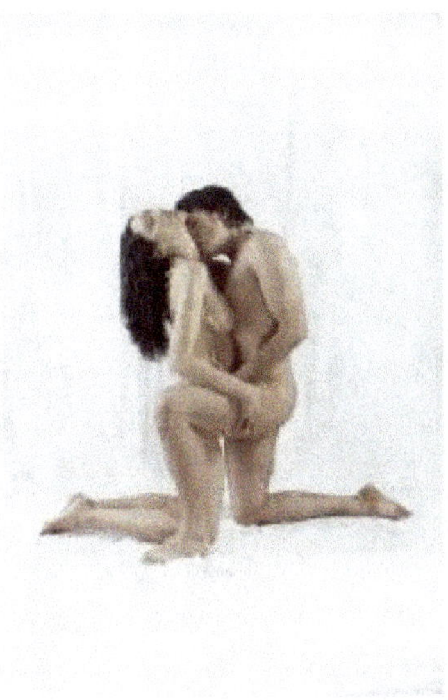

May 10

Precision Mastery

Here the couple is supported by the perfect blend of balance and pleasure. Should one of them give in totally to delight, both will fall. Love is at once fragile and solid.

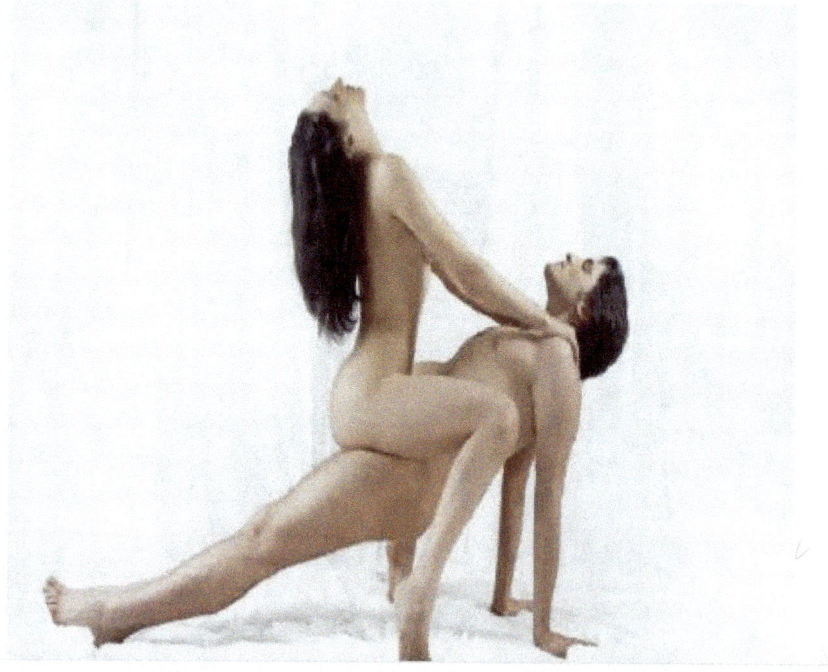

May 11

Self-Absorbed

The lovers carve out a place just for themselves. The ephemeral cocoon looks simple to make, but it does require some flexibility. The man wraps his arms around his partner, holding her tenderly but firmly.

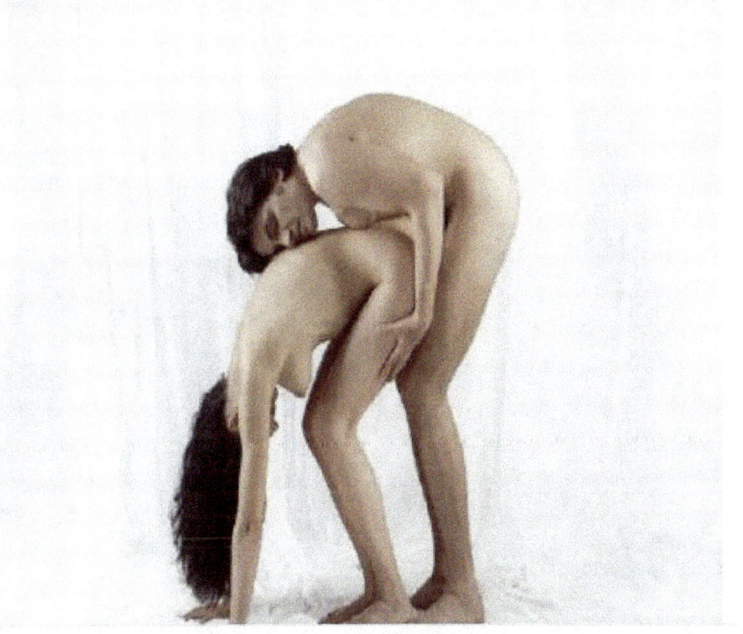

May 12

Straddled

The man offers himself, ready to begin this sensual journey. The woman sits astride him for their torrid trip. Don't start off too fast, you have to go the distance!

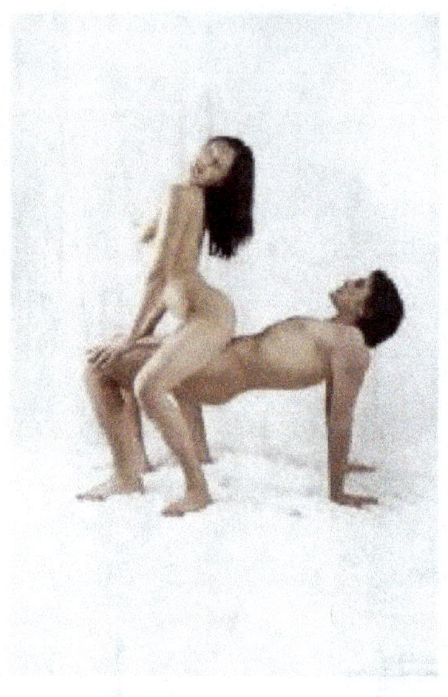

May 13

The Trident

The trident is the symbol of the dominion of the seas; here it takes on another meaning as in this case the woman shows her authority over man.

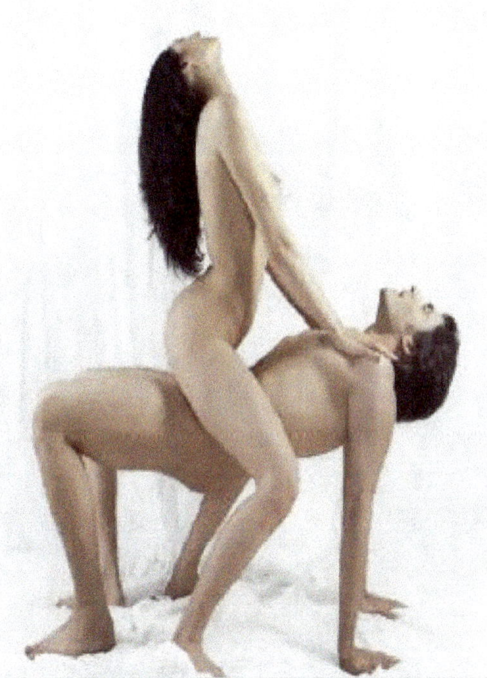

May 14

Acrobats

These acrobats for an evening have been training before trying out this number.
The main thing is not to let go too much or the man might loose his catch.

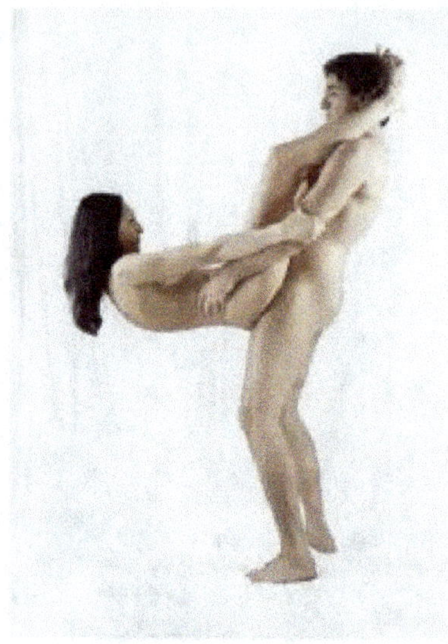

May 15

Rollercoaster

This rollercoaster guarantees a thrill! Round and round and upside down, the lovers are on a dangerous path, but one that is strewn with pleasures. Hold onto your hats!

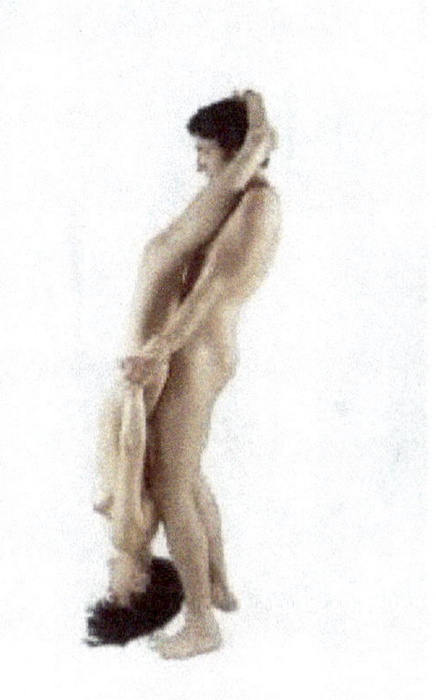

May 16

The Tango

The partners push and pull each other onward in this improvised dance. Here the man guides his partner but each change of position is a joint decision, made with their hips together.

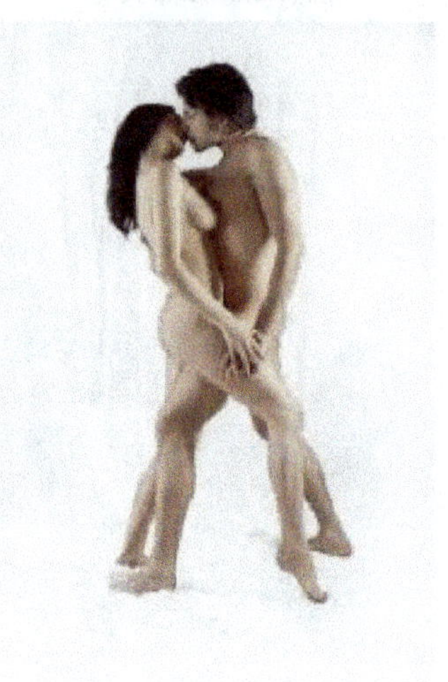

May 17
Embrace

Hanging on her beloved's neck, the woman gives herself to him, in an ecstatic jolt. Her lover's frenzy will soon give way to a languorous dance to the beat of their rhythmic hips.

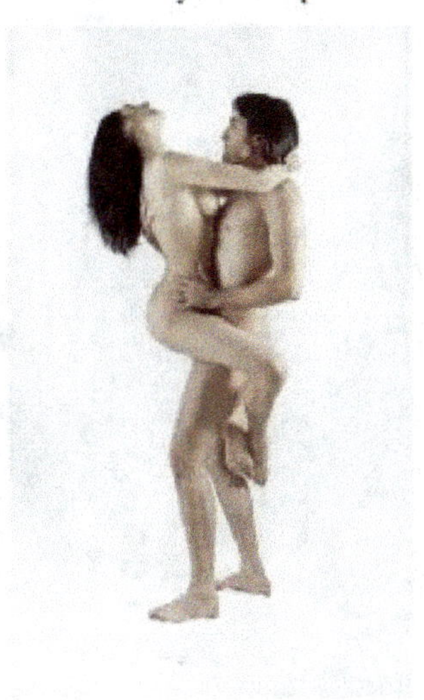

May 18

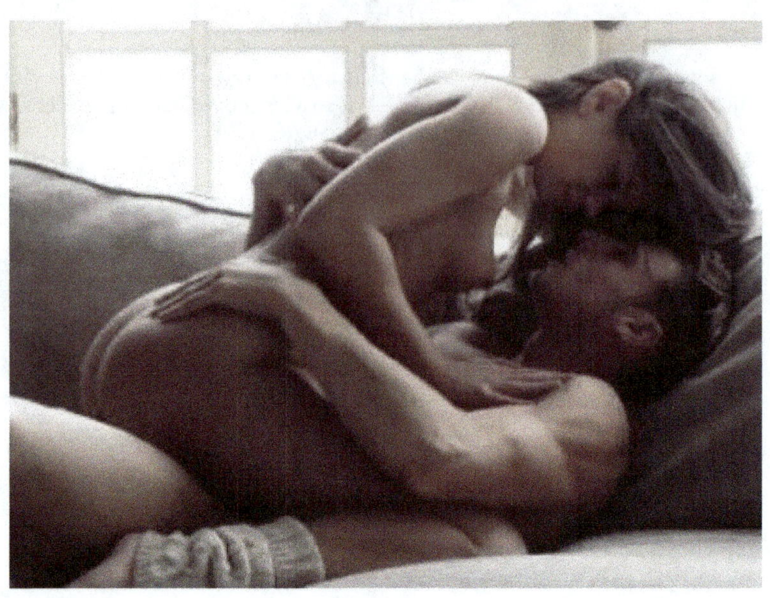

Rodeo

If you want to try this one, I guarantee you will not regret it. Hold on to your hat though, 'cause it's gonna be one wild ride.

May 19

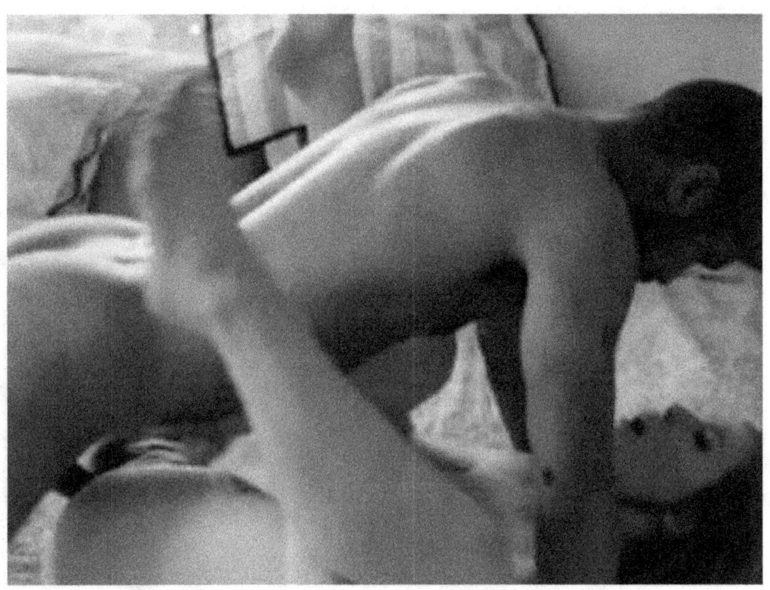

Backdoor Missionary

The Missionary position might have a reputation for being vanilla, but trust me, there's nothing plain about it when you go for the backdoor.

May 20

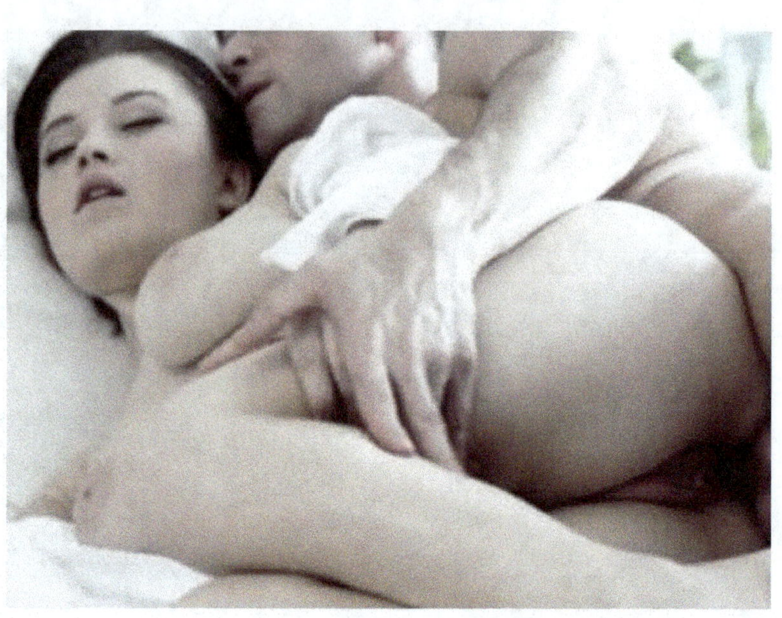

The Spoon

Combining the intimate and relaxed nature of spooning with the taboo thrill of anal, this position is sure to be a favorite!

May 21

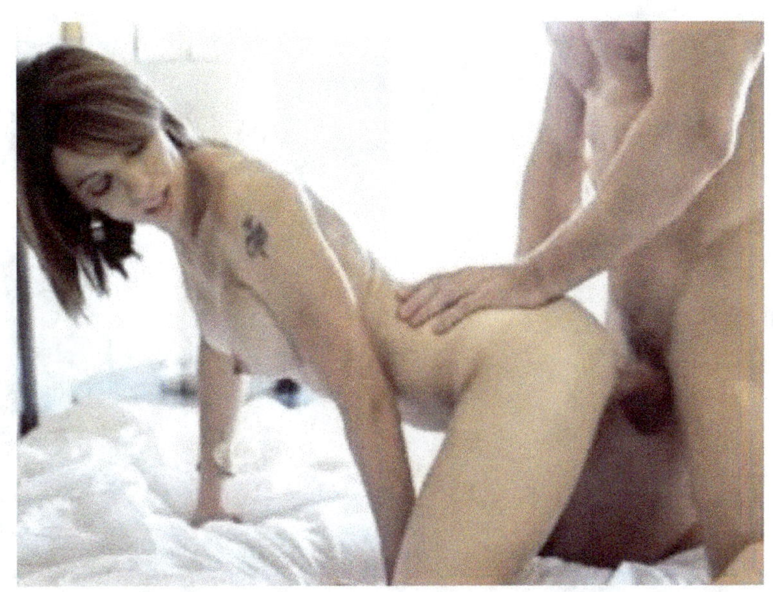

The Backdoor

According to our women readers, backdoor sex is the number one position their male partners ask them to try. Check out this video demonstrating how to enjoy anal sex

May 22

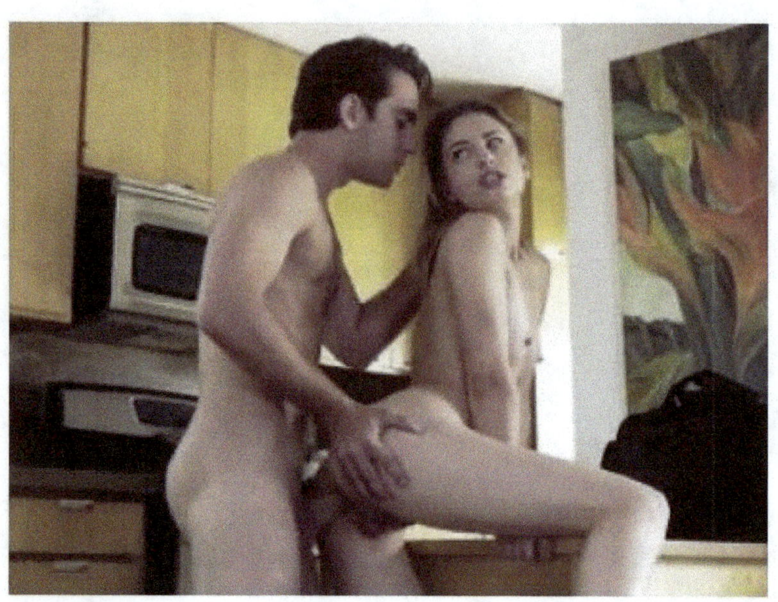

Tailpipe

If you're interested in trying a standing anal sex position the Tailpipe is a great choice.

May 23

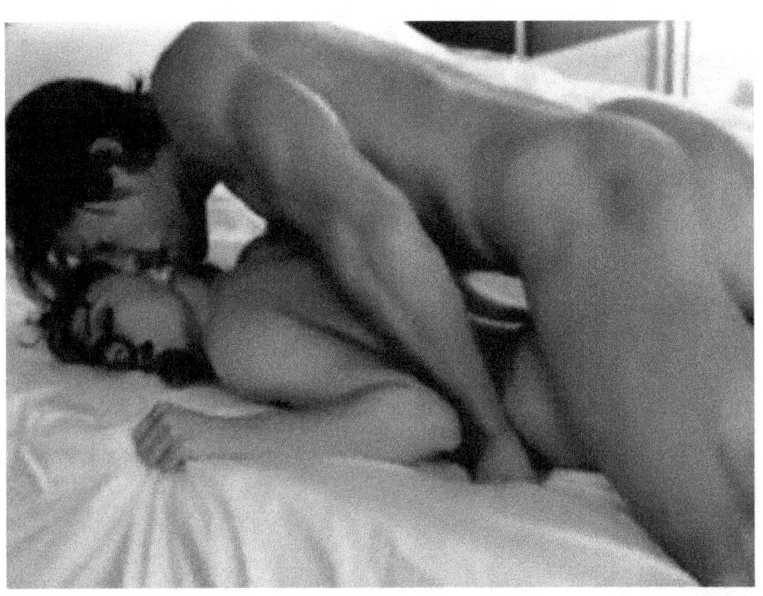

Flatiron

Perfect for g spot stimulation and deep penetration, the Flatiron creates a sensationally snug fit that makes your guy feel even bigger.

May 24

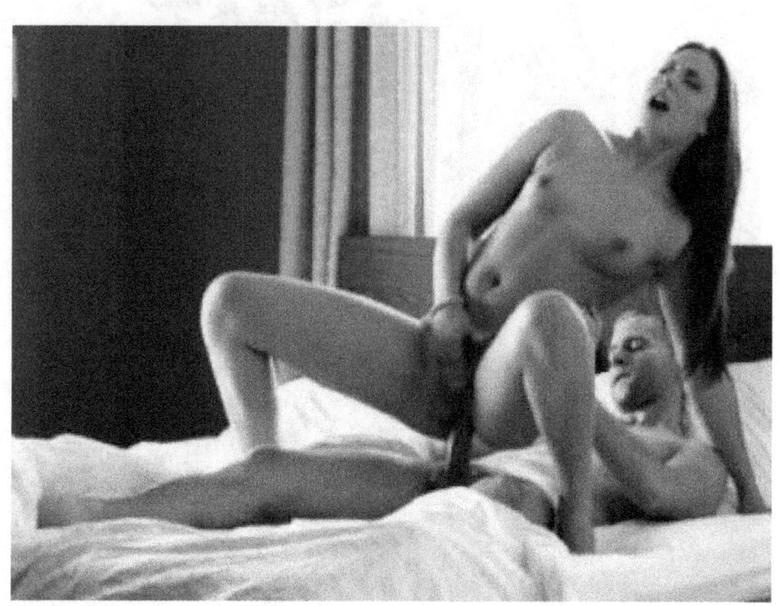

Anal Reverse Cowgirl

Because of the unique angle, the Rear View provides intense sensations for both partners, resulting in unforgettable pleasure.

May 25

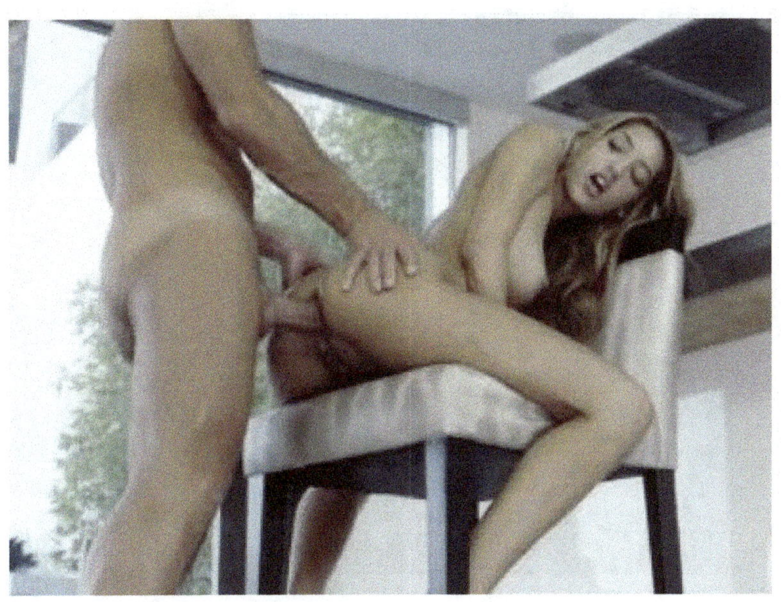

Back Seat Driver

If this one doesn't get you to hit the high notes, I don't know what will.

May 26

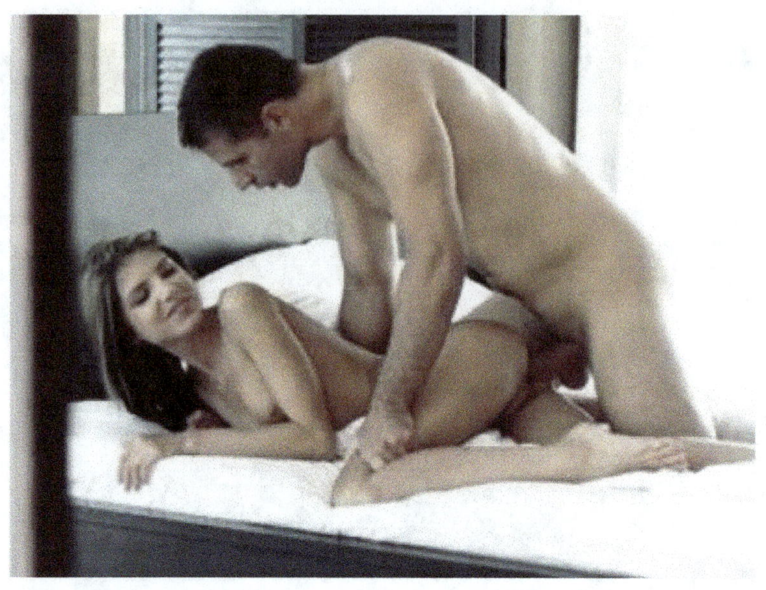

The Sphinx

This comfortable, side entry pose allows both partners to fully enjoy the surprising sensations that anal sex provides.

May 27

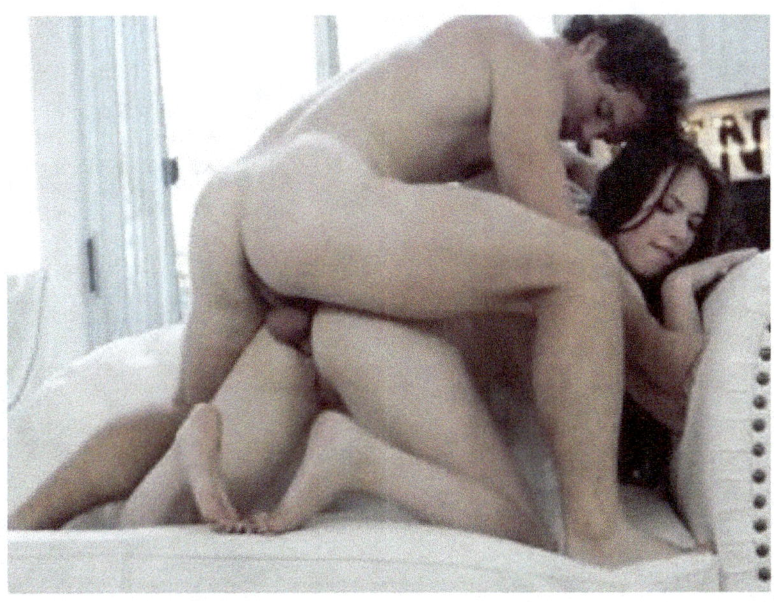

Bulldog

Looking for some hot anal moves that will have you feeling like you just stepped into your very own porno? The Bulldog is the best of them all.

May 28

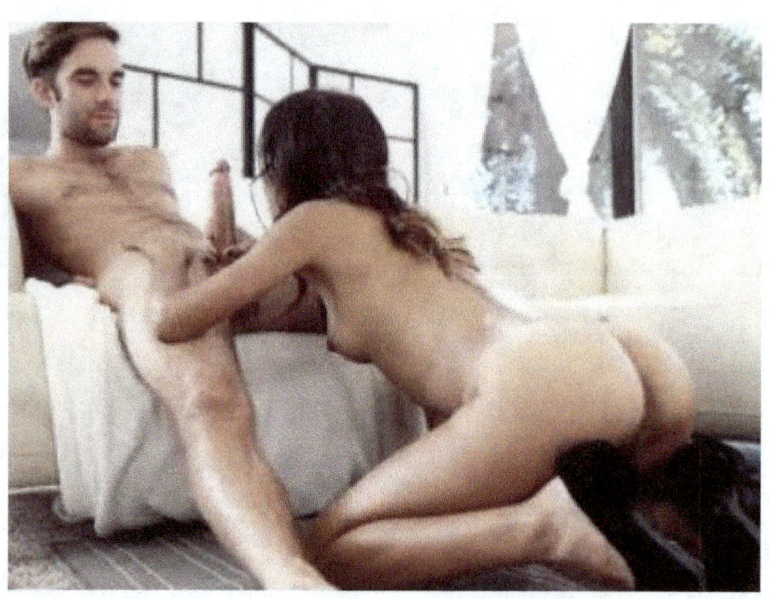

Boss's Chair

Make him feel like a boss with this beginner-friendly kneeling blow job position. The Boss's Chair is easy — and fun!

May 29

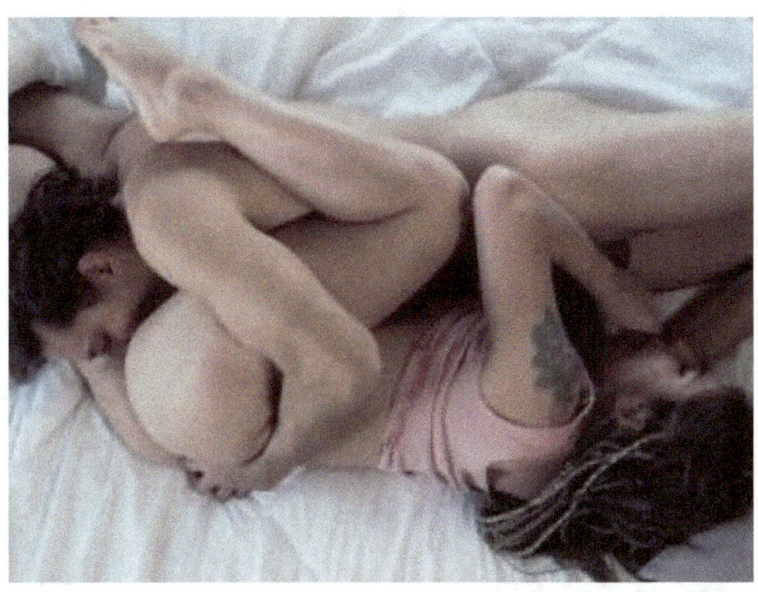

Sideways 69

Fans of reciprocity will surely appreciate this comfier take on 69. Instead of one person literally laying on top of the other, both partners lay on their sides.

May 30

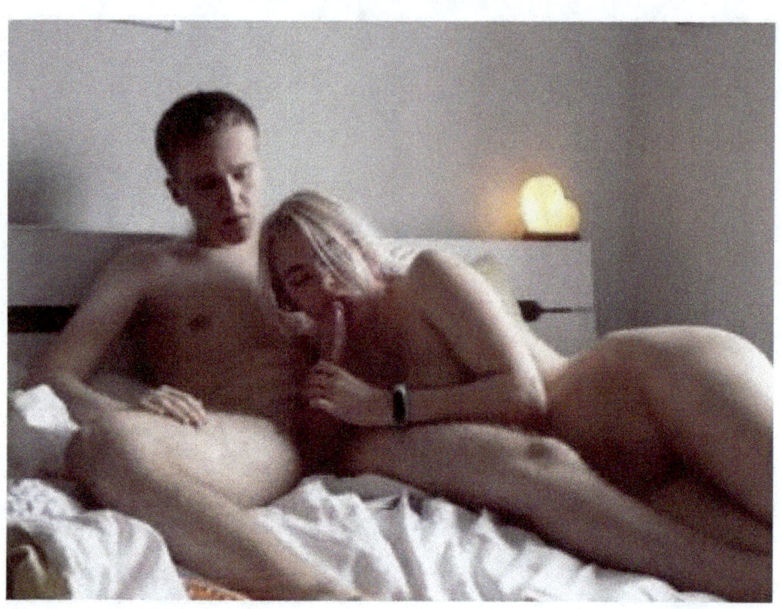

Lazy Sunday

Here's a proven fact: Surprising a guy with a morning BJ will lead to you getting your way the entire rest of the week.

May 31

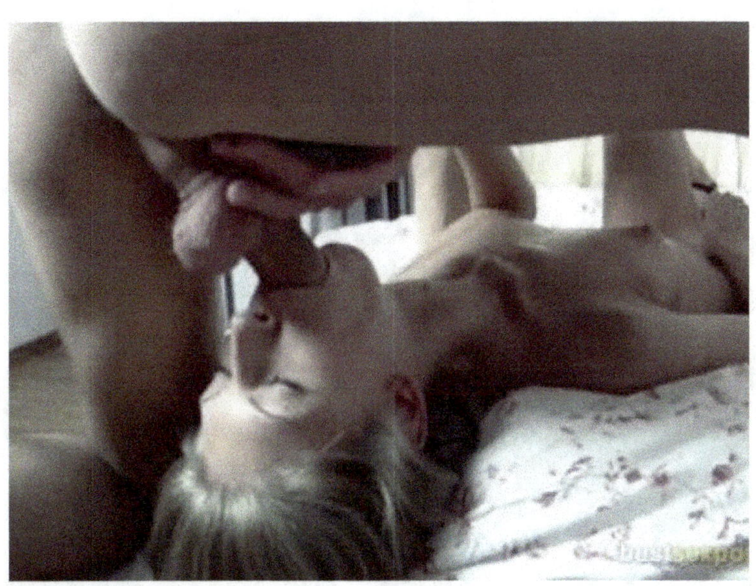

Over the Edge

"Open wide!" The Over the Edge blowjob position puts her at the ultimate angle for deepthroat.

June

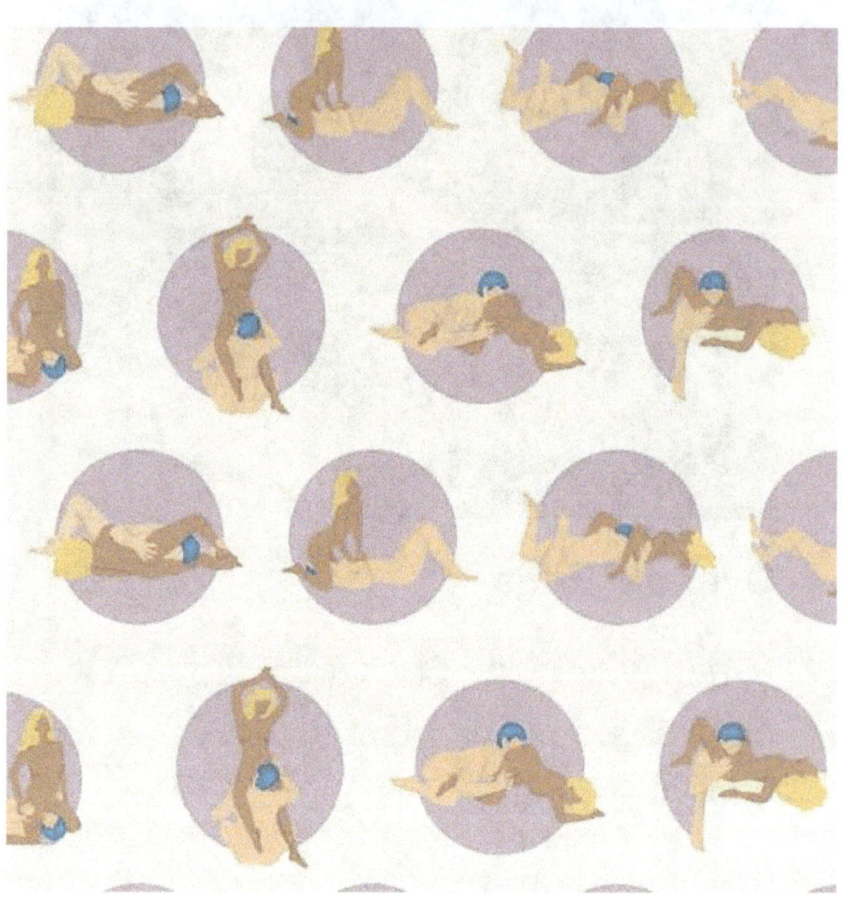

Key Techniques for Giving a Sensual Massage

- **Slow and Rhythmic Strokes:**

Use long, flowing strokes with consistent pressure to promote relaxation.

- **Focus on Underrated Areas:**

Pay attention to the ears, back of the knees, soles of the feet, nape of the neck, and other areas often overlooked in massages.

- **Aromatherapy:**

Incorporate aromatherapy oils to enhance the sensory experience and create a relaxing mood. Make sure it's not a scent the other person hates!

- **Soft Touches:**

Gentle, soft strokes can be very effective in creating a sensual and pleasurable experience.

- **Breathing:**

Encourage the recipient to breathe deeply and consciously, as this can enhance relaxation and body awareness.

- **Communication:**

Maintain open communication with the recipient throughout the massage to ensure comfort and pleasure.

- **Sensual Teasing:**

Use light, suggestive touches, such as feather-light strokes or using clothing as a barrier, to build anticipation and desire.

- **Use of Massage Oil:**

Massage oil helps to create a smooth, gliding sensation and can be chosen for its scent and moisturizing properties. Not using massage oil can be painful, itchy, and most definitely un-sexy.

If you didn't take my advice at the beginning of the book and load up on coconut oil, this is the perfect opportunity to do so.

Coconut Oil - https://amzn.to/4nZxPAm

June 1

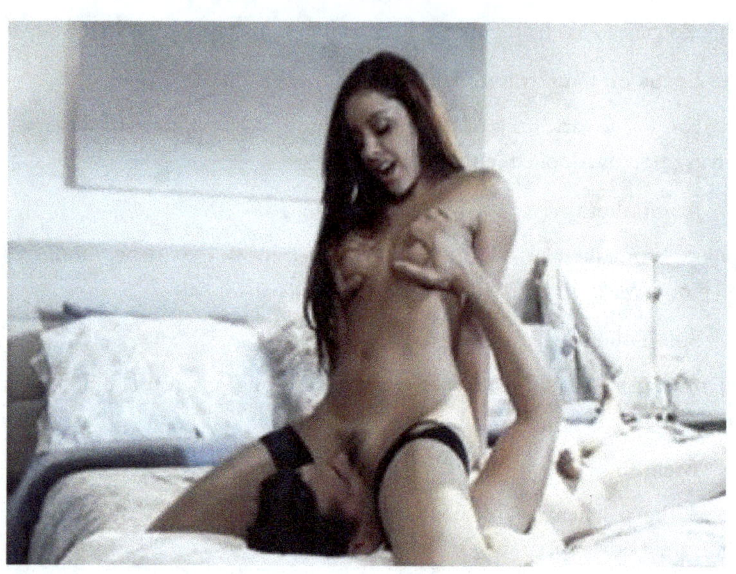

Facesitting

If you like feeling submissive, the facesitting sex position is the perfect move. The focus is 100 percent on her, and she really gets to dominate you as she rides your face.

June 2

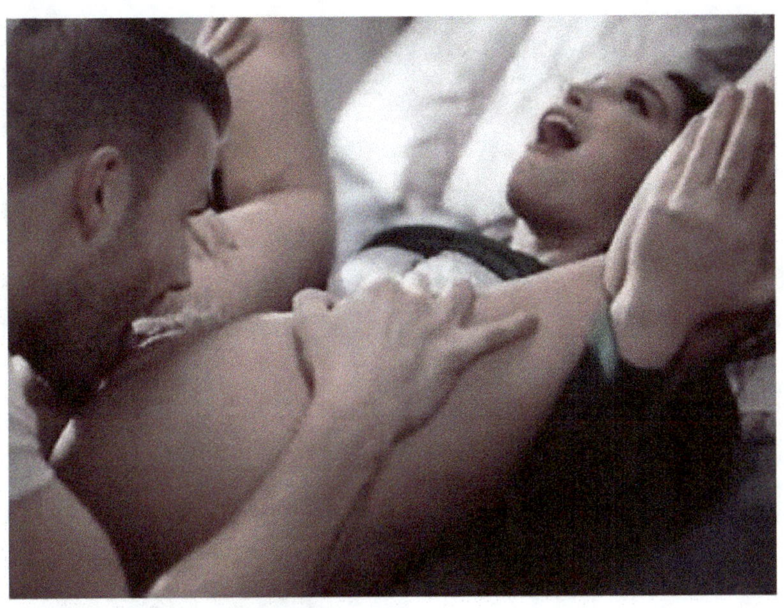

Under the Hood

It's the 'missionary' of cunnilingus, offering the most ease for oral sex action for both of you.

June 3

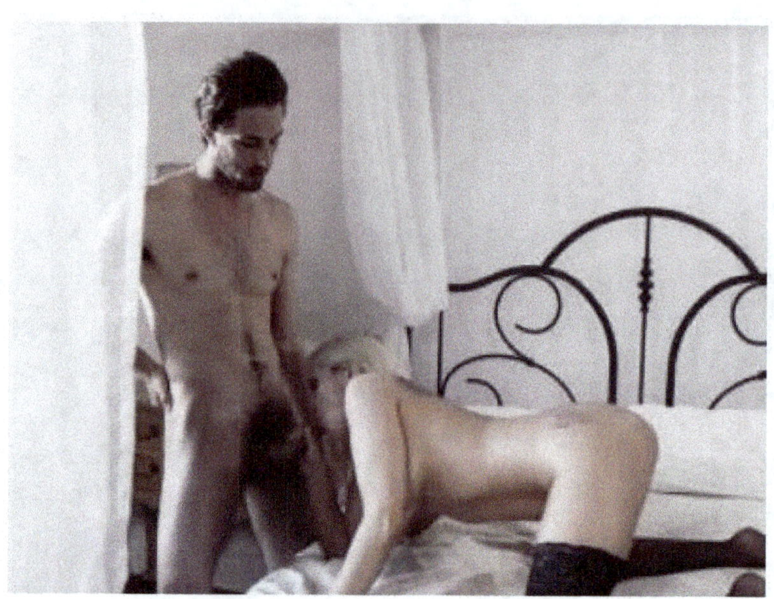

All Fours Position

Want to give your man the best blowjob of his entire life? The All Fours Blowjob position is the perfect move.

June 4

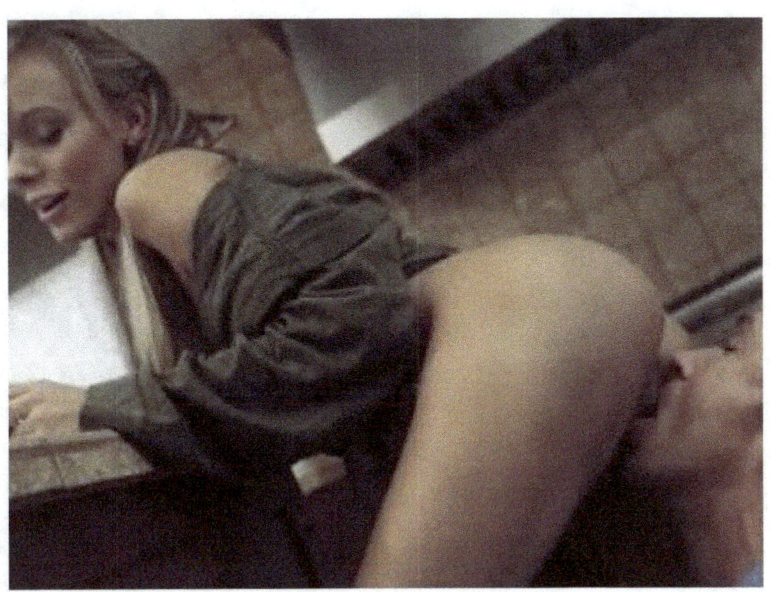

From the Back

If you're feeling adventurous, try bending her over a kitchen counter or the bathroom sink and tongue her to ecstacy.

June 5

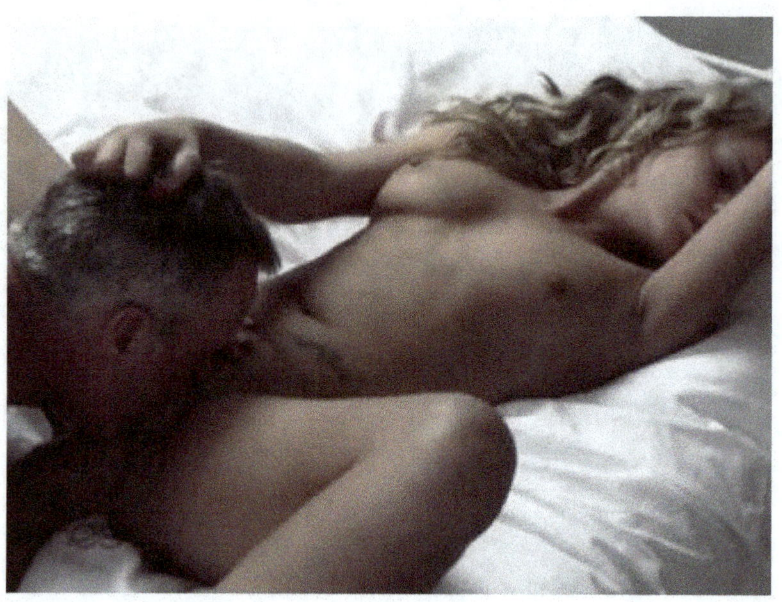

Muff Diver

Time to go on a diving adventure and dive deep into that sweet muff! You're searching for the golden treasure and it's there for the taking.

June 6

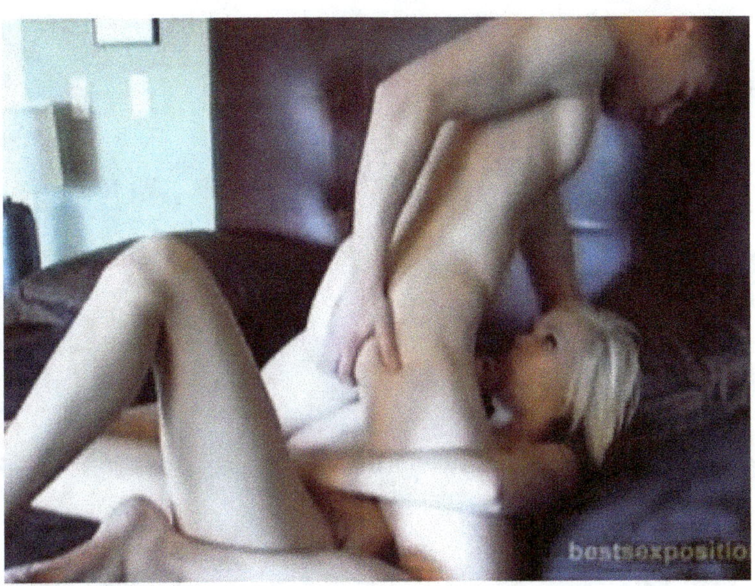

Face Fuck

If your man doesn't come from blowjobs, there is one way to change that. Let him fuck your throat like a pussy.

June 7

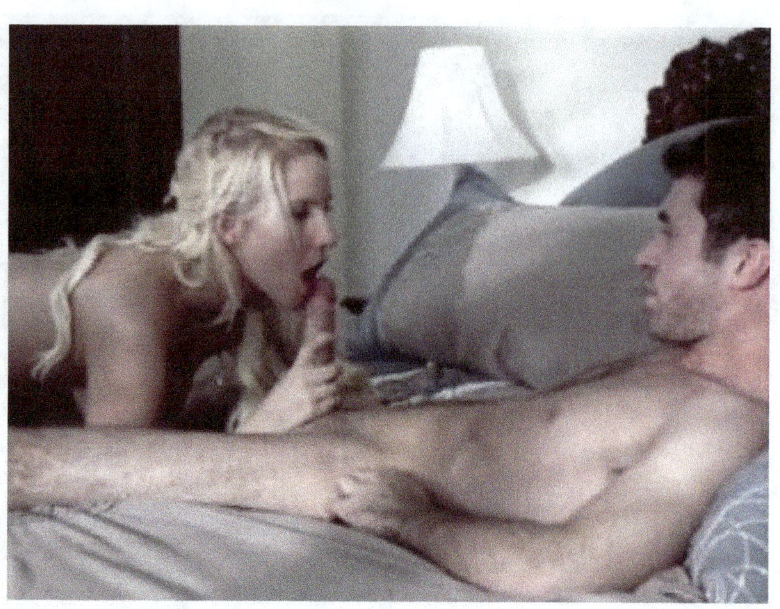

Lay Back Jack

In the Lay Back Jack (aka "The Usual") Position, the guy simply lays back while his partner performs oral from a lying position between his legs.

June 8

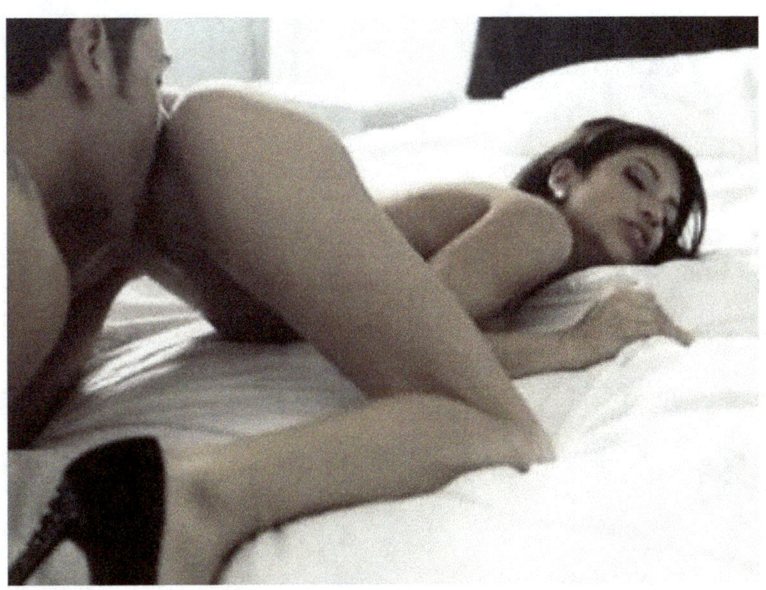

Downward Dog

Don't tell me you haven't thought about sex acts while watching women assume yoga poses. The Downward Dog, in particular, is a position practically designed to eat pussy.

June 9

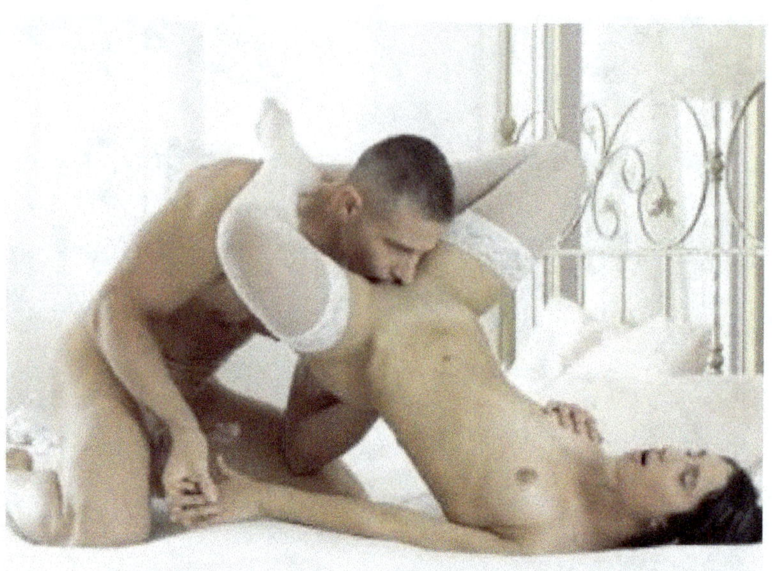

Head Rush

When you're in the mood for an exciting new pussy eating position, the Head Rush will give both of you a great thrill!

June 10

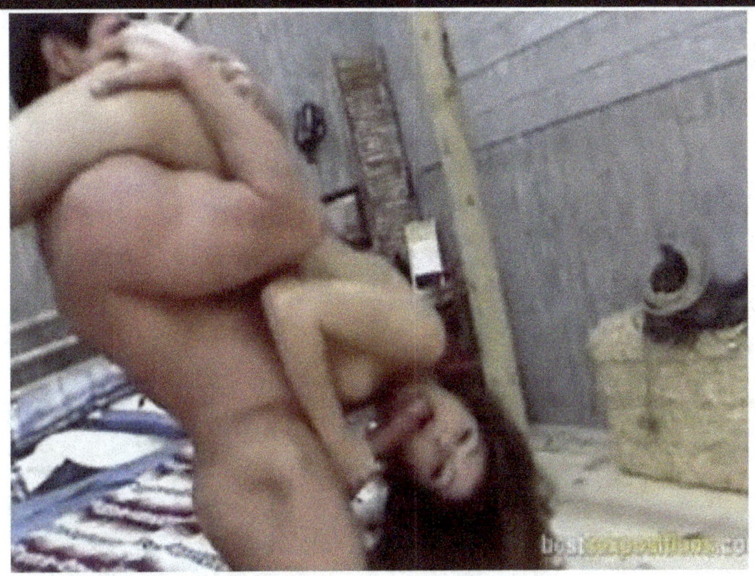

Standing 69

If you're feeling adventurous, try this acrobatic oral position. The man stands up and holds his gal upside down so she can stuff her face with his rod, while simultaneously macking down on her pussy.

June 11

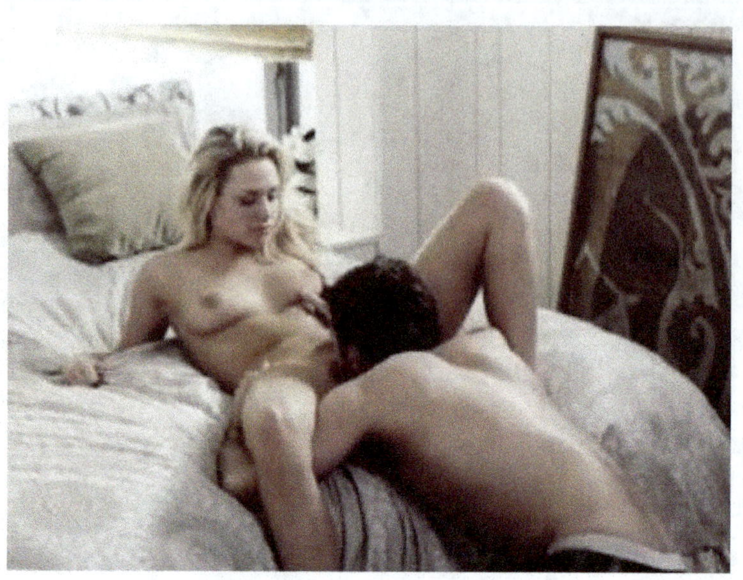

Spread Eagle

The perfect cunnilingus position for a quickie or a long slow road to orgasm, in the Spread Eagle she can lie back and truly indulge in the pleasure of oral sex.

June 12

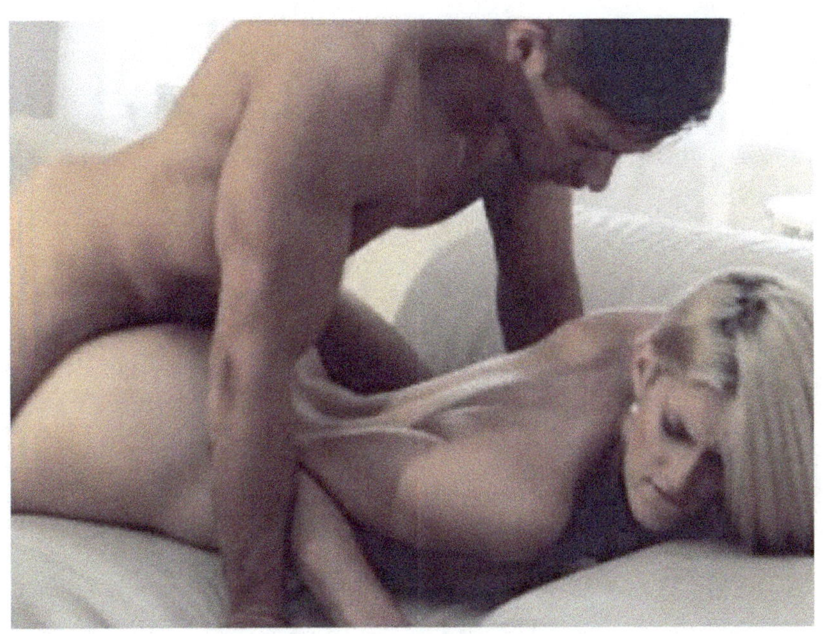

Prone Bone

With the woman facing down, her butt on the very edge of the bed and the man behind her leaning over. This is an excellent position for having rough sex. Men: Don't be afraid to get in there! Try pinning her wrists down on the bed.

June 13

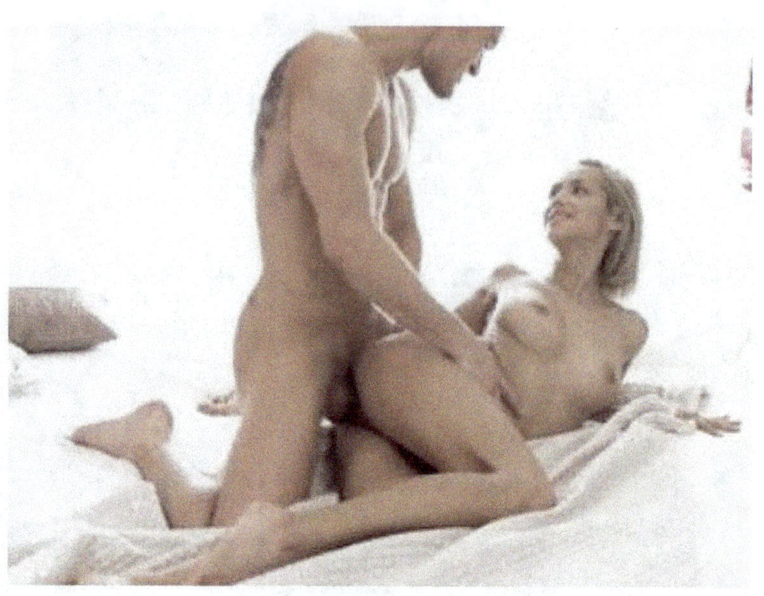

The Corkscrew

Another amazing position for rough vaginal or anal sex. The woman lays on her side while the man, on his knees, enter behind her, grabbing on tight at the hips. This a also a good transition from spooning position.

June 14

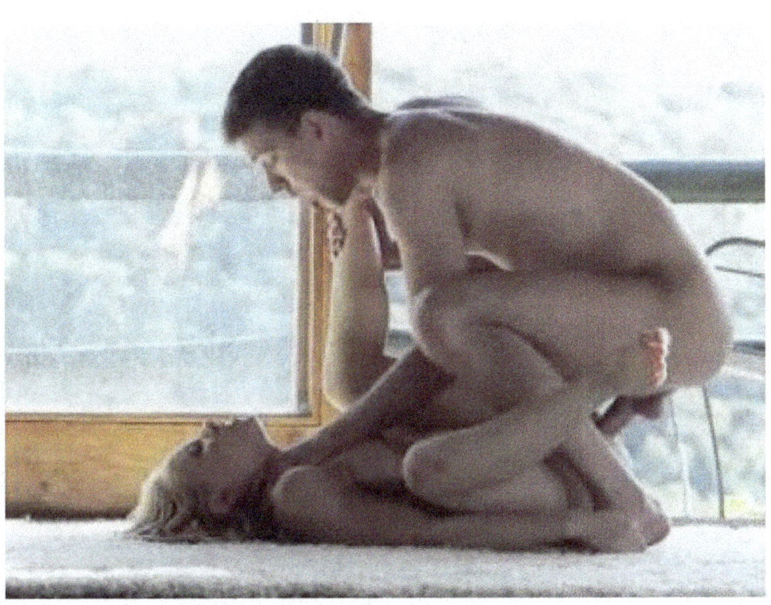

Cowboy Position

Cowgirl with the man on top, controlling her legs as for deep penetration. With her hands free, the woman can use a vibrator if desired.

Bonus points for choking.

June 15

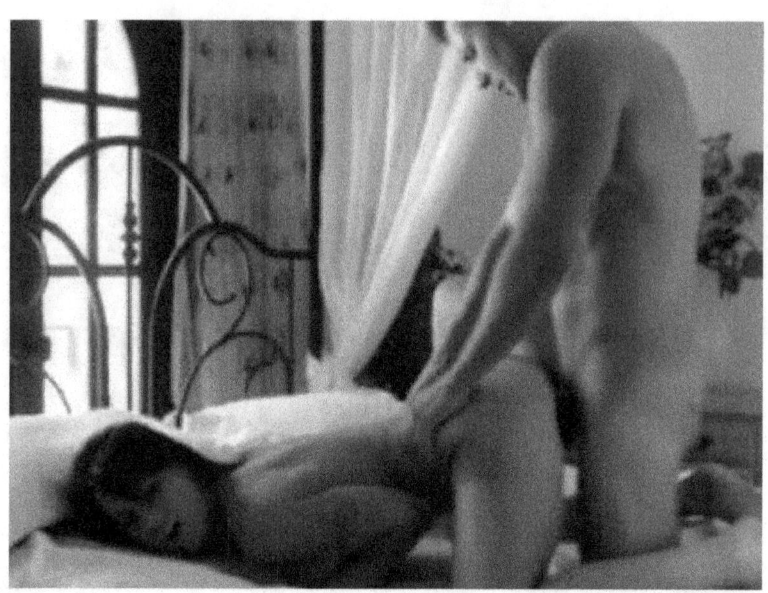

Face Down, Ass Up

The name says it all. Dealer's choice of vaginal or anal.

Men: You have a lot to grab onto in this position that will allow you to throw a lot of power behind each thrust.

Women: If he's not being rough enough with you, a words of encouragement will do wonders. You can also throw it back, matching his power.

June 16

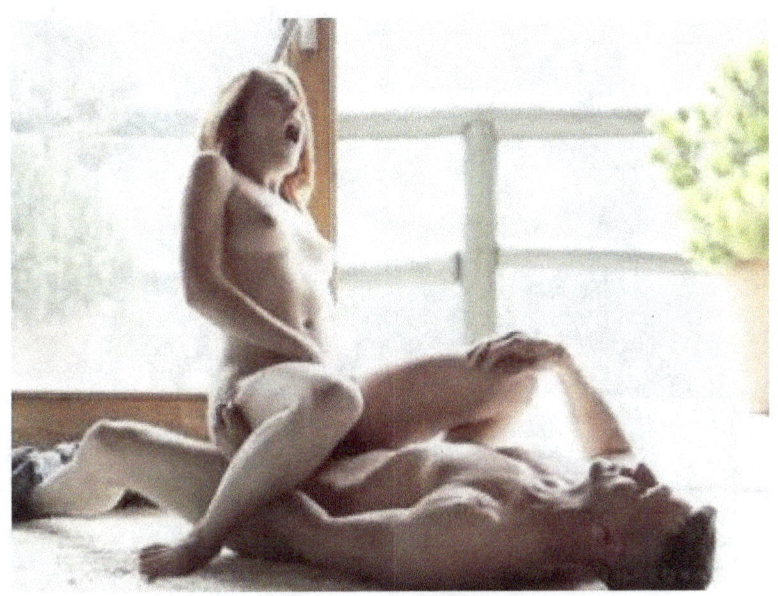

Vertical Cowgirl

With the woman on top, back arched, allowing her to control the pace and level of stimulation. In Vertical Cowgirl, she typically puts her hands behind her for balance, thrusting up and down at the hips.

June 17

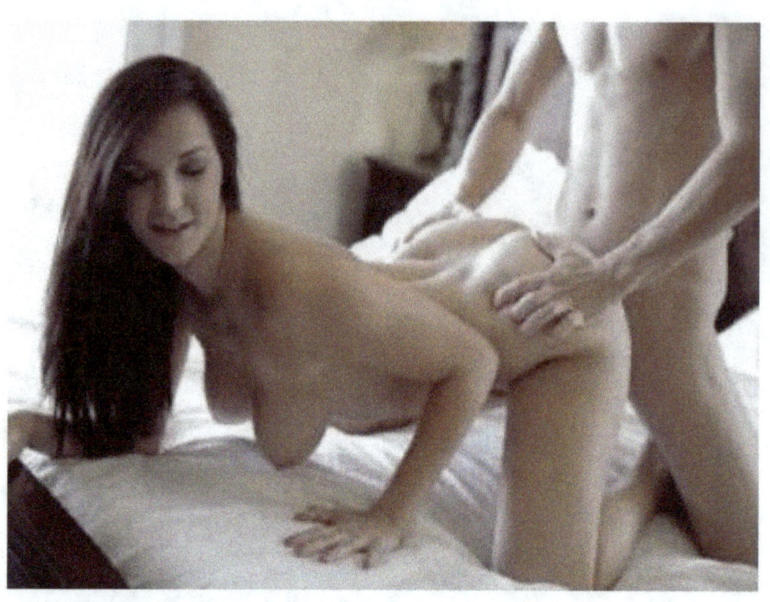

Doggystyle

There is nothing wrong with the classics.

Make it hotter:

- Introduce a vibrator for her. Or better yet, a vibrating cock ring.

- Her: Spread those cheeks so he can get in deeper. Add clitoral stimulation to the mix for an easy orgasm.

- Him: Rough play is definitely encouraged. Spankings are mandatory.

- Bored of Doggystyle already? Have you tried anal doggy?

June 18

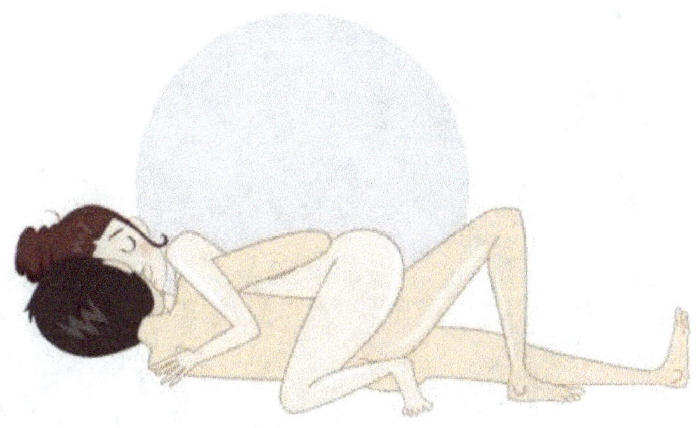

The Zen Pause

Difficulty level: Easy

Special features: Slow-going, romantic

This position is ideal if you need to slow down the pace during a long sex session.

The man and the woman both lay on their sides facing each other. The man enters the woman as she wraps her legs around him.

June 19

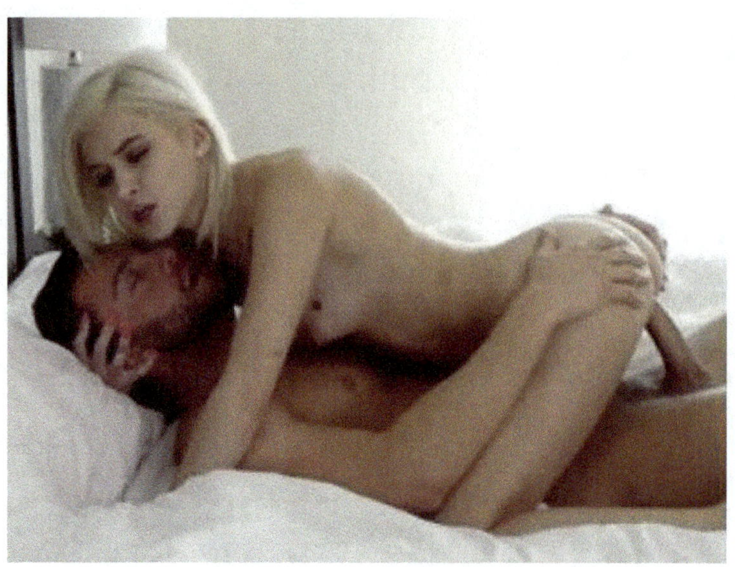

Fast Fuck

The Fast Fuck sex position is great for when you want a quickie with your man. As the name suggests, the Fast Fuck involves your man rapidly thrusting in and out. In a lot of ways, the Fast Fuck is quite similar to the Cowgirl, but with the added leverage of the woman on lunging on top.

To set it up, your man just needs to lie down on his back and bend his knees slightly with his feet planted on the ground. You then need to straddle him. You have a choice of being on your knees or on your feet. It's up to you. But you will be leaning forward, resting on your hands or elbows. You need to position yourself so that you are slightly raised above your man.

The Fast Fuck feels great for your man, no matter what angle he enters you at, but you need to do a little experimentation with how your position yourself (on your knees/feet/how far forward you lean over) to find a spot that you really enjoy.

The Fast Fuck usually doesn't feel great for anal sex unless you use large quantities of lube.

One drawback to the Fast Fuck is that it's not particularly intimate. You won't be making a lot of physical contact with your man during it.

June 20

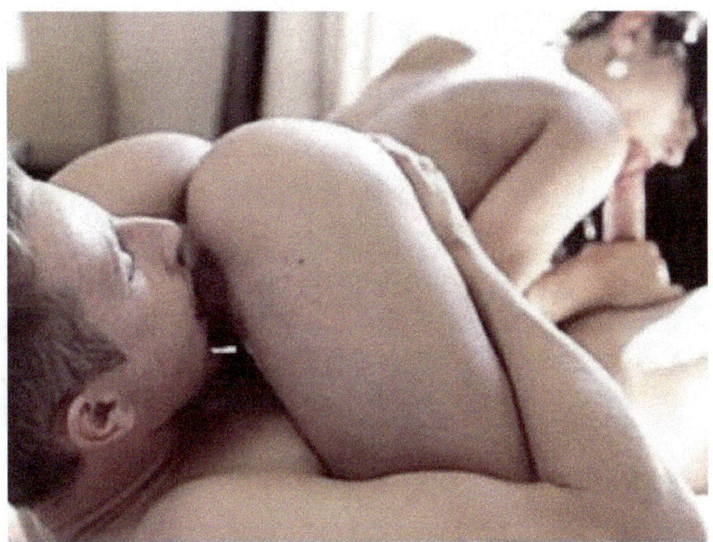

69 Position

The 69 is is perfect for during foreplay. You don't have to only lie on your side during the 69. If you like, you can lie on your back while your man is supporting himself above you on his hands and knees. Or he can lie on his back, while you are above.

When sucking your man's dick, you can try grabbing the base of it with one hand to prevent it from going too far into your throat.

It you want more intense stimulation from your man, get him to wrap his arms around your waist to pull you in on top of him.

If you don't like the idea of kissing your man right after performing the 69 on him, then make sure to keep some mints/gum close by to cover any tastes you don't want.

If you feel that you are about to climax, then take your man's penis out of your mouth. People often clench their jaws as they orgasm. **This is why you do not want to orgasm when his cock is in your mouth!**

If your man is usually quite quick to ejaculate, then it might be a good idea to let him eat you out for a while first, before you start giving him a blowjob. That way you both get a ton of enjoyment out of it and you're are not left wanting.

June 21

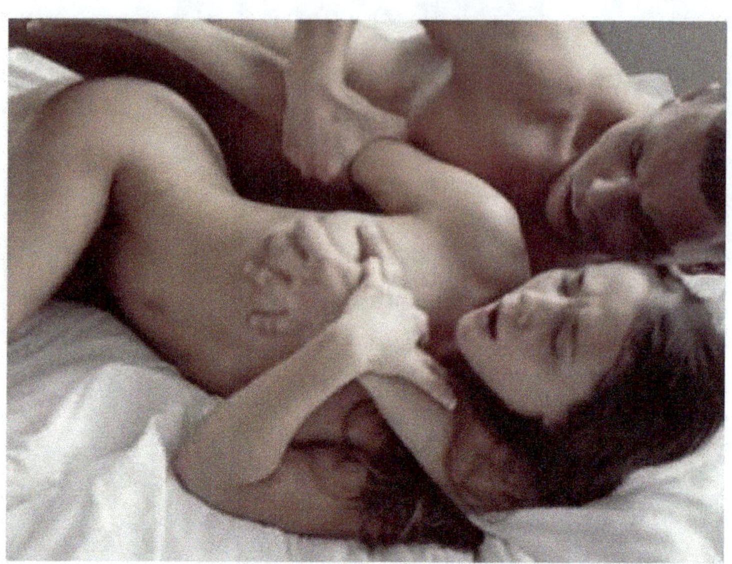

The Bouncing Spoon

The Bouncing Spoon sex position is a sort of pseudo-spooning position for you and your man. It's a fairly simple position to do which makes it great for spicing things up in the bedroom.

If you are looking for something really intimate, especially while watching a movie/TV in bed, then this is a great position, especially when you lean right back into your man and he wraps his arms around you

The Bouncing Spoon sex position is great to transition to from something like Reverse Cowgirl as all your man has to do is sit up.

As with a lot of positions I teach, you need to lean forward/backward to find that 'perfect place' that gives you maximum pleasure.

June 22

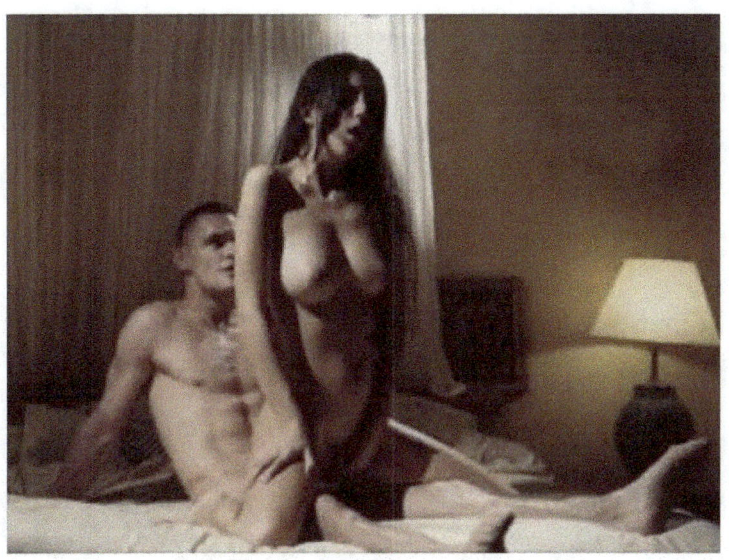

Twerking Cowgirl

This is one of my personal favorites. Its another one where the woman controls the pace and is easy to transition. Excellent for men who love to stare at your ass as you wiggle it

Make it hotter:

- Introduce a handheld vibrator.
- Knees getting tired? Lean forward and brace your hands on the bed, shifting your weight as you twerk your booty up and down his cock.
- Fuck in 4 dimensions: swivel your hips from side to side. It might not give you perfect clitoral stimulation, but your man will love it and consider you a pro, this I can guarantee.
- Lean back into a Acrobat position as he thrusts up into you.
- Try transitioning from reverse cowgirl to cowgirl without breaking penetration.

June 23

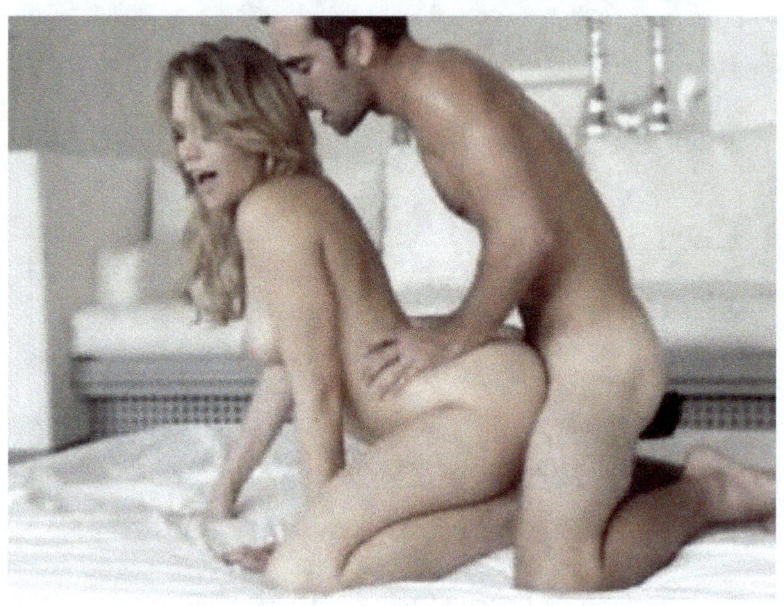

Camel Style

The G-spot activation of Doggy with added closeness and intimacy.

The woman must be positioned with her legs folded underneath her.

For the woman, try to sit up straight (unlike the couple in the picture). The right angle makes it easy to hit your G-spot every time.

The man gets a firm grasp on her hips, butt, back, anything he can hold onto to throw added power behind his thrusts.

June 24

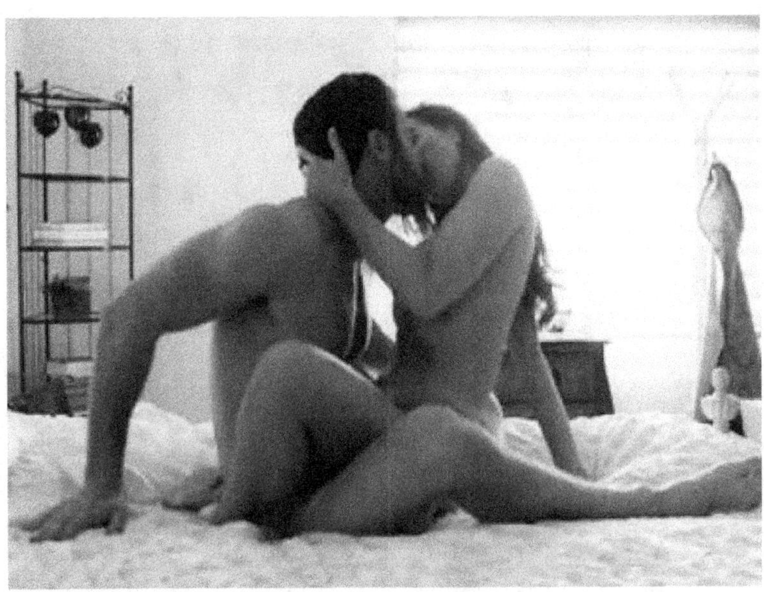

Lotus Position

To get into the Lotus sex position, your man needs to sit down on his butt with his legs crossed and pulled fairly close in front of him like the traditional yoga pose. You then need to sit down on his crotch while facing him and hold on to him quite tightly by wrapping your arms around his back and putting your legs around his back as well to pull him in to you. Your man will also hold on to your quite firmly as well by putting his arms around you.

It's an intimate position, not a 'hardcore sex position'. So use it for when you want to get closer and more intimate with your man.

Don't worry if your man can't cross his legs or finds it painful. It's just as pleasurable when he has them straight.

You may find that leaning backwards slightly during it allows your man to provide more stimulation to your G-Spot.

June 25

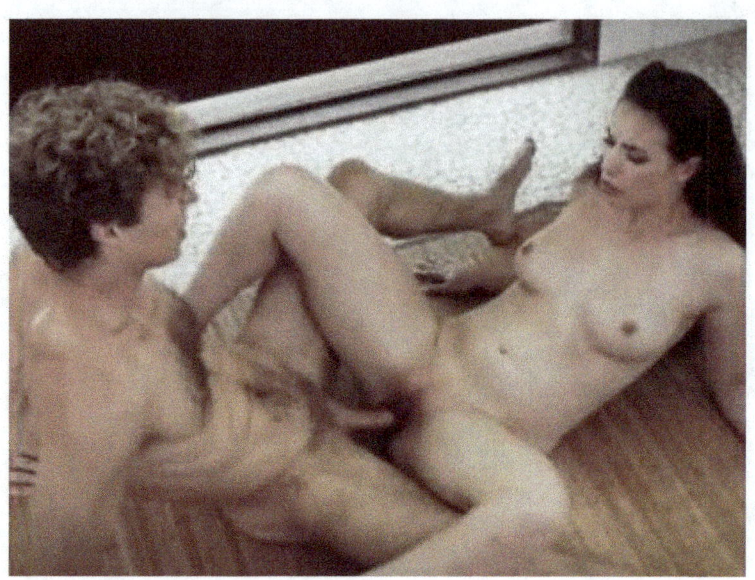

Spider Position

How to do it: Sit on a bed with both partners' legs bent toward one another, with your arms back to support yourselves. Now, move together so that the receiver goes onto the giver's penis or **strap-on**. The receiver's hips will end up between the giver's spread legs, the receiver's knees bent, and feet outside of the giver's hips and flat on the bed. Then, rock back and forth.

Benefits: "The spider position can be intimate, as you can look in to each other's eyes while having sex," explains Needle. Plus, you can easily control the giving partner's depth of penetration by moving your hips closer or further away.

Make it hotter: The receiving partner can grab the giver's hands and pull themself up into a squatting position while the giver lies back. Or the giver can remain seated upright and pull the receiver against their chest into the Lazy Man position.

June 26

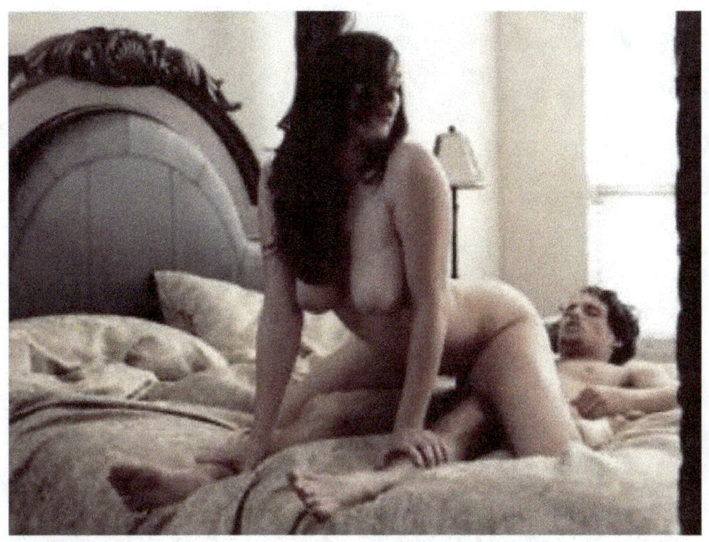

The Rider

The Rider is a move that has been around for long, long time, but only recently became really popular in adult films and even in our culture as a whole. The Rider goes by another name that you're probably more familiar with: The Twerk.

In my experience, twerking on a guy's dick is the fastest way to get him to cum. Period. You don't need a ridiculous rap video booty to twerk. Actually, you don't need any ass at all – I can testify to that. In fact, if your man likes big butts, but you have a tiny heiny, twerking in reverse cowgirl is a surefire way to get him to appreciate your rump.

Ladies, twerking is NOT easy. At least, it's not an easy thing to do really well. You WILL need to practice this move by yourself. First, try it out in front of a mirror – or if you're in your 20s, TikTok.

Expect his dick to fall out the first 10 times you try this move – but keep at it! Go slow at first, then work up a faster pace. Angle and rhythm are everything. He may be tempted to thrust upwards, but it's easier if the man just lies stationary while the woman does her thing. If you can master the reverse cowgirl twerk (They called it The Rider in the 70s), then you will never be lonely again for the rest of your life.

June 27

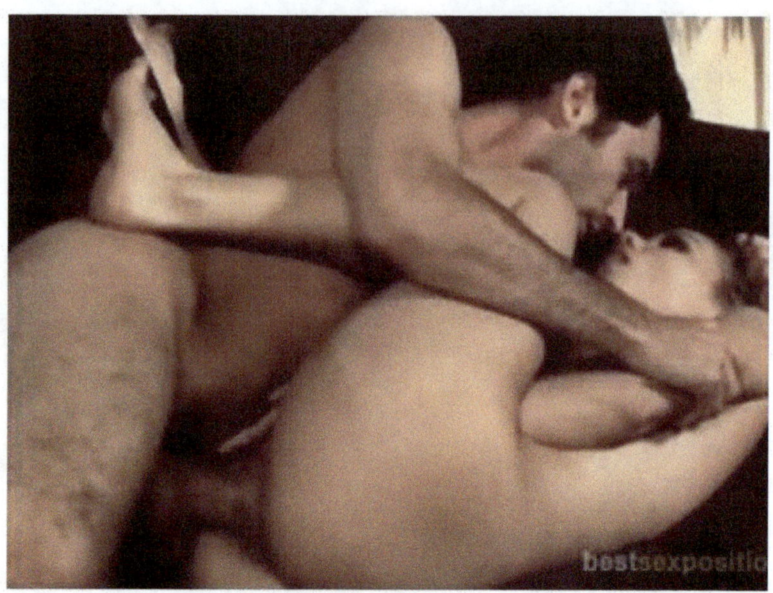

Love's Fusion

Think of Love's Fusion as reverse spooning. You get all of the benefits of face-to-face sex and, if done right, deep penetration with G-spot activation.

This position works best when the woman starts out on her side with one leg bent in the air and the other leg touching the bed extended straight.

The man enters by lying on his side, face-to-face with your partner. Unless the man is considerably taller than the woman, he will need to be lying staggered further down the bed.

If you're both lying face-to-face, and the man is slightly taller, have him lie eye-level with the woman's collarbone. If you're both the same height, his line of sight should be centered at the woman's breasts.

When you start out with a staggered height, with the woman higher up on the bed, it allows for the man to enter at the perfect angle for comfort, leverage, and g-spot intensity. The man can then manipulate the woman's leg for better positioning and deeper penetration.

June 28

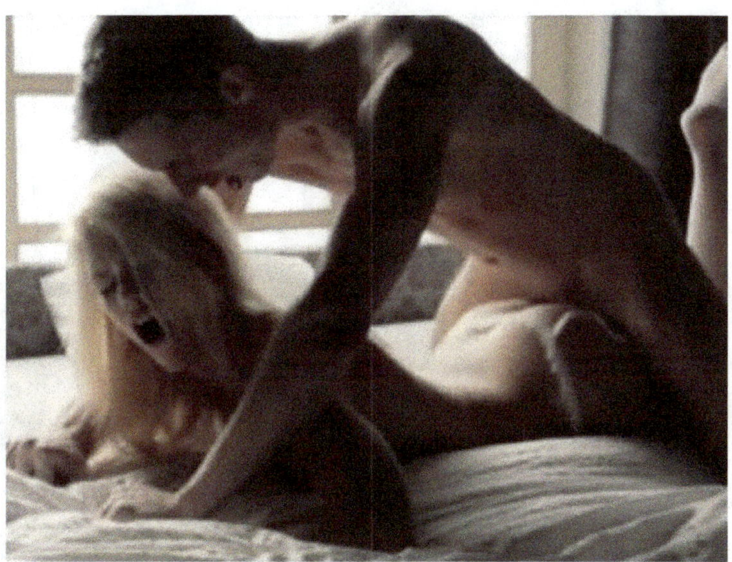

The Elephant

The Elephant is a sex game in which the receiver covers her ass in lube or oil, then lies flat on her stomach. The giver sits atop the receiver's upper thighs, sticking his meat in between the buns, using the receiver's slick and slippery cheeks to build friction.

The giver is supposed to lean over the back of the receiver, almost like in a Flatiron position, which thrusts between the receiver's cheeks until he scores a hole in one.

The kinky thrill of this game is that it can sometimes end with anal and sometimes end with vaginal intercourse. Some men will find it thrilling that the woman doesn't care which hole he puts it in. And that is Elephant.

The Elephant is a fun game for any man with a fetish for big butts.

June 29

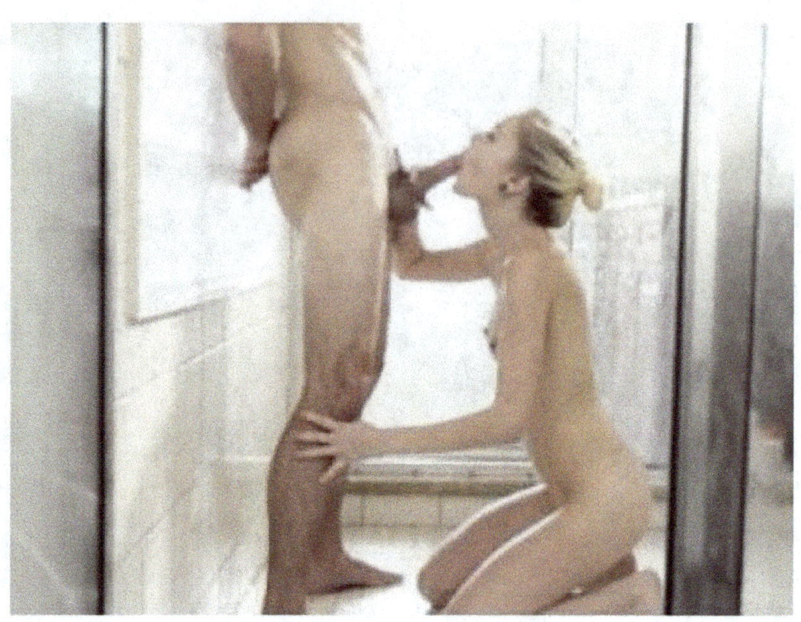

On Your Knees, Please

In this position the man stands up and the woman gets down on her knees – putting her head at just the right spot for the perfect blow job.

June 30

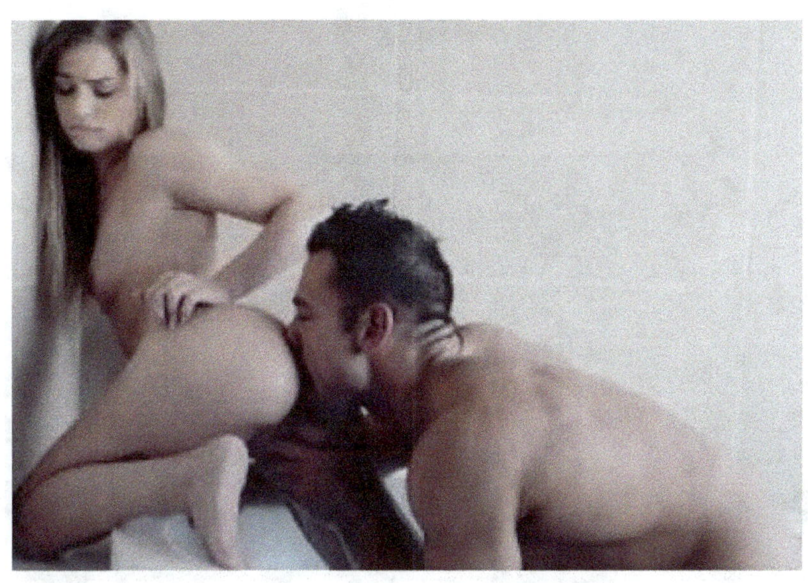

Rimming

Eating ass is more just an occupational hazard of going down on a woman. All women secretly love having their asshole licked – even if they don't know it yet. It's a wonderous sensation that will have you both coming back for more.

Rimming + a little clitoral stimulation = An orgasm that will have you screaming, "Don't stop! Don't you dare stop!"

July

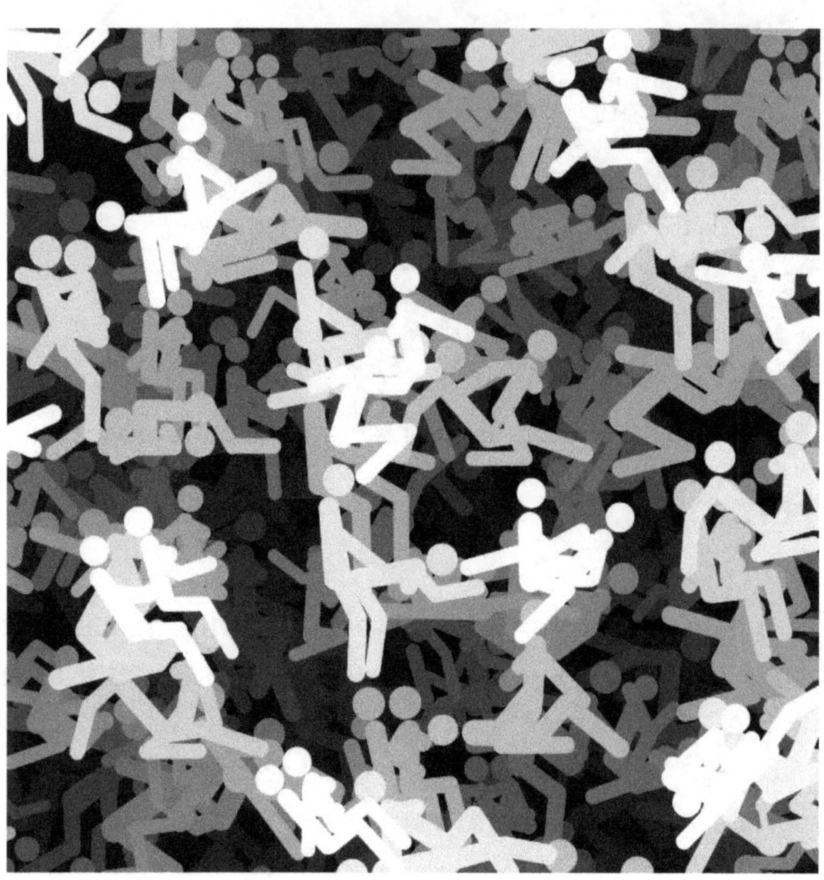

Ally's Sex Toy Recommendations

For limitless pleasure & intense orgasms, familiarize yourself with different handheld toys and the best positions in which they can be implemented.

FOR HER

- **Hits all the right spots:**
  Classic Rabbit Vibrator for Women - https://amzn.to/3TPOEjD
- **Waterproof Kinky Set:**
  Beginners Kinky Plug Trainer Set - https://amzn.to/3IJtOzT
- **Remote-controlled fun:**
  Remote controlled clit stimulator vibrator- https://amzn.to/4eZAje0
- **For "alone time":**
  Vibrating Didlo for Women - https://amzn.to/44Jo1TB

FOR HIM

- **6 Size Classic Cock Ring Set:**
  Soft silicone cock ring for men - https://amzn.to/44ZClWR
- **Guys with a little kink:**
  Cock Ring for For Sex Men Vibrant Pennis Ring Prostate Massager - https://amzn.to/4lItWyv
- **Guys solo play:**
  App Controlled Male Heated Masturabator Pleasure Toys - https://amzn.to/44VKgEF

HIM OR HER

- **The unbeatable classic:**
  Hitatchi Magic Wand personal massager - https://amzn.to/3Uo8CSG
- **The holy grail:**
  G-spot vibrator for men and women - https://amzn.to/46kiUKV
- **For tingling electric sensations:**
  TENS 7000 Digital TENS Unit with Accessories - https://amzn.to/4f81Wlg

July 1

Anal Missionary

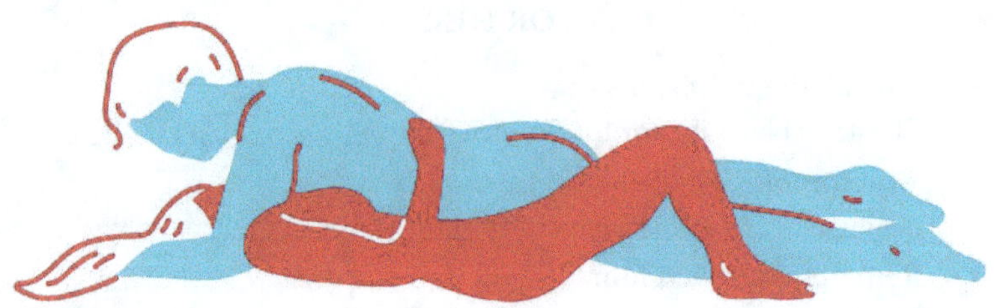

How to do it: The receiver lies on their back, while the giver lies facedown on top.

Benefits: It's kinky twist on a classic. The missionary sex position is simple, elegant, effective, and surprisingly versatile.

Make it hotter: The bottom partner can switch up the sensations for both parties by shifting the angle of their legs.

July 2

Power Doggy

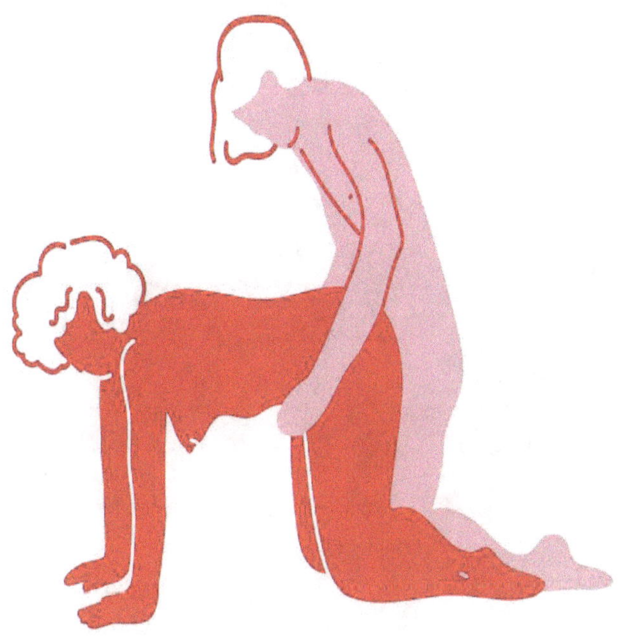

How to do it: The receiver gets on all fours. Then, the giver kneels behind them, with their upper body straight up or slightly draped over the receiver.

Benefits: This sex position allows for deep penetration and easier **G-spot stimulation**.

Make it hotter: The Woman can **stimulate the clitoris** with one hand, or ask their partner to do the finger work for them. Temperature play can happen here, too. Grab an ice cube and slowly run it down the spine of your partner.

July 3
Power Cowgirl

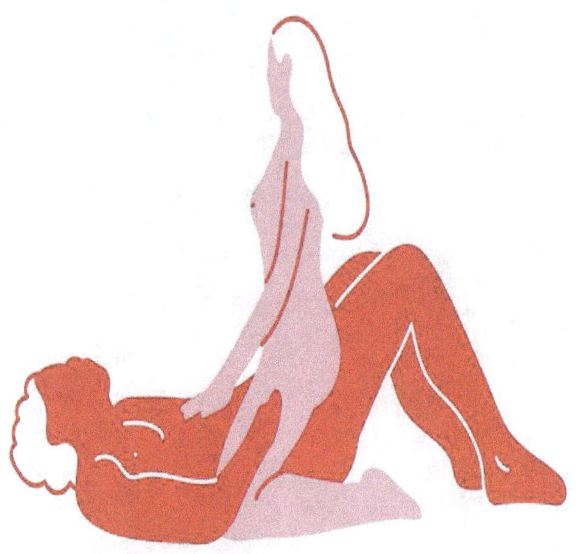

How to do it: The receiver kneels on top, pushing off the giver's chest and sliding up and down their thighs. The receiver can relieve some of the weight from their partner's pelvis by leaning back and supporting themself on their thighs.

Benefits: By being the dominant force in this sex position, the receiver delays their partner's climax *and* intensifies their own.

Make it hotter: Change the depth and pressure by bringing your chests closer together, a.k.a. lean in. While you're leaning forward, take the time to add in some nipple play and neck kisses. Alternatively, she recommends grinding in directions that slightly differ from what you normally do. Tend to go back and forth? Channel your inner Ariana Grande and go side to side.

July 4
Cowgirl's Helper

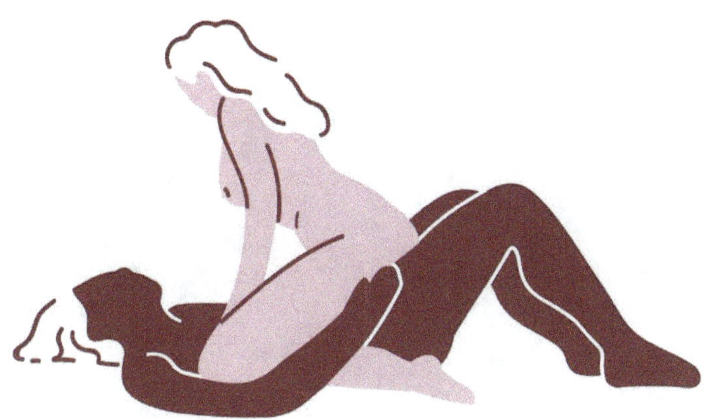

How to do it: Similar to the popular cowgirl sex position, the receiver kneels on top, pushing off the giver's chest and sliding up and down the thighs. But the giver helps by supporting some of the receiver's weight and grabbing their hips or thighs while they rise to meet each thrust.

Benefits: This sex position puts less stress on the receiver's legs, making climaxing easier. Plus, if the giver is a penis owner, it can delay their climax—extending the pleasure sesh.

Make it hotter: Alternate between shallow and deep thrusting to stimulate different nerve endings.

July 5

Rider Astride

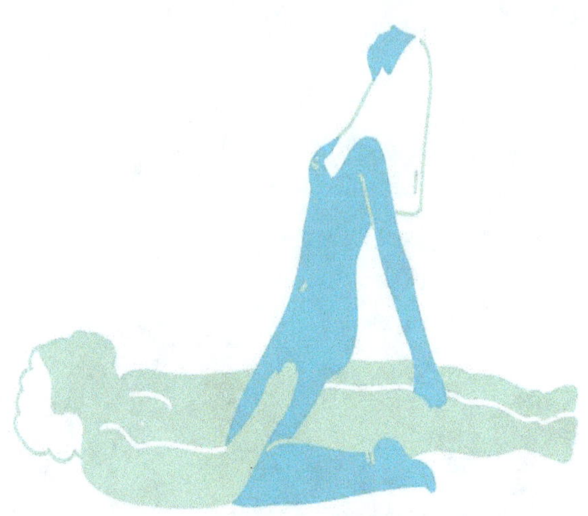

How to do it: This position is just like cowgirl, but with a twist. The receiver climbs on top, while their partner enters them from a lying down position. Then, the receiver leans back and places their hands on the bed for support, creating a 45-degree angle with the giving partner's legs.

Benefits: For vulva owners, this change in angle helps target the G-spot even more, and gives more control over the speed and depth of thrusts. Plus, giving partners have easy access to the clitoris.

Make it hotter: If you have a vulva, give yourself a hand with the "V stroke": Make a V with the index and ring finger of one hand and place the fingers on either side of the clitoris with the giving partner's penis, strap-on, or a dildo in between. Push your fingers down in a rocking motion.

July 6
Easy Rider

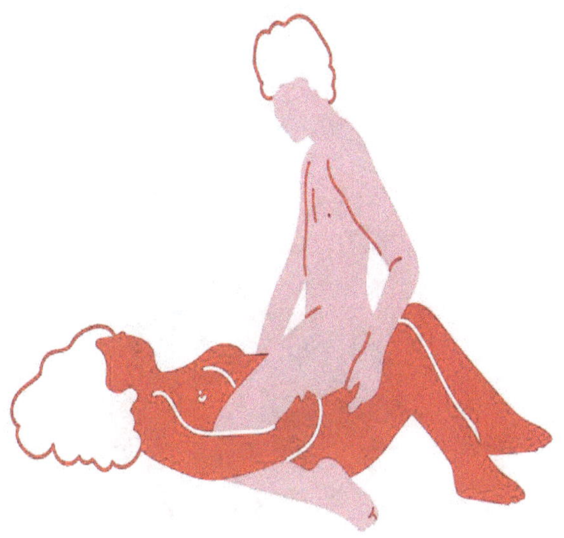

How to do it: The receiver lies on their back while the giving partner straddles them. The giver then gently inserts their penis, strap-on, or finger through the tight opening created by the receiver's semi-closed legs.

Benefits: The tightness afforded by this position increases the intensity of the penetration.

Make it hotter: Have the giver gently hold down the receiver's wrists for a **little bondage action**. If you're into **BDSM**, this is a great opportunity for some light choking or nipple play using nipple clamps that have adjustable pressure. Plus, the same toys used on clits, like the viral Hitachi Magic Wand can also be used on your nipples, she adds. (Blossoming sex life, right this way!)

July 7

Mind Melt

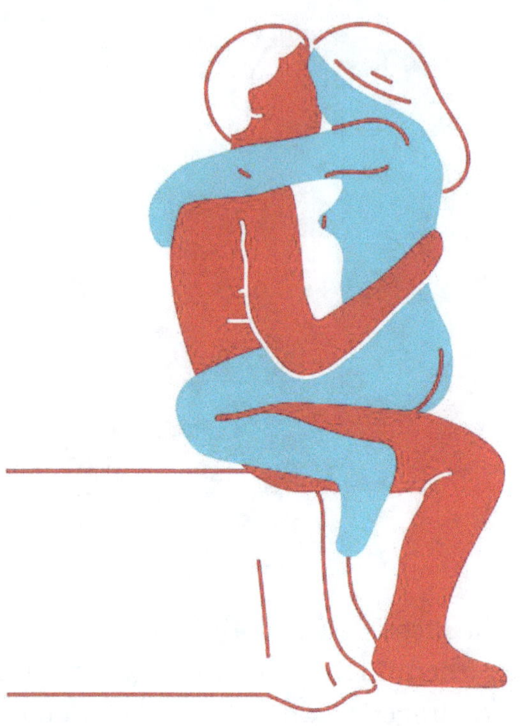

How to do it: The giving partner sits on a chair or the edge of the bed; the receiver faces them while seated on their lap. Benefits: This sex position allows you to control the pace and depth of penetration. Plus, being seated adds support, so it's great for marathon sex sessions.

Make it hotter: Let your fingers (and hands) do the talking. Once seated, you both can put your hands anywhere on each other's bodies to make things more interesting. (Nipple play, anyone?)

July 8
Pretzel Dip

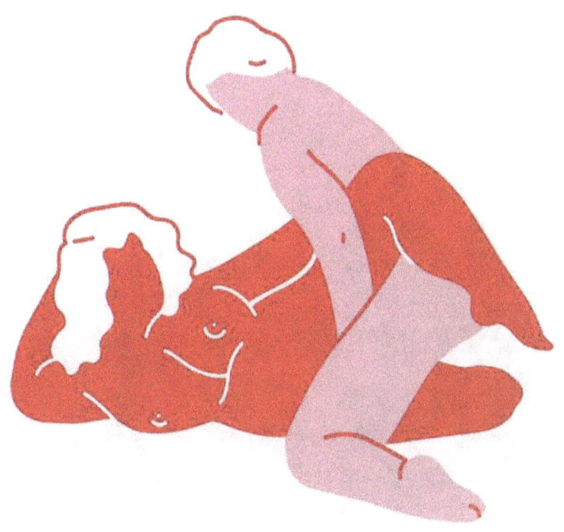

How to do it: The receiving partner lies down on their side. Then, the giving partner kneels between their thighs, straddling their bottom leg. The receiver's top leg then rests on one of the giver's thighs.

Benefits: With the **pretzel dip position**, you get the deeper penetration of doggy style while still being able to make eye contact with your partner. Vulva owners who don't love a ton of penetration can, alternatively, have the giver grind up against them, stimulating their clit.

Make it hotter: Add nipple clamps into the mix or grab an ice cube and use it on your or your partner's nipples.

July 9

G-Whiz

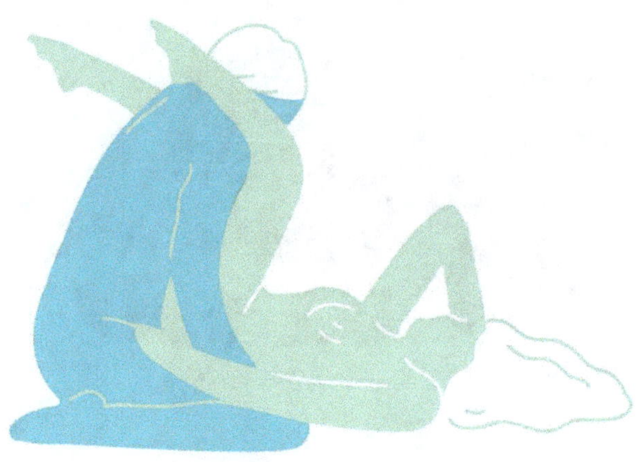

How to do it: The receiver lies on their back with one leg resting on each of the giver's shoulders. The giver can enter as they would from the front.

Benefits: For receivers with vulvas, this sex position is awesome because raising the legs narrows the vagina and helps **target the G-spot**.

Make it hotter: The giver can rock the receiver in a side-to-side or up-and-down motion.

July 10
Coital Alignment Technique

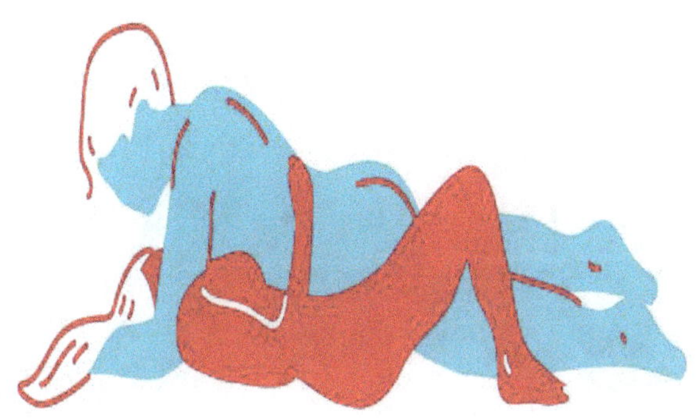

How to do it: The receiver lies on their back and wraps their ankles around the giving partner's calves. Then, the receiver should flex their legs to bring their partner closer.

Benefits: This position is meant to pull the giving partner's penis or **dildo** up closer towards the genitals for extra pleasure.

Make it hotter: Taking it slow will give you and your partner an opportunity to talk dirty, gaze into each other's eyes, and all that good stuff.

July 11

Magic Mountain

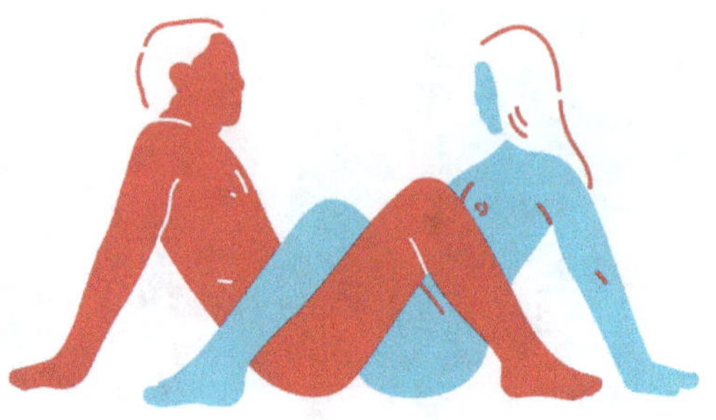

How to do it: The giver sits, legs bent, leaning back on their hands and forearms. The receiver does the same and then inches toward the giver until contact is made.

Benefits: This position allows for tons of eye contact, which can be extremely intimate. Plus, vulva owners can grind their clitoris against the giver's pelvis for some added stimulation.

Make it hotter: Temperature play, anyone? Slide ice cubes down one partner's chest and let the cold water collect at the base of their pelvis.

July 12

Cross-Booty

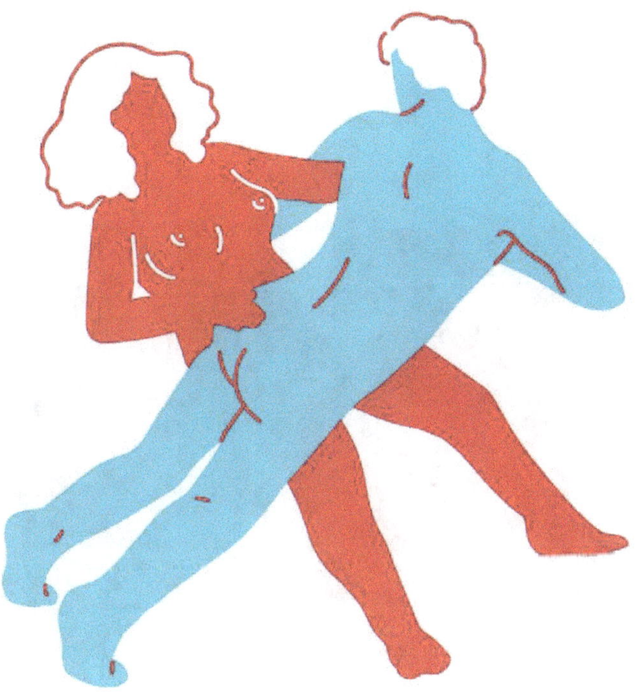

How to do it: The giving partner enters the receiver from the missionary position, then slides their chest and legs off the receiver's body so their pelvis is in the same location but the limbs form an "X" together.

Benefits: You feel more of your partner's body in motion with this sex position.

Make it hotter: If you're the bottom partner, take advantage of this unique angle to massage their back, butt, or legs. They'll go crazy (as will you, watching them).

July 13

Reverse Scoop

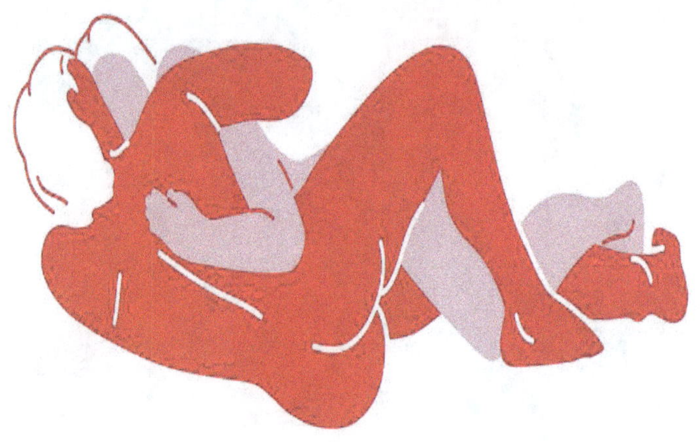

How to do it: From the missionary position, without disengaging, turn together onto your sides, using your arms to support your upper bodies.

Benefits: You get a really nice full-body press, and you can gaze into each other's eyes.

Make it hotter: Try intertwining your legs together or fondling them down below.

July 14

Spork

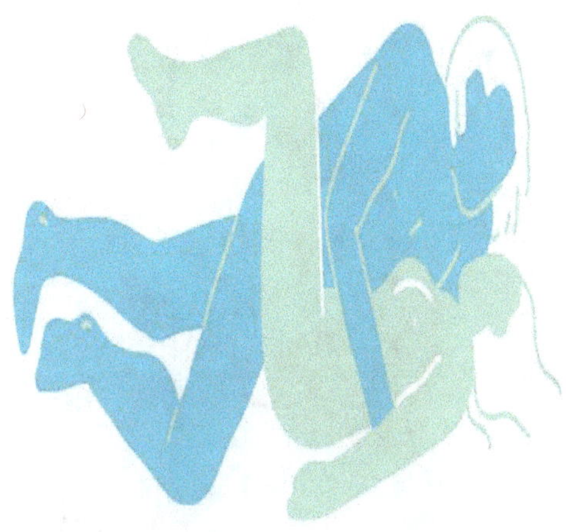

How to do it: The receiver should lie on their back and raise their right leg so the giving partner can position their body between their legs at a 90-degree angle and enter. The receiver's left leg can lie straight out on the bed or they can bend it to manipulate depth of penetration. For a rear-entry option, the receiver can lie on their stomach, bend one leg, and have the giving partner position themselves in between their legs.

Benefits: From the spork position, the receiver can lift their top leg and support it by resting it on the giving partner's shoulder. From here, vulva owners can easily stimulate their clitoris.

Make it hotter: Synchronize your breathing. One of you takes the lead and the other follows so that you inhale and exhale together. The coordinated rhythm opens an unspoken dialogue of intimacy.

July 15

Love Pretzel

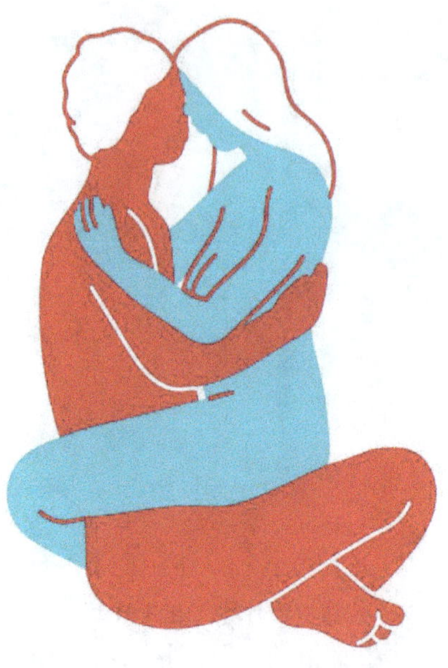

How to do it: The giving partner sits cross-legged (yoga/pretzel-style), while the receiver sits in their lap facing them. The receiver should wrap their legs around the giver and hug each other for support.

Benefits: This configuration is best for **tantric sex**. Rocking, not thrusting, is the key when it comes to this very intimate position.

Make it hotter: Lock into each other's deep gaze to put some extra "oh" into the big O.

July 16
Wrapped Lotus

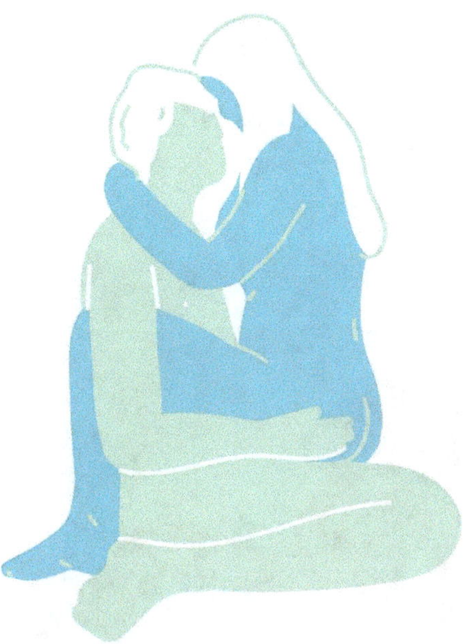

How to do it: The giving partner sits cross-legged and the receiver climbs into their lap, facing them, with the receiver's legs wrapped around the giver's back. The giving partner enters, and the receiver grinds up against their pelvis.

Benefits: This position allows for some major face-to-face intimacy. Plus there's plenty of room for creativity in this position—like stimulating **different erogenous zones** on each others' upper bodies, like the head, neck, and face.

Make it hotter: Ask them to **lick your nipples** and let their hands roam. And roam...and roam. (You get the idea.)

July 17
The Spider

July 18
Diagonal Scissoring

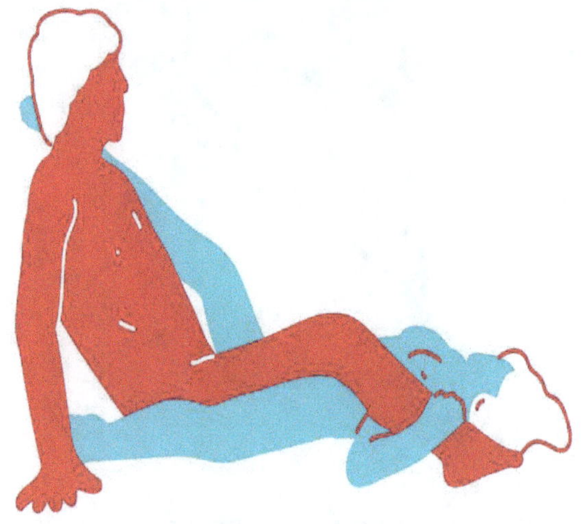

How to do it: Sit on the bed facing each other with legs forward. The giving partner's right leg goes over the receiver's left, and the receiver's right leg goes over the giver's left. Come together so the giver can enter. Now both of you lie back, your legs forming an X. Slow, leisurely gyrations replace thrusting.

Benefits: Prolonged slow sex will build your arousal. Shallow thrusts can also stimulate the nerve endings in the head of their penis (if a sexual partner has one). Better yet, this position also works as a grinding, **non-penetrative move**.

Make it hotter: Reach out and hold hands to pull together for pelvic thrusting. Also, take turns alternatively sitting up and lying back without changing the rhythm.

July 19
The Lazy Man

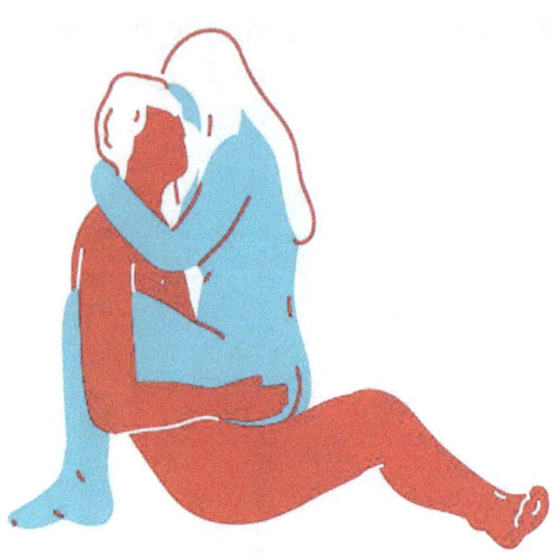

How to do it: Place pillows behind the giving partner's back and have them sit on the bed with legs outstretched. (Got a sex pillow? Break it out!) Now, the receiving partner can straddle the giver's waist with their feet on the bed. The receiver should bend their knees to lower themself onto their partner, using one hand to direct the penis or strap-on in. Just by pressing on the balls of their feet and releasing, they can raise and lower themself onto the shaft as slowly or as quickly as they please.

Benefits: This position puts the receiver in control, and maintains plenty of intimacy. For vulva owners, think of the giver's penis or strap-on as a masturbatory tool, something to rub and stimulate your clitoris with and against.

Make it hotter: From this position, you both can lie back into the Spider position.

July 20
Twerking Cowgirl

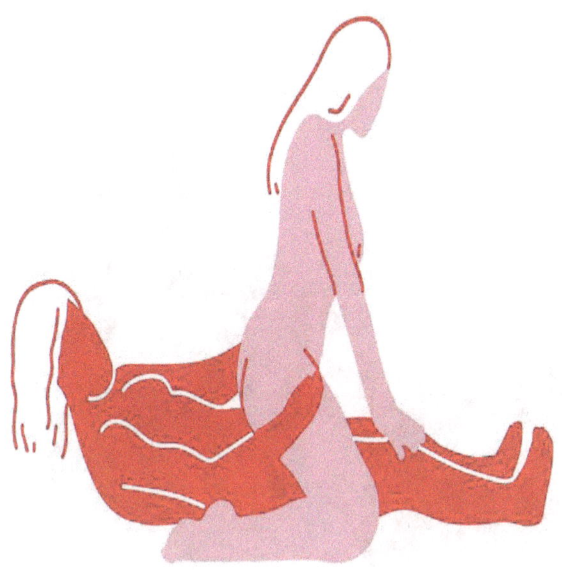

How to do it: The giver lies on their back; the receiver straddles them, facing their feet.

Benefits: The beauty of this cowgirl position is that it lets the receiver take control and show the giver the pace and rhythm they like.

Make it hotter: To get more leverage, the receiver can put their knees and shins inside their legs and under the giver's thighs.

July 21

The Snake

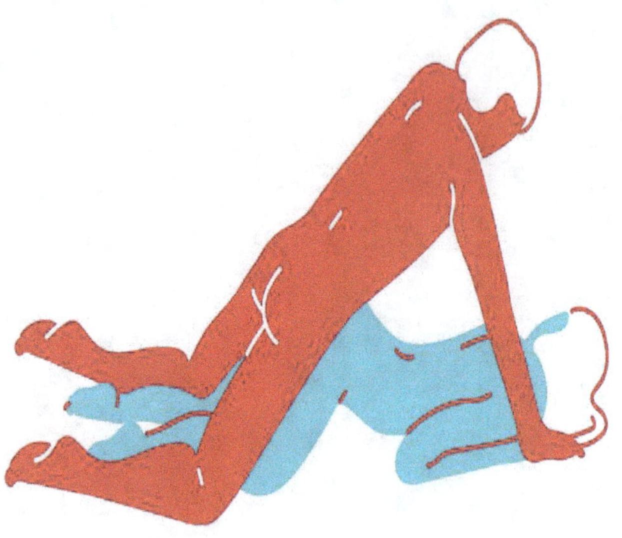

How to do it: The receiver lies down on their stomach, lifting up their butt. (They can also use a wedge or sex pillow to get the angle just right.) Then, the giving partner lies down on top of them and slides in from behind.

Benefits: This position allows for super-deep penetration, and a snug fit which can feel great for both parties.

Make it hotter: Receivers can reach back and wrap their hand around the shaft to help control how deep the giver gets, or they can change up the angle of their butt for the same effect.

July 22
The Chairman

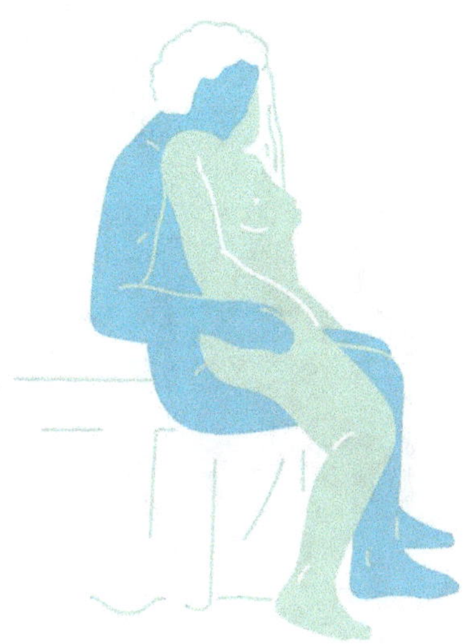

How to do it: The giving partner sits on the edge of the bed and the receiver sits on them, facing away. The receiving partner leans back on the giver, creating full body-to-body contact.

Benefits: For vulva owners, this sex position will hit the spot… as in, the G-spot. Meanwhile, you can use your hands to stimulate the scrotum, perineum, or clitoris.

Make it hotter: The receiver can bring their knees closer to their chest, supporting their feet on the bed.

July 23
Champagne Room

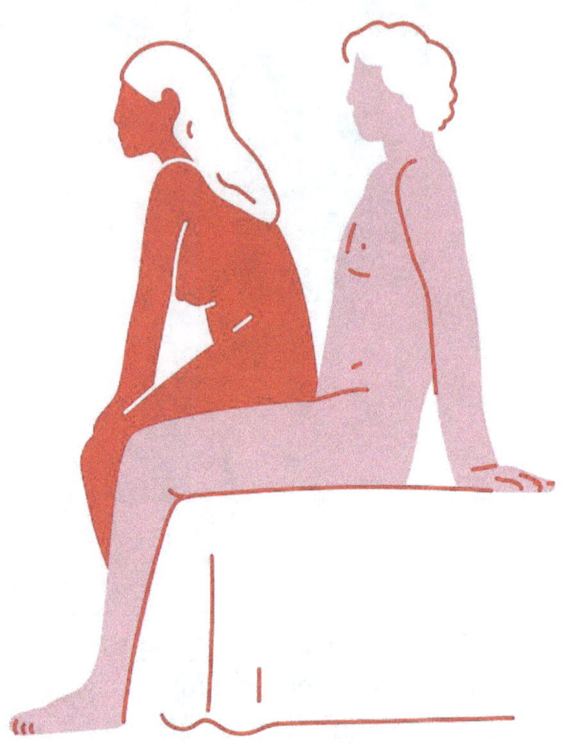

How to do it: The giving partner sits and the receiver sits on top of them, facing away. The receiving partner leans forward, rather than back on their partner (as seen in The Chairman).

Benefits: It helps the receiver regulate the pace and intensity of the thrusts.

Make it hotter: Try doing it on the stairs or the edge of the tub. Takes a bit of talent...but hey, practice makes perfect, am I right?

July 24

Full Press

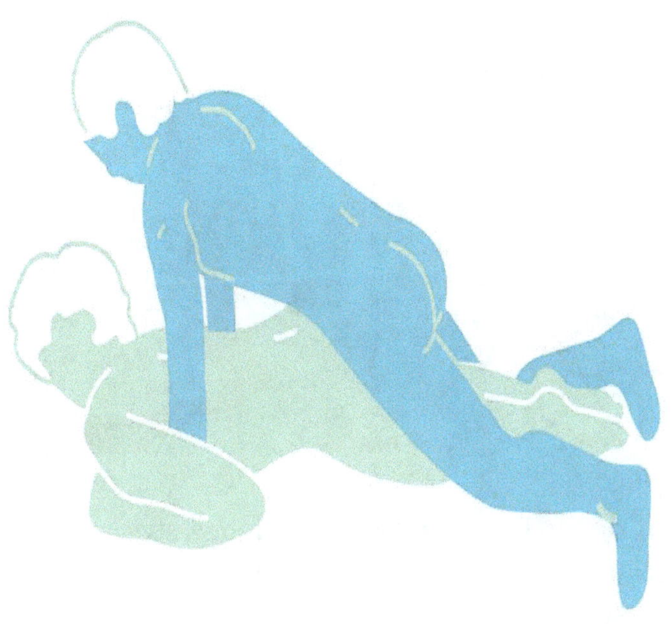

How to do it: The receiver lies facedown on the bed, legs straight, hips slightly raised. The giver can enter from behind.
Benefits: This sex position creates a snug fit, so the giver's penis or strap-on will feel even larger.
Make it hotter: This is a great opportunity to nibble or bite on your partner's shoulders and the back of their neck to add additional sensations..

July 25

Leapfrog

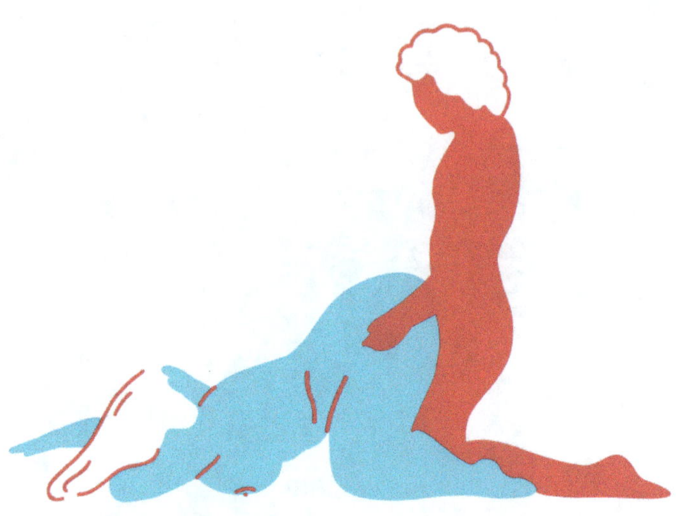

How to do it: This is a modified doggy style position. The receiver gets on their hands and knees, then, keeping hips raised, rests their head and arms on the bed. The giver can enter from behind.

Benefits: This sex position creates **deeper penetration—** and gives the receiver a chance to rest on a pillow.

Make it hotter: Vulva owners can use their hands or a toy to stimulate the clitoris. They might even choose to don a wearable or **hands-free vibrator.**

July 26

The Caboose

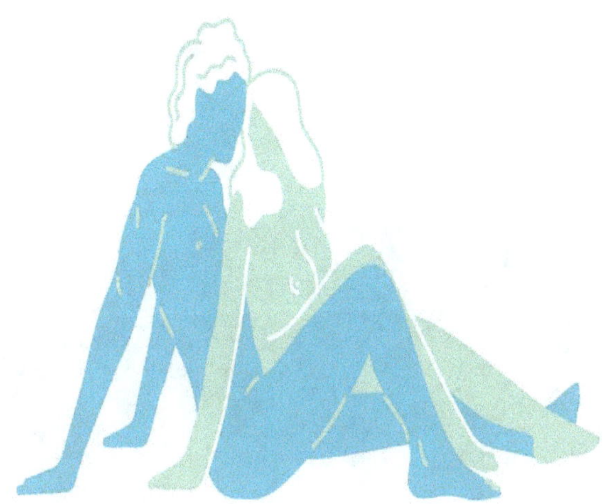

How to do it: While the giver sits on the bed or a chair, the receiver backs into the giver's lap and spoons while seated.

Benefits: You can't see your partner's face during this sex position, which means fantasizing is easier and can add to the excitement.

Make it hotter: Vulva owners can tighten the muscles of their pelvic floor so they can grip the giver. They can also stimulate their clitoris with their fingers, their partner's fingers, or a toy.

July 27
Scoop Me Up

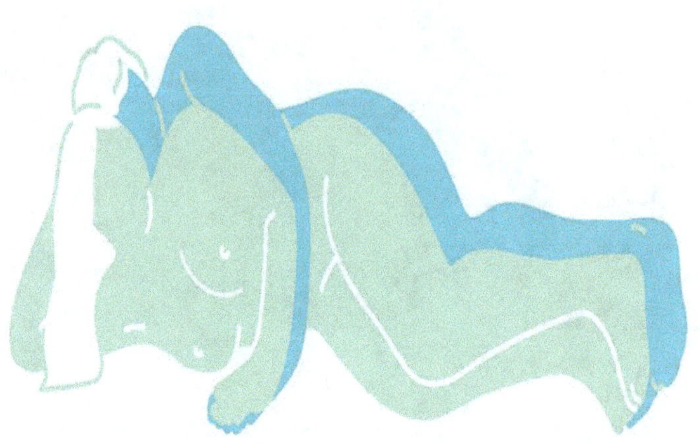

How to do it: Both partners lie on their sides, facing the same direction. The receiver brings their knees up slightly, while the giving partner slides up behind their pelvis and enters them from behind. (You may also know this as spooning.)

Benefits: This sex position allows for more skin-to-skin contact, increasing overall stimulation.

Make it hotter: The giving partner can place their hands on the receiver's shoulders to increase the intensity and deepness of the thrust.

July 27
The Seashell

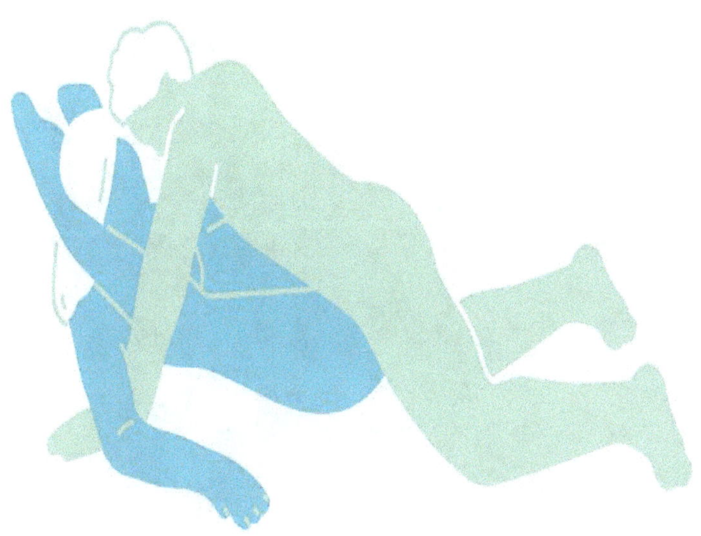

How to do it: The receiver should lie back with their legs raised all the way up and their ankles crossed behind their own head. The giver enters from a missionary position.
Benefits: Vulva owners are free to work their clitoris.
Make it hotter: For vulva owners, have the giver "ride high," rubbing their pubic bone against your clitoris, or "ride low," directly stimulating your G-spot with the head of the penis, the strap-on, a dildo, or a finger.

July 28
The Pinball Wizard

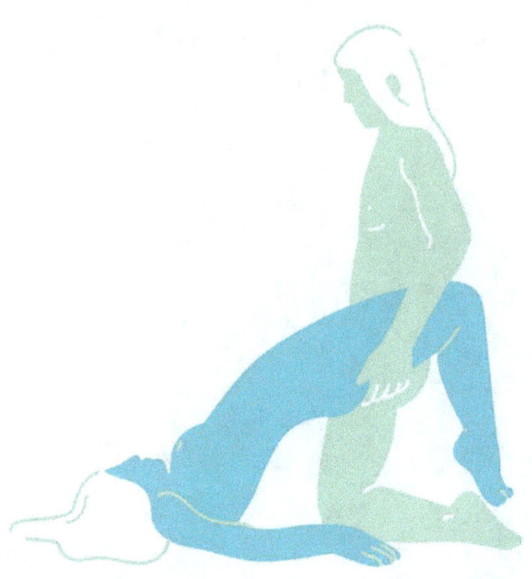

How to do it: The receiver gets into a partial bridge position (like a pinball machine), with their weight resting on their shoulders. The giving partner enters the receiver from a kneeling position.

Benefits: If the receiving partner has a vulva, this position allows the giving partner easy access to stimulate the clitoris and massage the mons pubis.

Make it hotter: The receiver can throw one leg up against their partner's shoulder for deeper penetration.

July 29

Valedictorian

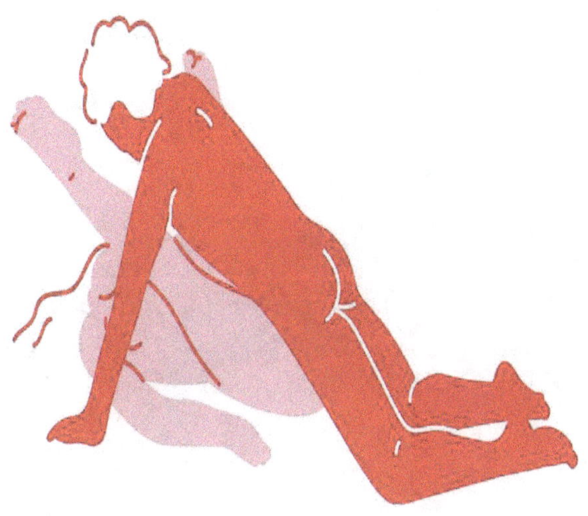

How to do it: From missionary position, the receiver raises their legs and extends them straight out (forming a "V").

Benefits: This allows for some good genital-to-genital contact, and even clit stimulation, too.

Make it hotter: Receivers can try grabbing their own ankles. That can give them stability and an added stretch to boost the sensation.

July 30

Seated Wheelbarrow

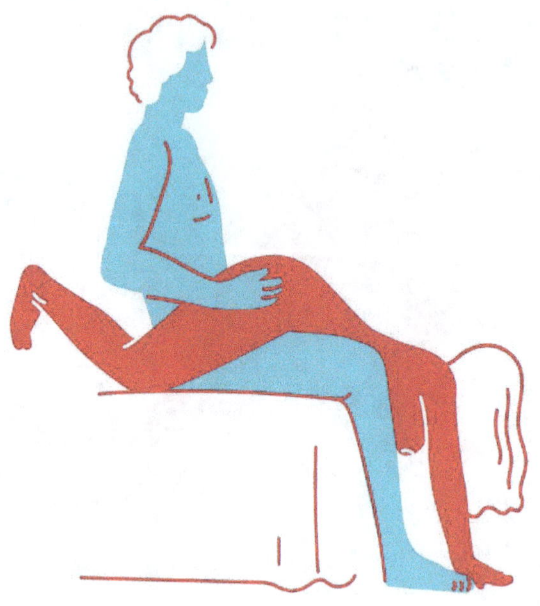

How to do it: The giving partner sits at the edge of a bed or chair, while the receiving partner positions themself so their butt is in the giver's lap. Then, the receiver plants their hands firmly on the floor, stretching their legs out behind the giver's waist (it'll probably work better if the giver supports their partner's thighs) as they pump away.

Benefits: This position allows for some super-deep penetration.

Make it hotter: Try rhythmically **squeezing your pelvic floor muscles**, to help you both reach a strong climax.

July 31

Table Top

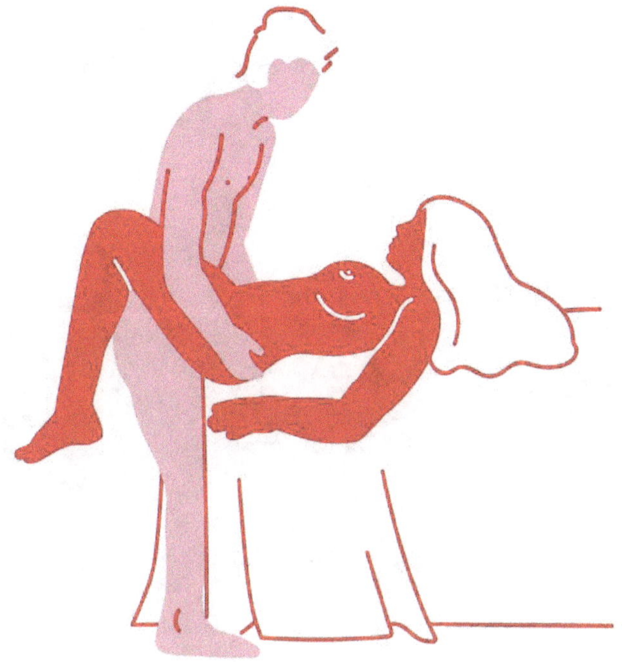

How to do it: You don't have to do this one on a table—any surface that hits your partner at crotch height will do. Have the giver enter while the receiver sits or lies at the edge of a table, counter, or bed.

Benefits: This position is great for face-to-face action. Plus, if you two are drastically different heights, this is a great option, since it puts you both at the same level.

Make it hotter: The receiver can bring their legs down and place their feet on their partner's chest, in front of their shoulders. This allows the receiver to control the tempo and depth of thrusts.

August

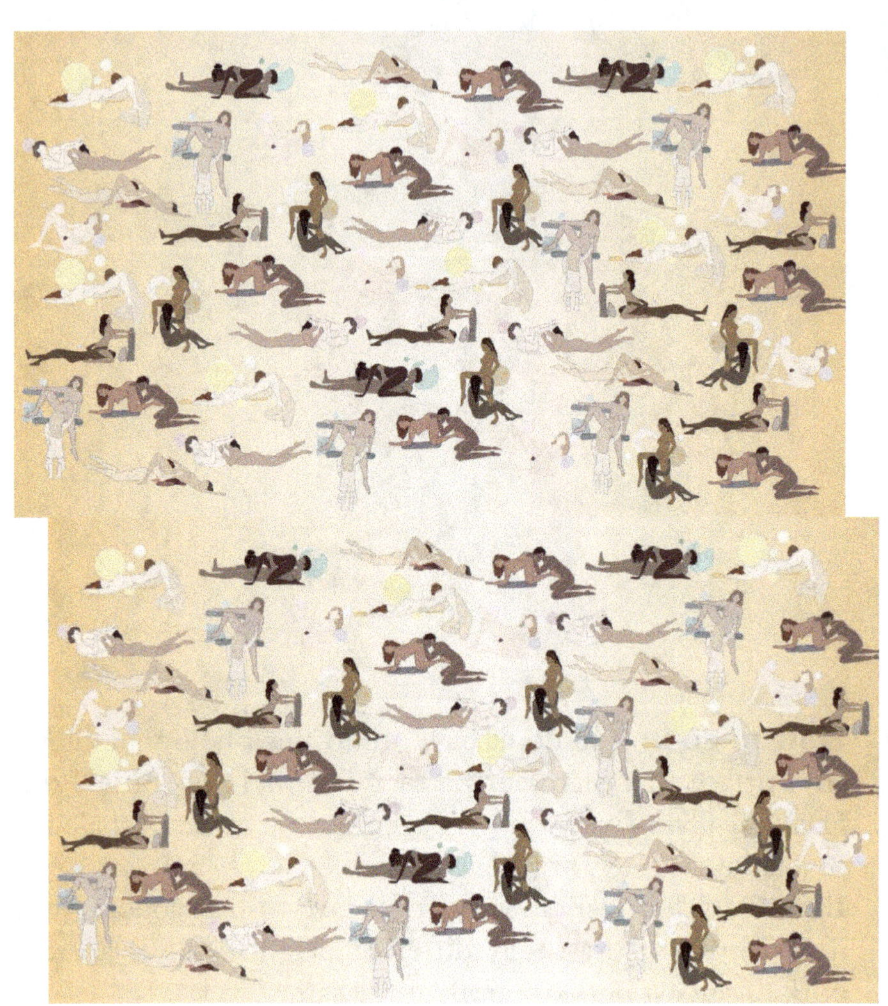

Are you a Dom or a Sub?

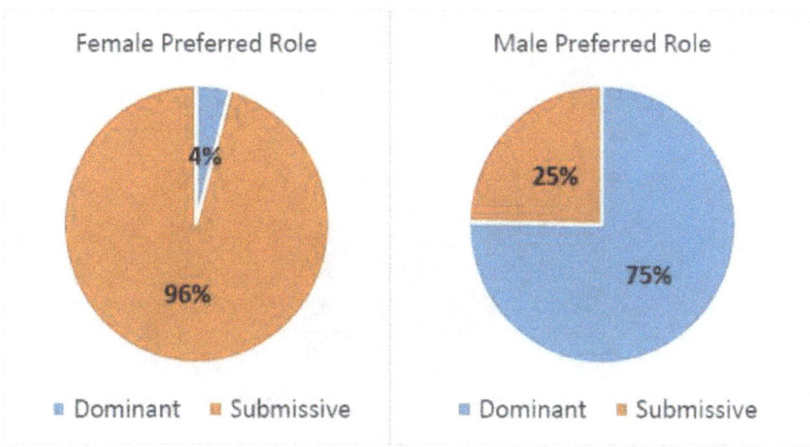

Percentages of female and male BDSM participants who preferred particular roles

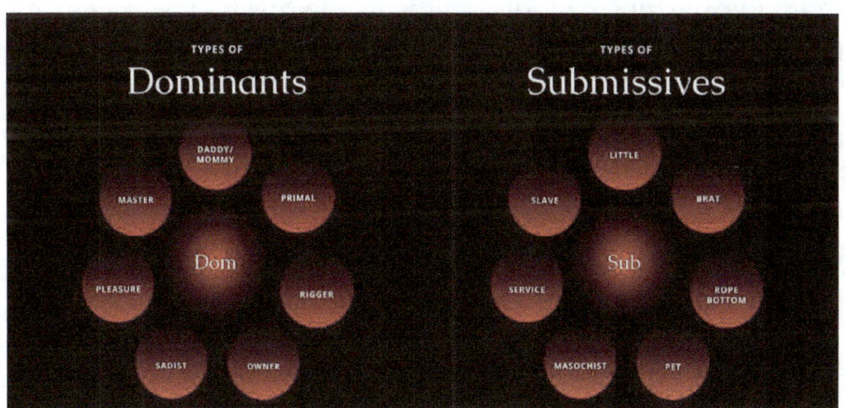

August 1

Snow Angel

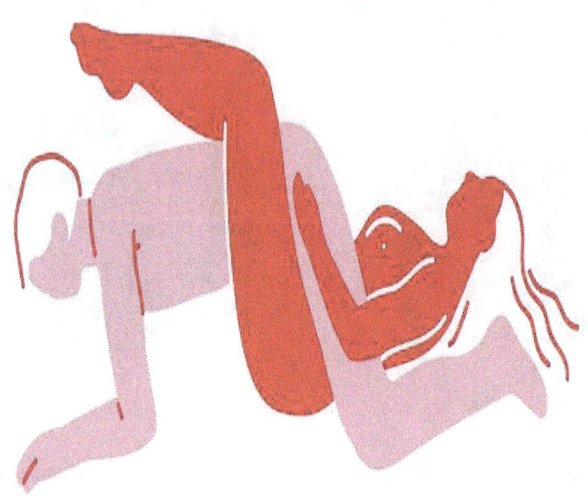

How to do it: The receiver should lie on their back and have the giving partner straddle them, facing away. The receiver lifts their legs and wraps them around the giver's back to elevate their pelvis so the giver can enter. Grabbing the giver's butt can help them slide up and back.

Benefits: The receiver gets a prime view of the giver's cute butt. Plus, from this position, you have easy access to fondle their testicles or clitoris. Not to mention, their pelvis is perfectly positioned for grinding.

Make it hotter: Have the giver spin around into missionary style to face the receiver while trying to stay inserted. Then, switch positions, this time with the receiver on top and facing away.

August 2

Golden Arch

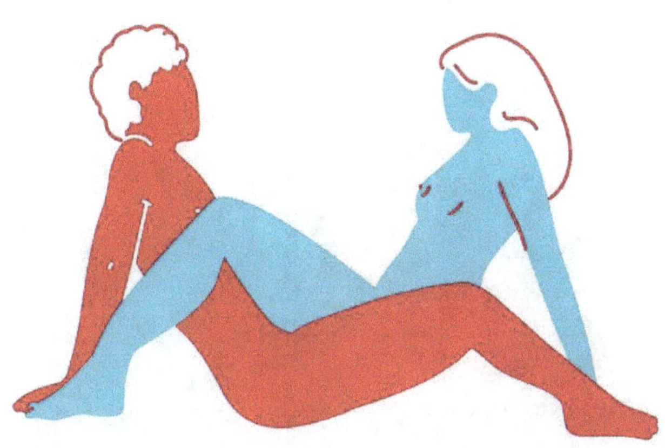

How to do it: This position is similar to Magic Mountain but turned up a notch. The giving partner sits with their legs straight, and the receiver sits on top of the giver with bent knees on top of their thighs. Then, you both lean back.

Benefits: This position gives you both nice views of each other's full bodies. You'll also have control over the depth, speed, and angle of the thrusts.

Make it hotter: Vulva owners can have their partner use their hand to rub their clitoris, or use your own. Lean back farther for extra G-spot stimulation.

August 3

Face-To-Face

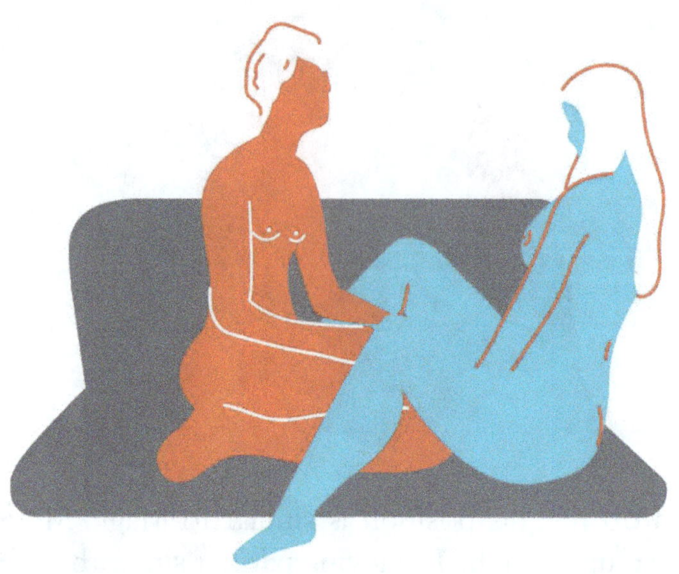

How to do it: No bed? No problem. This do-anywhere position simply involves both people sitting across from one another. From here, you can use your hands on each other's genitals, or even move closer to grind.

Benefits: This is a great move for couples who aren't interested in penetrative or oral sex (or are working their way towards that). Plus, you get tons of eye contact.

Make it hotter: Try this one in the backseat of a car for some spontaneous, semi-public fun.

August 4

Corkscrew

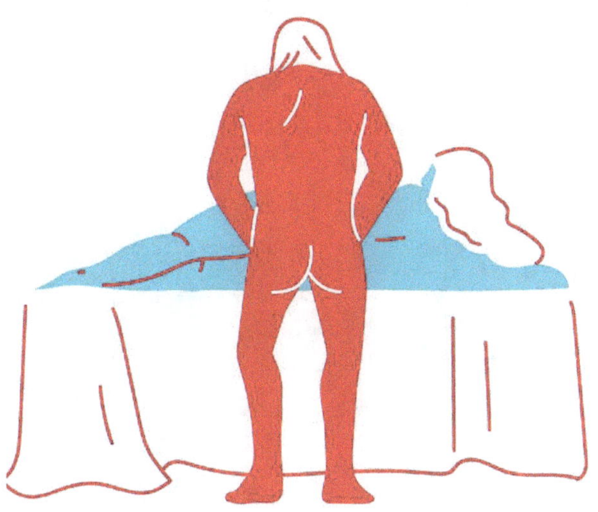

How to do it: Near the edge of a bed or bench, the receiver should rest on their hip and forearm and press their thighs together. Then, the giving partner stands and straddles the receiver, entering or grinding from behind.

Benefits: By keeping their legs pressed together during this **sex position**, the receiver allows for a tighter hold on the giver as they thrust.

Make it hotter: Instead of letting the giver do all the work, the receiver can try thrusting their hips slightly to match the tempo.

August 5

Wheelbarrow

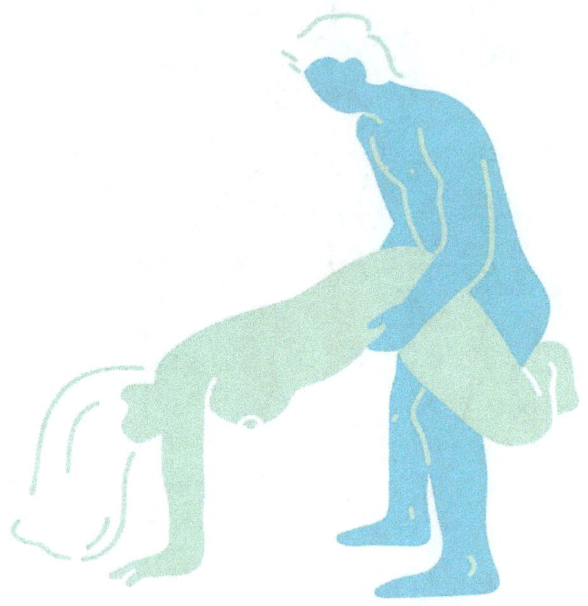

How to do it: The receiver gets on their hands and feet and has the giver pick them up by the pelvis. Then, the receiver grips the giver's waist with their thighs.

Benefits: Aside from being a fabulous arm workout, this sex position can allow for super-deep penetration. (After all, the receiver's legs are literally wrapped around the giver.)

Make it hotter: Arm strain can seriously kill the mood, so if you're enjoying a longer session, the receiving partner can try resting on a table or the side of the bed to give their arms a break.

August 6
Ballet Dancer

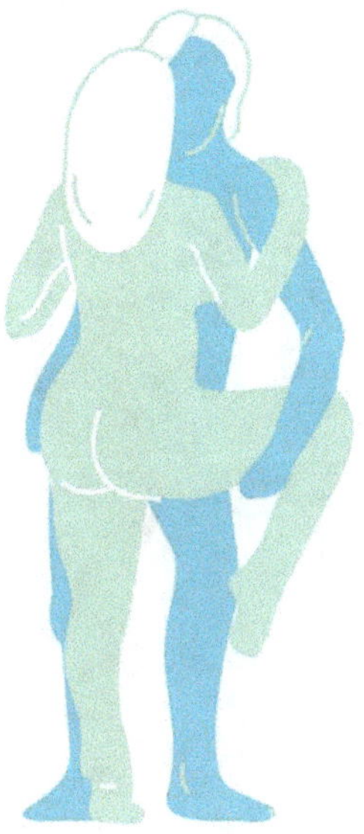

How to do it: Standing on one foot, the receiver should face the giving partner and wrap one of their legs around the giver's waist while the giver helps support.

Benefits: This sex position allows for some quality face-to-face time and connection.

Make it hotter: If the receiver is really flexible, they can put their raised leg on the giver's shoulder for even deeper penetration or **clitoral stimulation** during outercourse.

August 7
Standing Missionary

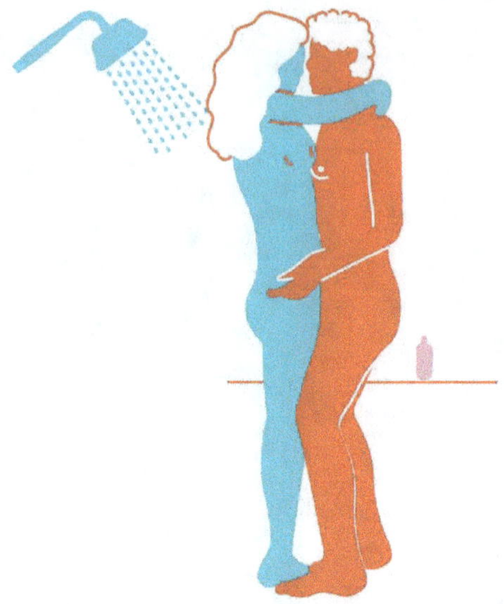

How to do it: This one's fairly straightforward. The giving partner enters the receiver from a face-to-face, standing position.

Benefits: Here, you get all the eye contact benefits of missionary. Plus, both partners have *tons* of opportunities to touch each other's erogenous zones.

Make it hotter: Try this position against a wall for support—or enjoy some new, sexy sensations in the shower.

August 8

Butter Churner

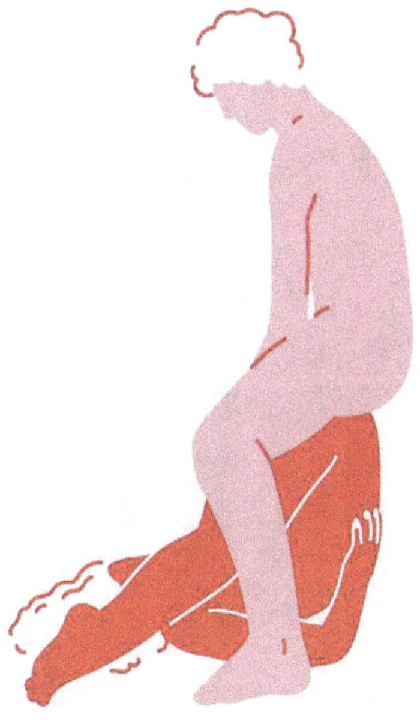

How to do it: The receiver should lie on their back with their legs raised and folded over so that their ankles are on either side of their head, while the giver squats and dips their penis, strap-on, dildo, or finger in and out.

Benefits: Aside from getting that eye contact, the extra rush of blood into your head will increase the ecstasy.

Make it hotter: The top partner can dribble chocolate syrup or something sweet into the receiver's mouth (yes, really). It gets more of your senses involved, amping up the entire experience.

August 9

Upstanding Citizen

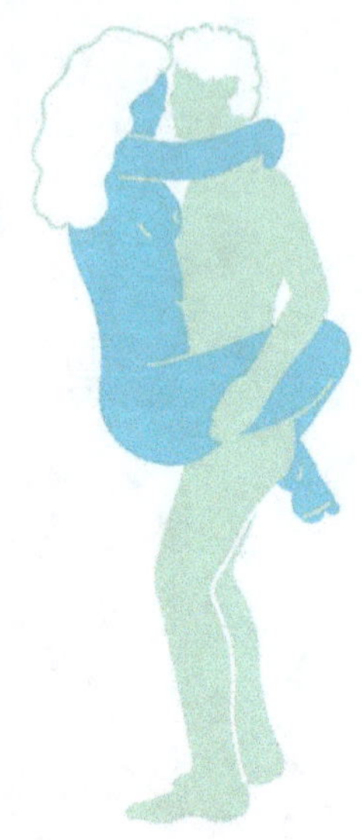

How to do it: The receiver straddles the giver, wrapping their legs around the other's body (the giver keeps their knees unlocked and thighs spread slightly). The giver stands and supports the receiver in their arms. You can start on the bed and move around without disengaging. (Or, for the truly bold, receivers can hop aboard from the standing position!)

Benefits: This is the position seen in every **steamy romance movie**... so, it's definitely worth a try, especially if you're trying a little roleplay.

Make it hotter: Have the giver push the receiver up against a wall—very carefully.

August 10

Stand and Deliver

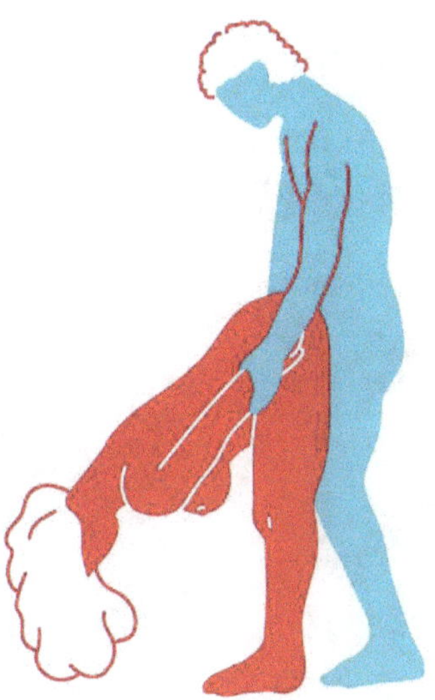

How to do it: With both of you standing, the receiver bends over at the waist; the giver enters from behind.

Benefits: For vulva owners, bending over during this sex position helps make the vaginal walls tighter and increases the intensity of the friction.

Make it hotter: Those with vulvas can ask for clitoral stimulation, or the giver can loosely tie their partner's hands together with a silky scarf.

August 11

Classic Oral

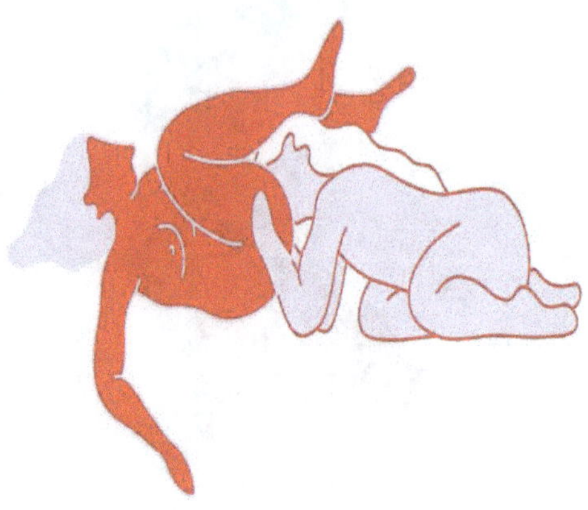

How to do it: On a bed or couch, the receiving partner lies on their back with their legs slightly spread apart and their knees up. From here, the giver can kneel or lie down—whichever feels more comfortable—in front of the receiver's genitals. If the receiving partner has a penis, the giver may choose to kneel or lie beside them for maximum comfort.

Benefits: This beginner-friendly position is great for people who are new to having sex with each other. There's a lot of opportunity for eye contact, which can help the receiver provide verbal and nonverbal feedback (and a sexy visual). Plus, the giver has total control over what they're doing here, which can be especially useful during **fellatio** (i.e. oral sex on a penis)—after all, if the giving partner has a sensitive gag reflex, they can choose the depth and pace at which they're performing oral.

Make it hotter: If you're giving a blow job, bring in a helping hand. Meaning, grasp the receiver's shaft, put your mouth over the penis head, and move them both up and down in rhythm together. If you're trying this position during **cunnilingus**, the receiver can try keeping their legs closed together once their partner is firmly in place for a different sensation.

August 12

96

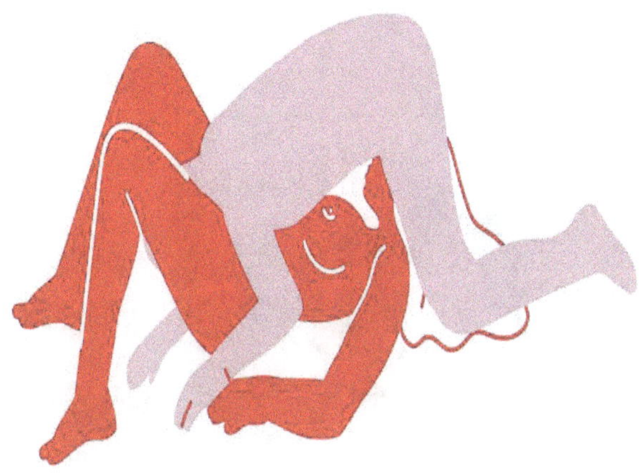

How to do it: For this position, one partner lies down, flat on their back. The other climbs on top, so they're facing away from the other person's upper body. This creates the illusion of the number 96. (Get it?) Your genitals should be lined up with your partner's mouth, and vice versa. Alternatively, try it in a side-by-side position.

Benefits: This position is one of the best for dual pleasure, as both partners can give and receive **oral sex** at once.

Make it hotter: Sure, the mouth-to-genitals stuff is the main attraction, but don't shy away from getting handsy, too. Folks on the bottom can get a better angle to their partner's genitals by using a sex wedge.

August 13

Sideways 69

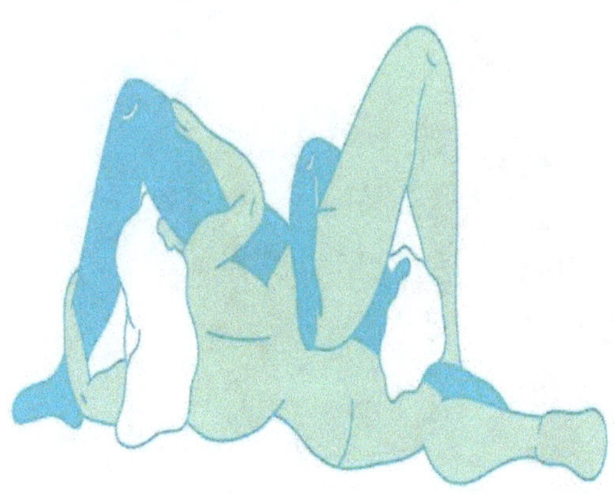

How to do it: Both partners lie on their sides, with their mouths facing each other's genitals. You can also lift one another's thighs for easier access, if you catch my drift...

Benefits: If you enjoy **spooning sex** and 69-ing, this position is the best of both worlds: You can enjoy all the comfort of resting on your side with some mutual oral action. What's not to love?

Make it hotter: With this position, **sex pillows** are your best friend. Place one between your thighs to keep your legs spread apart, or place one under your neck so your head doesn't get tired.

August 14

Seated Oral

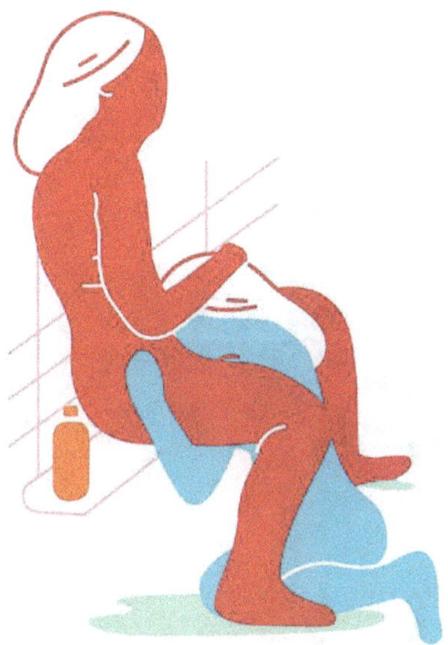

How to do it: Looking to mix up your oral routine? With this position, the receiving partner sits down (on the edge of a bed or bathtub, chair, or bench in the shower) and spreads their legs for the giver.

Benefits: This oral position is super-comfortable, and especially great for **shower sex**: If the receiving partner is facing the shower head, both parties get to enjoy the warm water, but it likely won't get in the giving partner's mouth as they're going down.

Make it hotter: From here, the receiving partner can easily play with or pull the giving partner's hair. If you're in the shower, maybe the receiver can even massage their head with some shampoo? Your options are limitless.

August 15

Pleasure Chair

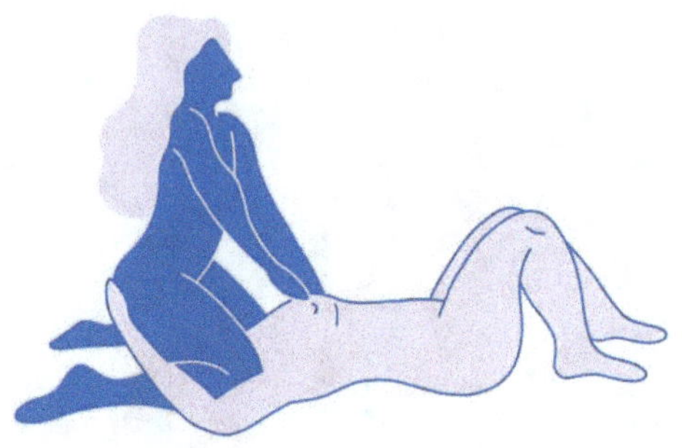

How to do it: The receiver straddles their partner's face, aligning their genitals with the giver's mouth.

Benefits: This position works whether the receiving partner has a penis or vulva, and either way, the receiving partner is in control of the speed, pace, and sensations they receive. That said, if the receiver has a penis, they should make sure they're not hurting their partner by thrusting in *too* quickly or deeply.

Make it hotter: This is a great move for a little power play if you and you're partner are looking for ways to try some light BDSM in the bedroom. Pro tip: Have a nonverbal equivalent of a safeword, or some kind of hand signal the giver can use if they need to stop. You want to make sure that the [giving] person has a way to tap out or take a breath Usually, this can look like a little tap on the thigh.

August 16
Reverse Face-Sitting

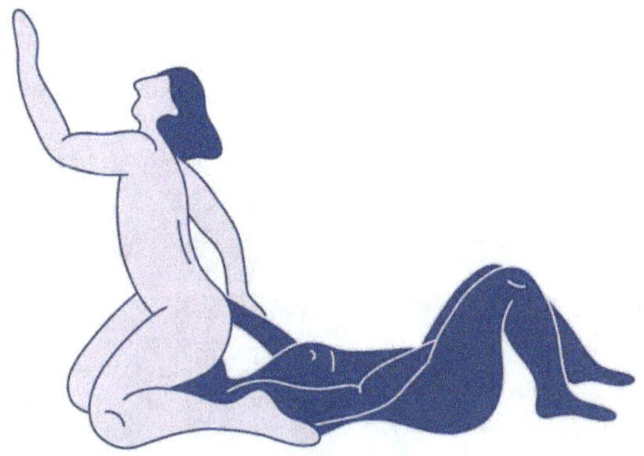

How to do it: This is exactly the same as face-sitting, but with the receiving partner facing away from the giving partner. And once again, just remember to have a nonverbal safeword in place.

Benefits: This position also works well for **analingus** (a.k.a. rimming). Just make sure you don't move from the anus to the vulva or penis because that can spread STI-causing bacteria.

Make it hotter: If you want to incorporate some anal play while *also* performing oral sex on a penis or vulva, the receiving partner can insert a butt plug before they assume the reverse face-sitting position.

August 17
Bullseye

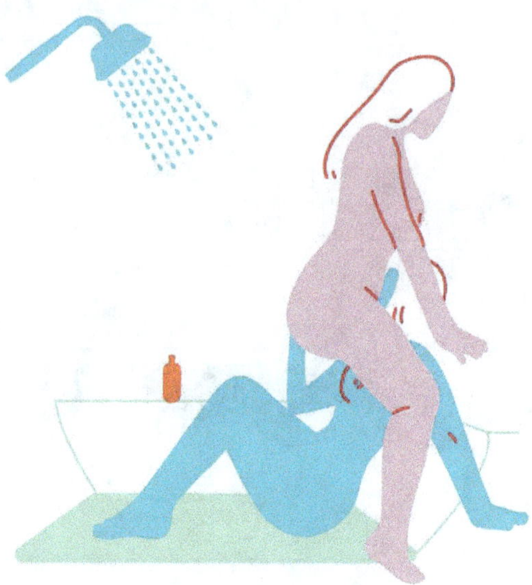

How to do it: For another seated oral option that lets the giver sit back and relax, try this. The giving partner leans against a wall or surface, and the receiver stands in front of them, spreading their legs out. The "bullseye" here is, of course, the clitoris.

Benefits: This is a great way for both parties to enjoy the sensations of face-sitting while helping the receiver stay more comfortable.

Make it hotter: The giving partner can easily use a vibrator on themself in this position. Or, if you're trying it in the shower, the giver might also enjoy the sensation of warm water between their legs.

August 18

Swinging 69

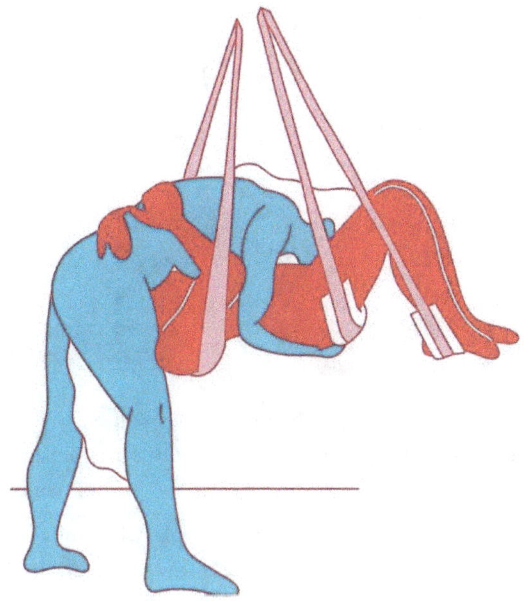

How to do it: First, you'll want to invest in a high-quality **sex swing**. Then, use it for (you guessed it!) some mutual oral. One partner climbs into the swing and lies on their back, while the other leans over them until both parties are face-to-genital.

Benefits: This variation on 69-ing can take some weight off the top partner's knees and elbows. Plus, picking out a piece of **sex furniture** together can be an ultra-hot bonding activity!

Make it hotter: Don't be afraid to get handsy. From here, both partners can easily grab each other's thighs and butt.

August 19

The Eiffel Tower

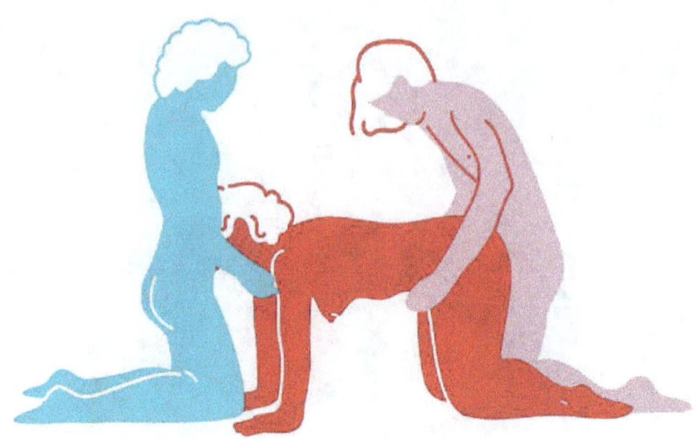

How to do it: In a **throuple**, or just **having a threesome**? Meet your new favorite position. Partner #1 gets in a doggy style position while performing oral sex on Partner #2, and then Partner #3 penetrates Partner #1 from behind.

Benefits: This is a great position for three people who enjoy different types of stimulation. After all, someone gets to thrust, someone gets to receive oral, and someone gets to receive vaginal or anal penetration—and everyone wins.

Make it hotter: For even more intimacy, Partner #2 and Partner #3 can reach across and touch each other, too.

August 20
Oral-Penetrative Train

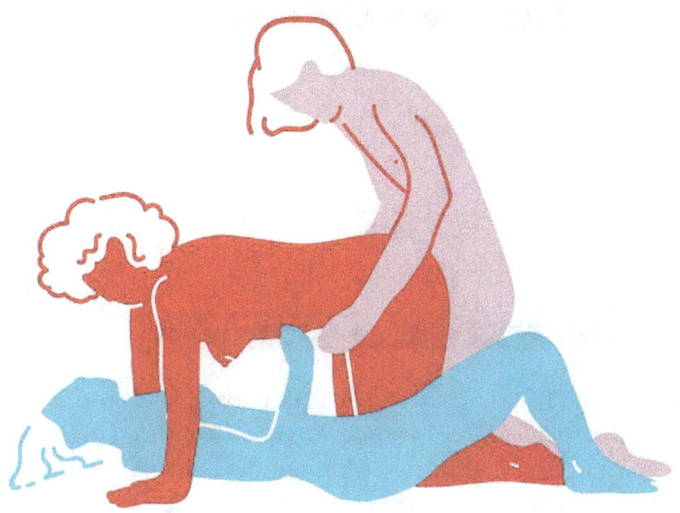

How to do it: Like The Eiffel Tower, this three-way position combines oral and penetrative sex. Person #1 lies on their back while Person #2 leans over and performs oral sex on them. Then, Person #3 thrusts into Person #2.

Benefits: This position works easily for three people with all kinds of genitals. If the penetrating partner has a vulva, they can use a strap-on or a toy.

Make it hotter: Partner #1 can use their hands to touch both of their partners at once. Hot, hot, hot!

August 21

Virtual Threesome

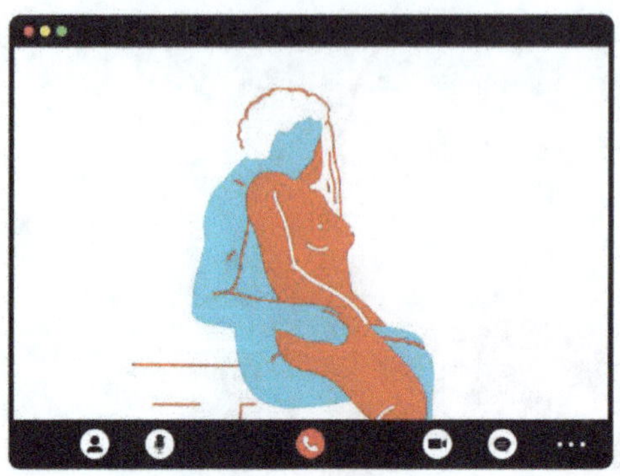

How to do it: You don't need to have a third person with you in order to have a threesome. Here, two partners can have sex via video-chat while a third person watches on and masturbates. The two people who are physically together might want to try the Champagne Room or The Chairman, so they can both get a good view of their partner on-screen.

Benefits: This one's great for long-distance partners.

Make it hotter: The third person can tell their partners exactly what to do to one another. Warning: Things might get really kinky, really fast.

August 22

Sex Position: Stand and Deliver

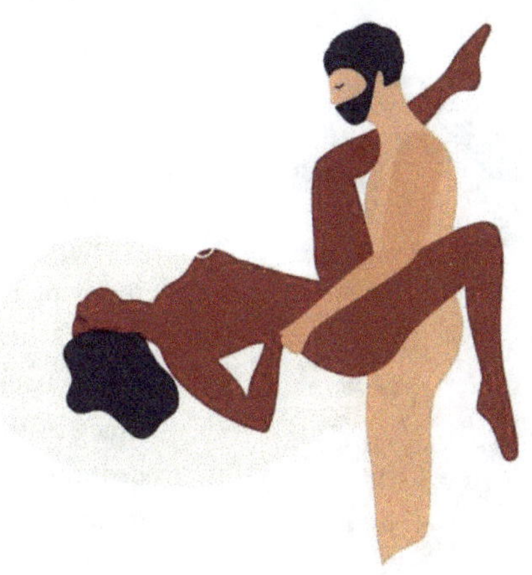

Also known as: The Bicycle

Benefits: The giver (a.k.a. the partner who's doing the penetrating) can enjoy the view of their penis or dildo thrusting.

Technique: The giver stands at the edge of a bed or desk while the receiver (a.k.a. the partner who's being penetrated) lies back and raises their legs to their chest. The receiver's knees are bent as if they're doing a "bicycling" exercise. The giver grabs their partner's ankles and enters them. The giver should thrust slowly, as the deep penetration may be painful for the receiver.

Also try: The receiving partner can place their heels on the giver's shoulders, which will help open their hips.

Hot tip: If you're the giver, encourage your partner to play with their clitoris or penis in this position. Also, show them that they can control your penetration by flexing their thighs.

August 24
Face Off

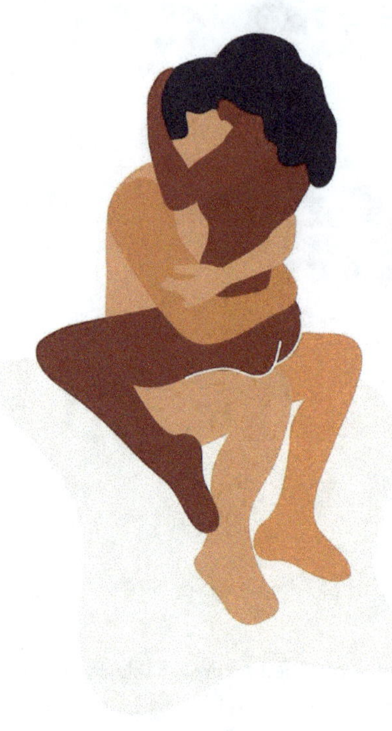

Also known as: The Lap Dance

Benefits: Allows for face-to-face intimacy; cozy for long sessions.

Technique: The giver sits on a chair or at the edge of a bed. The receiving partner faces the giver, wraps their arms around the giver's back, and sits in their lap. Once in the saddle, the receiver can ride up and down on the giver's shaft by pressing with their legs or knees. Want to go faster? The giver can grab the receiving partner's buttocks to assist with lifting and bouncing.

Also try: The receiver can sit facing the giver on a rocking chair. Old wooden rockers on hardwood or stone floors provide extra movement.

Hot tip: There's lots of room for creativity in this position for stimulating erogenous areas of the upper body, head, neck, and face. If the receiver likes having their nipples licked, go for it!

August 25
Pearly Gates

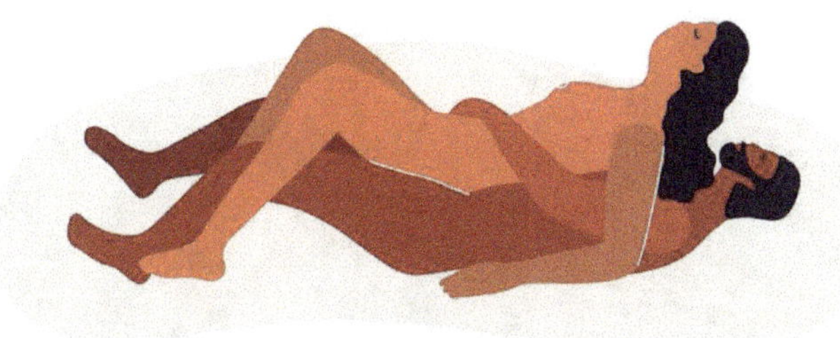

Benefits: Great for **G-spot stimulation**.

Technique: The giver lies on their back. The receiver can straddle them in a reverse cowgirl position before carefully leaning backward until their back is on their partner's chest.

Hot tip: The giver can reach around and play with the receiver's nipples or clitoris. (The receiver can also **use a vibrator** in this position.)

August 26

The Socket

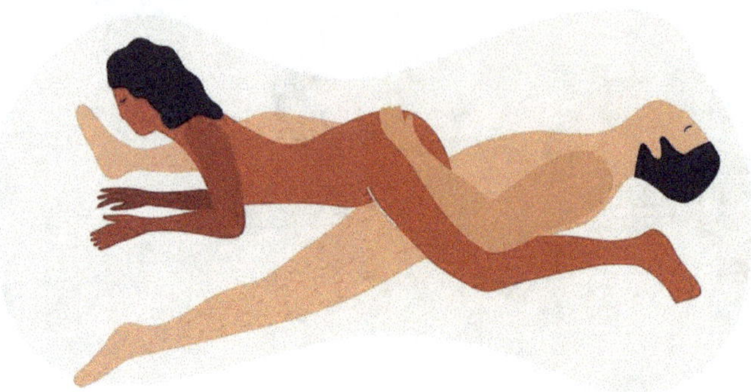

Benefits: "This looks like it's a nice position to fantasize a little and get a new view of your partner's behind. It's a chance to get absorbed in the sensations.

Technique: From reverse cowgirl, the receiving partner bends all the way forward, extending their legs all the way back. They should be supporting their body by resting on their elbows, as if they're holding a plank.

Hot tip: In this position, a vulva-owning receiver can easily touch their clitoris while being penetrated. And if the two of you are into **spanking**, have at it.

August 27

Happy Baby

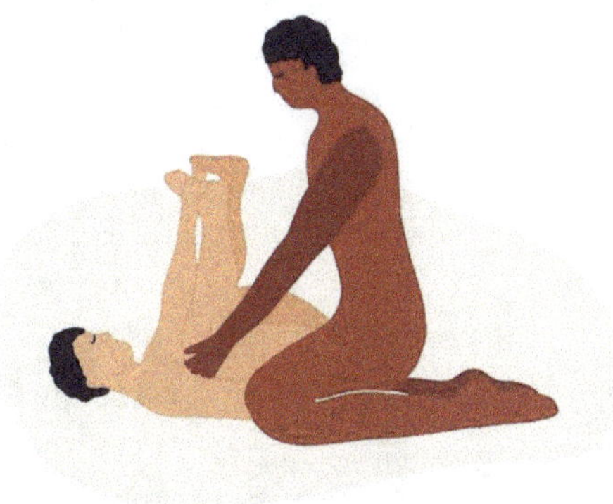

Benefits: This position works for both vaginal and anal penetration—and it's perfect for G-spot stimulation. It's also a more comfortable option for receivers with lower back pain.

Technique: The receiving partner assumes the "happy baby" pose, a yoga position where you lie on your back, bend your knees into your chest, grip the outer edges of your feet, and roll side to side like, well, a happy baby. In this case, instead of rolling around, the receiver stays put so the giver can enter them from a kneeling position.

Also try: Tweaking your angles by sliding a **sex pillow** underneath the receiving partner's hips.

Hot tip: If the receiver doesn't have much flexibility or balance, the giver can help hold their legs up and apart.

August 28
Standing O

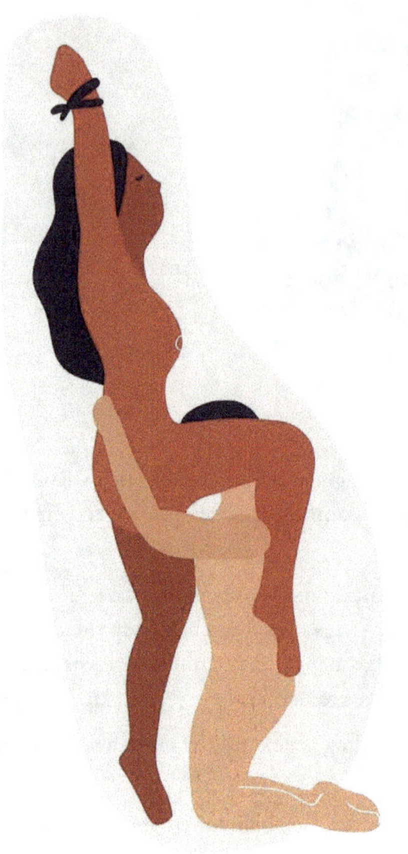

Benefits: Ideal position for all things cunnilingus and any forms of vulva or vaginal stimulation you want to throw in: clit sucking, rubbing, digital penetration, and G-spot stroking.

Technique: The giving partner should be on their knees, with the receiving partner standing upright. The receiver should drape one of their legs around the giver's shoulders—then, let the eating out begin!

Hot tip: Ideally, the receiving partner should have their hands above their head. This can be accomplished by using some **BDSM restraints**. If restraints aren't their thing, see if you can find an anchored bar or beam for them to grasp.

August 29

The Little Dipper

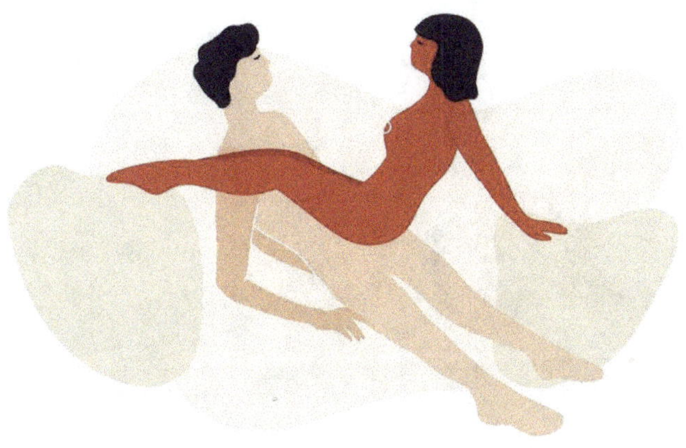

Benefits: A great position that allows for clitoral stimulation with both your mouth and fingers.

Technique: FYI, the receiving partner will have sore triceps once you both finish. For the Little Dipper, the receiving partner uses either a bed, couch, or chair to hoist themselves over their partner. The giver then inserts their penis or dildo into their partner's vagina or anus. The receiver then does tricep dips to move up and down on their partner's shaft. If done correctly, you should be in a T-shape formation.

Make it Hotter: The giver can play with the receiver's clitoris or penis for extra stimulation.

August 30

Golden Gate

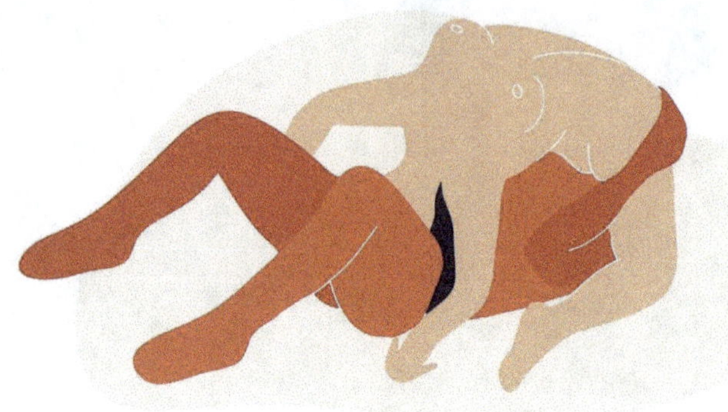

Technique: This just looks impossible to me. But if you're able to do it, go for it. I think it's just a victory in being able to pull this position off."

Make it Hotter: If you're the person lying on your back, you may need to help out your partner by thrusting your pelvis up, so their mouth can actually reach your genitals.

August 31
The Cat

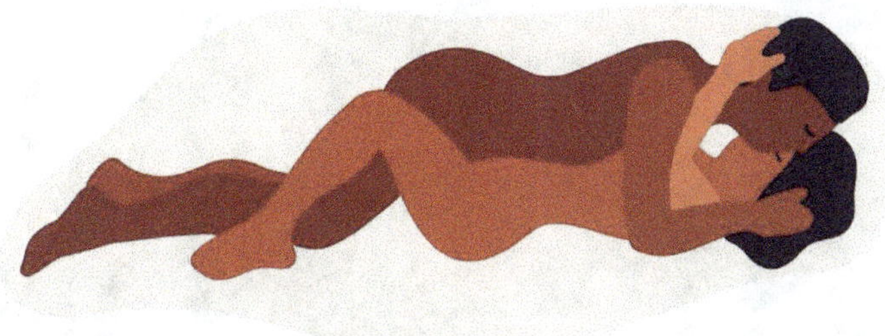

Benefits: This position offers strong clitoral stimulation for partners with vulvas. **A study** published in the *Journal of Sex and Marital Therapy* found that the CAT significantly increases the likelihood that a vulva-owning partner will orgasm during sex.

Technique: The CAT is very similar to the missionary position, except the giver is positioned farther up and to one side. Instead of being chest to chest, the giver's chest is near the receiver's shoulders. The receiving partner should bend their legs about 45 degrees to tilt their hips up. This causes the base of the giver's shaft to maintain constant contact with the receiving partner's clitoris.

Also try: The giver can push their pelvis down a few inches while the receiver pushes up for extra pressure.

Hot tip: Instead of thrusting up and down, the giver can try rocking forward and back or grinding their pelvis in a circular motion, depending on what feels best for their partner.

September

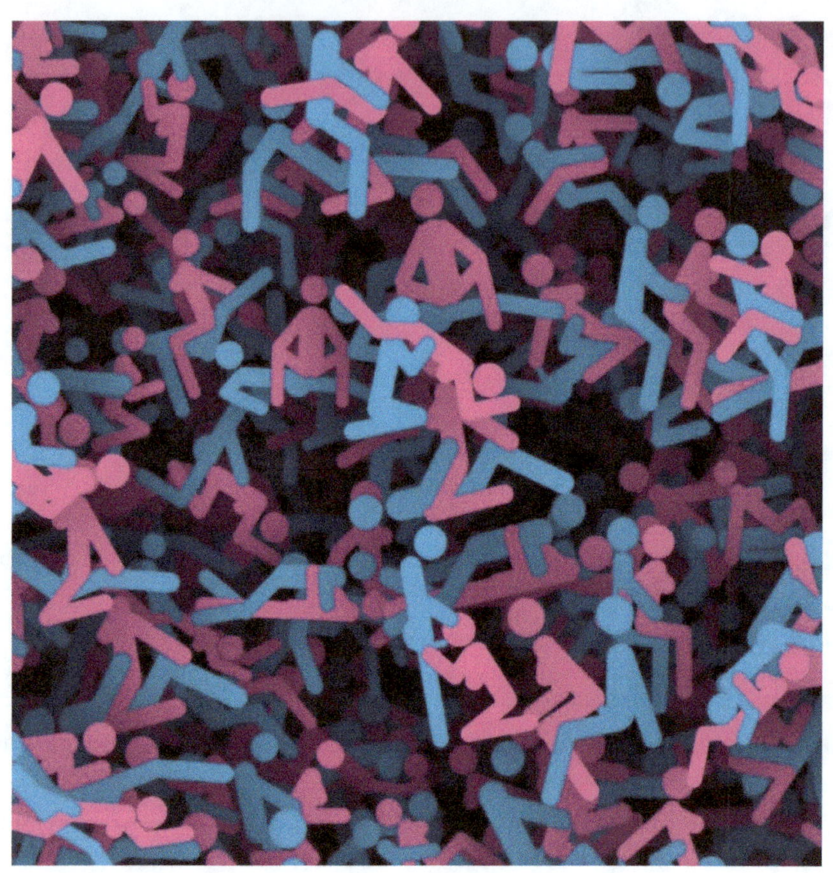

This is the bingo card that inspired the events in [The Exhibitionist Bingo Challenge.](#) How many have you done? How far are you willing to go?

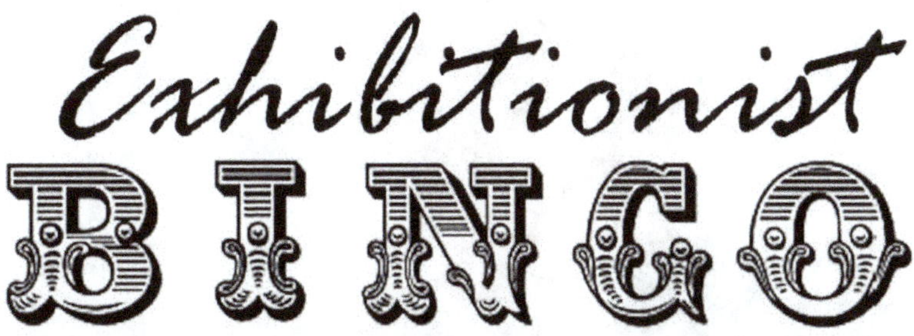

BALCONY	RESTAURANT	PARKING LOT	BEACH	MOVIE THEATER
LIBRARY (SHHH...)	ELEVATOR	GYM	NIGHT-CLUB	BUS / TRAIN
SAUNA	CHURCH	FREE	FITTING ROOM	PARK
BAR	CARNIVAL	POOL / HOT TUB	MUSEUM	BALCONY
CONCERT	DRIVE-THRU	GROCERY STORE	CAFE / COFFEE SHOP	STREET CORNER / ALLEY WAY

September 1

The Captain

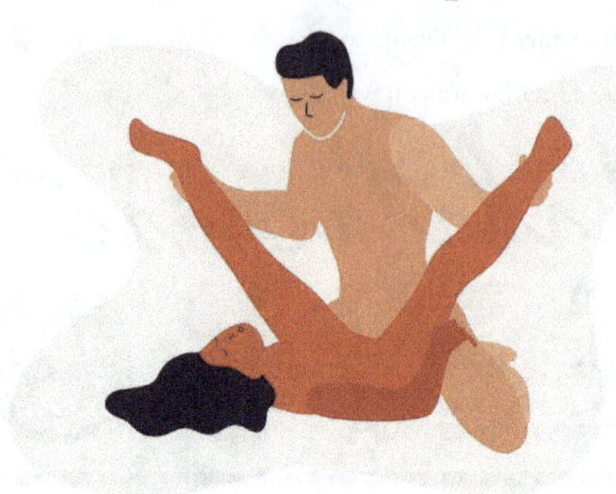

Also known as: V is for Victory

Benefits: Deep penetration, G-spot or prostate stimulation, and access to the clitoris.

Technique: The receiving partner lies on their back and raises their legs in the air. Kneeling, the giver holds the receiver's ankles and spreads their legs into a V shape before entering them.

Hot tip: Since the giver's hands are busy holding the receiver's legs in place, the receiver can hold a vibrator if they want to add some clit stimulation to this position. Don't forget to make sure the receiving partner stretches their hamstrings first.

September 2

Waterfall

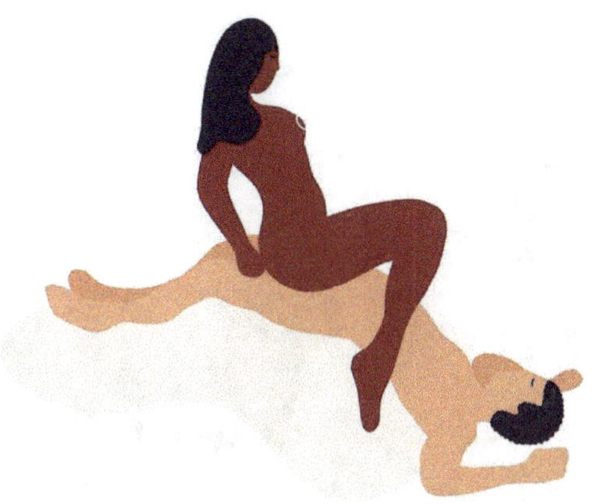

Benefits: The blood will rush to the giver's *other* head, too.

Technique: The giver moves to the edge of the bed and lies back with their head and shoulders on the floor as their partner straddles them. The blood will rush to the giver's head, creating mind-blowing sensations upon orgasm.

Hot tip: Make sure the giver has a pillow under their head for a safer, more comfortable experience.

September 3
One Up

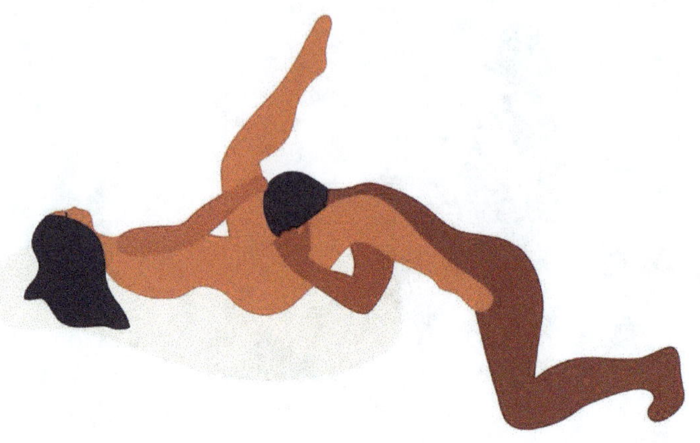

Also known as: Over Your Shoulder, The Hamstring Stretch

Benefits: This is a great sex position for vulva-owners who are particularly sensitive along one side of the clitoris.

Technique: The giver kneels on the floor with their mate lying on the edge of the bed. The giver then raises one of their partner's legs and asks their partner to support it by wrapping their hands around their thigh. With one hip raised, the receiving partner will be able to add some movement to aid in the giver's stroking or to help move the giver to the perfect spot.

Also try: The receiver can wriggle a little to help their partner get the right rhythm.

Hot tip: During cunnilingus, the giver can allow the knuckle of their finger to trail behind their tongue. The contrast between soft flesh of the tongue and hard bone of the finger will create a pleasing sensation. (For more oral pleasure positions, check out **Your Ultimate Guide to Oral Sex.**) The receiver can also show their partner the tongue pressure and technique they prefer by demonstrating with their mouth on their partner's earlobe.

September 4
Sublime Supine

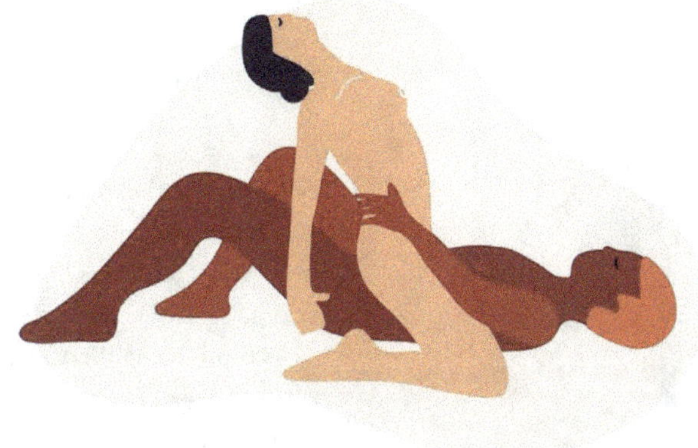

Benefits: There's going to be G-spot stimulation, clitoral stimulation, and cervical stimulation. It's a nice position for the person on top to really control their orgasm. It also gives you a great view of everything that's happening.

Technique: Cowgirl is one of the best sex positions because it allows for a variety of interesting sights and sensations, especially for vulva-owning receivers. It allows the receiver to take charge of the pace and depth of penetration. Alternate between shallow and deep thrusts. Shallow will stimulate the front third of the vagina, which is the most sensitive.

Also try: Lie chest to chest. The receiving partner should brace their feet on the tops of the giver's feet and push off to create a rocking motion that will rub the vulva and clitoral area against the giver's pubic bone.

Make it Hotter: It will be easier for the receiver to climax in this position if the giver stimulates them manually and orally until they're extremely aroused.

September 5
The Love Seat

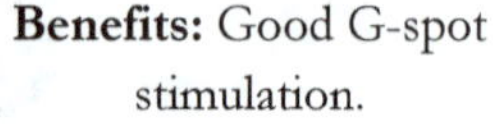

Benefits: Good G-spot stimulation.

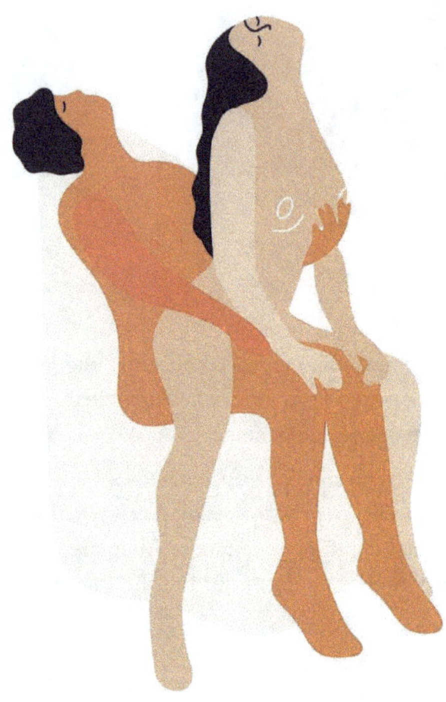

Technique: The giver sits on the edge of the bed or on a chair with their feet on the floor. The receiving partner turns away and backs up, sitting between their partner's legs. They can ride the giver's shaft by pushing off the chair arms or pressing up with their feet. While doggy style is about the giver's dominance, The Hot Seat puts the receiving partner in the driver's seat. And that makes it one of the best sex positions for both of you.

Also try: The receiving partner can reach under and stimulate the base of the penetrating partner's penis, scrotum, and perineum. Meanwhile, the giver can reach around and stimulate the receiver's nipples.

Hot tip: The receiver can control the angle of entry by arching their back and pressing their buttocks into the giver's groin.

September 6

Spin Cycle

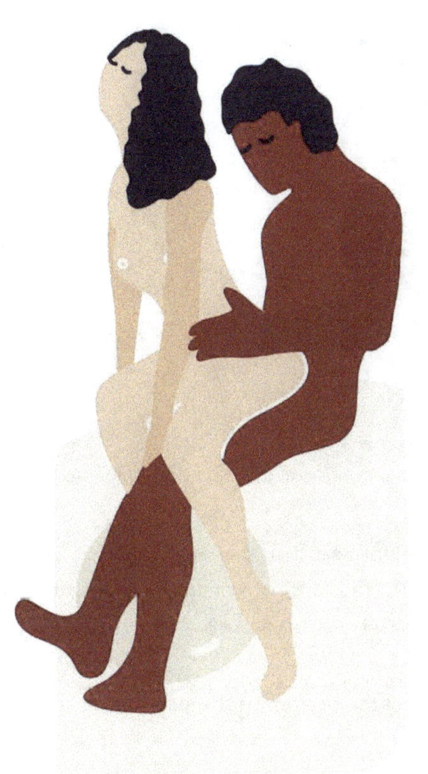

Also known as: Maytag Repair Man

Benefits: Extra vibes.

Technique: This is a variation on the Hot Seat with the receiving partner sitting in the penetrating partner's lap, but this time, you plant yourselves on top of a washing machine set at the highest agitator cycle.

Hot tip: The partner sitting on the washing machine can spread their buttocks and enjoy the vibration against their perineum.

September 7

Step Lively

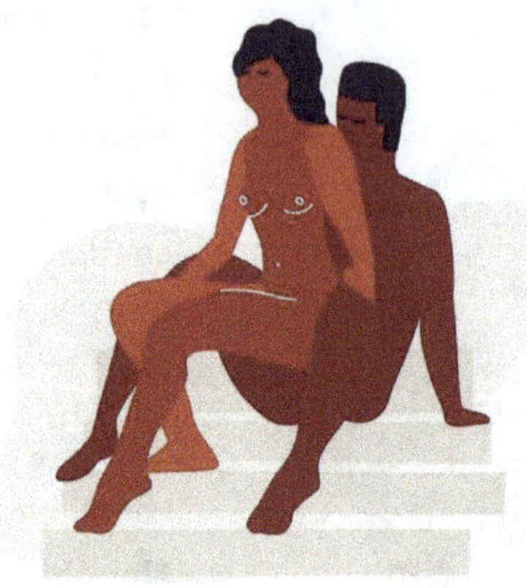

Benefits: Good hand holds for the receiving partner, and you don't have to wait until you reach the bedroom.

Technique: This is a variation on The Hot Seat with the receiver sitting on top of their partner while the giver sits on one of the stairs of a staircase. Stairs offer good seating possibilities, and a hand rail for extra support and leverage.

Hot tip: For a safer experience, try this at the bottom of the steps rather than at the top.

September 8

Halfway Around the World

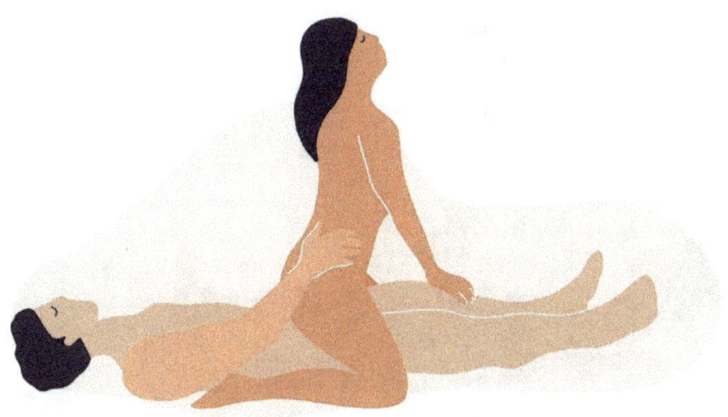

Also known as: Rodeo Drive, Halfway Around the World

Benefits: With a pillow under their head, the giver gets an awesome view of their mate's backside. The receiving partner can also control depth of penetration and pace with this sex position.

Technique: The giver lies on their back with their legs outstretched. The receiving partner kneels next to the giver and then turns and spreads their legs, straddling the giver's hips and facing their feet. Kneeling, the receiver lowers down onto the giver's shaft and begins riding.

Also try: The receiving partner can lean forward or back to change the angle of penetration.

Hot tip: From this position, the receiver partner can easily reach down to touch themselves or direct the penis or dildo where it feels best.

September 9

Thighmaster

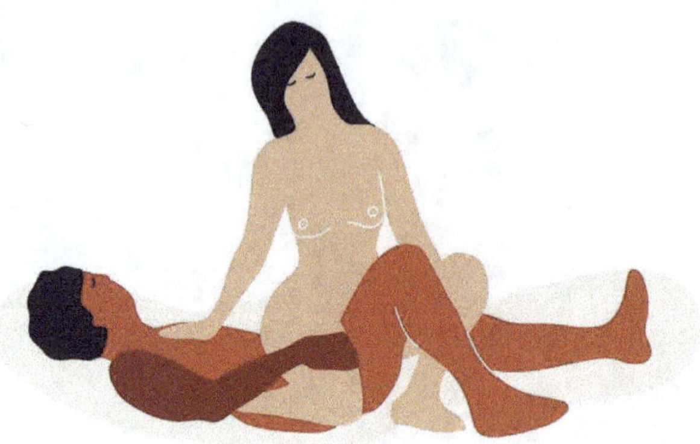

Benefits: Dual stimulation for the receiving; for the giver—a great view of the receiver's rear and your penis or dildo entering them.

Technique: The giver lies on their back and bends one of their legs, keeping the other outstretched. The receiving partner straddles the raised leg with a thigh on either side and lowers themselves onto the giver's member so that their back is facing the giver. They should hold the giver's knee and use it for support as they rock up and down.

Also try: A vulva-owning receiver can press their vulva hard against the giver's upper thigh, rubbing as the feeling dictates.

Hot tip: From Pole Position, the receiver can massage the giver's raised leg during the action or reach down and touch the giver's perineum.

September 10

Squat Thrust

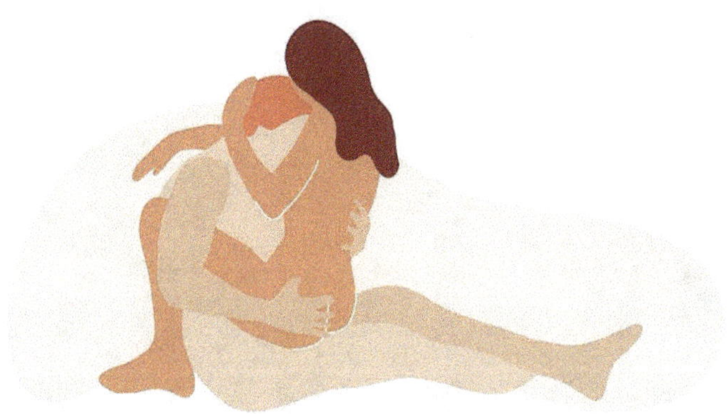

Benefits: Puts the receiver in control, maintains intimacy.

Technique: The giver places pillows behind their back and sits on the bed with legs outstretched. The receiving partner straddles the giver's waist with their feet on the bed. They then bend their knees to lower themselves onto the giver, using one hand to direct the shaft in. Just by pressing on the balls of their feet and releasing, they can raise and lower themselves on the giver's penis or dildo as slowly or quickly as they please.

Also try: From this position, you both lie back into the Spider position or its more challenging variation, The X.

Hot tip: The giver can easily lick the receiver's nipples in this position.

September 11
David Copperfield

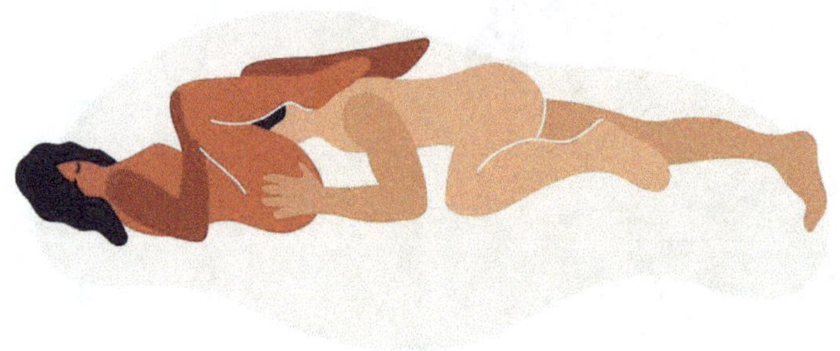

Also known as: Trick & Treat

Benefits: This sex position is the *piece de resistance* for partners who prefer a strong, upward stroking motion during cunnilingus.

Technique: Place a pillow under the receiver's hips to tilt their pelvis up. The receiver should bend their knees so they can place their feet on the giver's shoulder blades.

Also try: The giver can amplify their oral efforts with a simple sleight-of-hand trick: While lapping away, try using your hands to push gently upward on the receiver's abdomen, stretching their skin away from their pubic bone, to help coax the head of the clitoris out from beneath the hood.

Hot tip: The giver can let their tongue rest firmly and flat against the full length of the vaginal entrance and have the receiver grind against their tongue.

September 12

Heir to the Throne

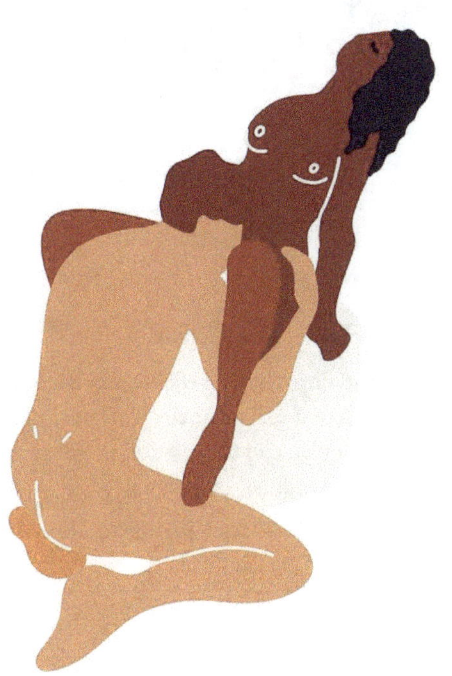

Also known as: Lazy Girl

Benefits: The ultimate sex position for oral on the go.

Technique: The receiver sits on a chair with their legs wide open. This is a good sex position for either beginning the slow build-up with loose, broad, strokes, or ending with strong suction. In this position, the receiver can easily guide the giver, and the giver gets a full view between the receiver's legs, which is a turn-on for many people.

Also try: Switch to a swivel chair—the giver can turn it left and right as they hold their tongue stationary.

Hot tip: The giver can insert one or two fingers and stroke in a "come hither" motion to wake up their partner's G-spot in this sex position. With either their tongue or other hand, the giver can also apply pressure to the receiver's pubic bone. This dual stimulation executed just right will send the receiver over the edge.

September 13

Closed for Business

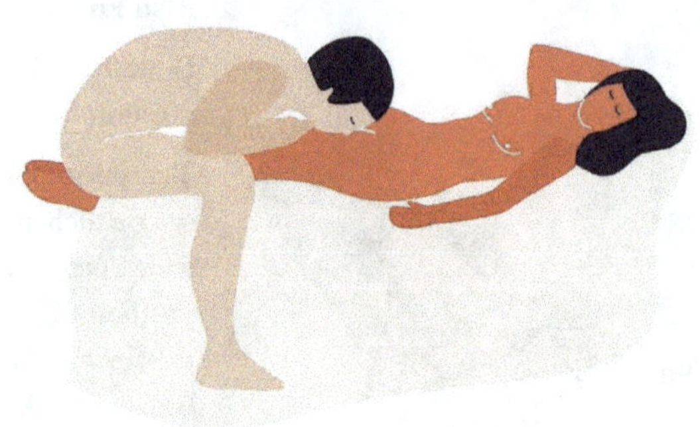

Benefits: A variation of One Up that allows for slow buildup.

Technique: Some people with vulvas find direct clitoral stimulation uncomfortable. Having the receiver close their legs during oral sex may help. The giver places their hand above the receiver's public mound, applying light pressure, and then rubs their tongue on the area around the clitoris to add indirect stimulation.

Hot tip: The giver can also try keeping their tongue still while the receiver rocks their pelvis back and forth.

September 14
The Incline Wedge

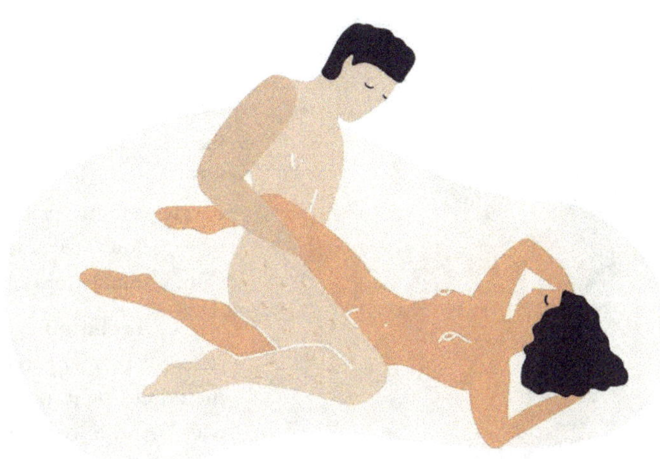

Benefits: The deep penetration of doggy-style while face to face.

Technique: The giver kneels and straddles the receiver's left leg while they're lying on their left side. The receiver then bends their right leg around the right side of the giver's waist, which will provide access to their vagina. For many people with vulvas, rear entry hurts their backs. This sex position allows them to lounge comfortably while enjoying deep penetration.

Also try: The giver can manually stimulate the receiver using their fingers in this position. They can also withdraw their penis or dildo and, holding their shaft with their left hand, rub the head against their partner's clitoris to bring them to the brink of orgasm.

Hot tip: The giver should be gentle with the clitoris. Some people even prefer gentle pressure around it rather than direct stimulation. Go soft, then increase speed and pressure.

September 15
Yourself on the Shelf

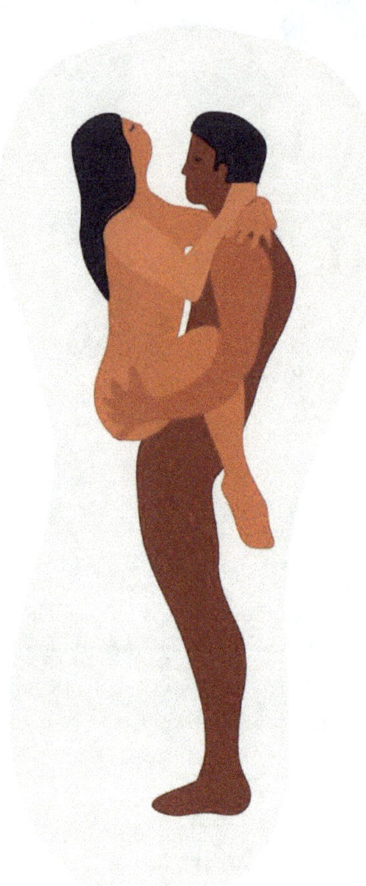

Also known as: The Bicycle

Benefits: You can enjoy the view of your penis thrusting inside of your partner, and this position really allows for direct clitoral stimulation.

Technique: The receiving partner perches their butt right on the edge of the bed. The giver enters them while standing. Then the receiver can wrap their legs around the giver while the giver wraps their hands around the receiver's back for extra support.

Also Try: If you're the giver and you don't have the quad and glute muscles to pull this position off, just keep your partner on the edge of the bed, penetrating them there.

Hot Tip: It's a great way to finish having sex. Since the position is strenuous, try doing it 30-60 seconds before you or your partner are about to orgasm.

September 16

The Shoulder Holder

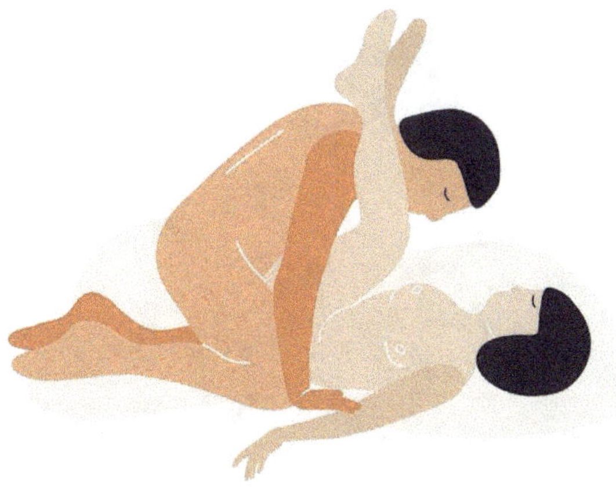

Benefits: Allows deep penetration and targeting the G-spot or P-spot.

Technique: The receiving partner lies on their back. The giver kneels between the receiver's legs and raises them, resting the receiver's calves over the giver's shoulders. The giver should rock the giver in a side-to-side and up-and-down motion to bring the head and shaft of their penis or dildo in direct contact with the front wall of the receiver's vagina or anus. Because this angle allows for deep penetration, thrust slowly at first to avoid causing discomfort.

Also try: The receiver can place their feet on the giver's chest This allows the receiver to control the tempo and depth of thrusts.

Hot tip: If you're the giver, notice your partner getting close to orgasm. You can do that by listening for their breath to become short and shallow. Flushed skin and slightly engorged breasts also indicate they're nearing the peak of arousal.

September 17

Man's Best Friend

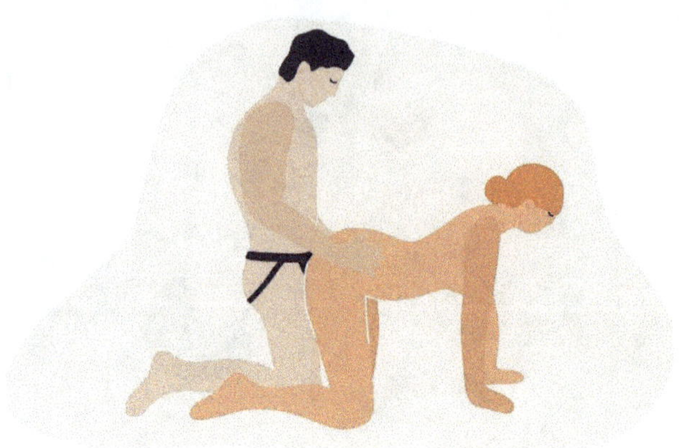

Benefits: Deep penetration and an erotic view.

Technique: This could be your next move after starting in The Flatiron sex position. By entering their partner from behind, the giver is able to thrust deep—and if they're entering vaginally, the tip of their penis or dildo might touch their partner's cervix, an often-neglected pleasure zone. But you should do this slowly and gently. Some people with vulvas find it painful.

Hot tip for her: The receiver may be able to increase the intensity of their orgasm by pushing their pelvic floor muscles outward, as if trying to squeeze something out of their vagina. This causes the vaginal walls to lower, making the G-spot more accessible.

September 18
Belly Flop

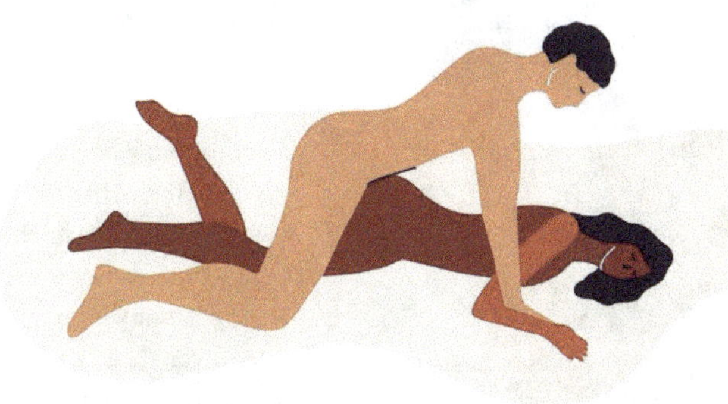

Benefits: Intensifies vaginal pleasure.

Technique: The receiver lies face down on the bed with their knees slightly bent and hips slightly raised. For comfort, and to increase the angle of their hips, they can place a pillow under their lower abs. The giver enters them from behind and keeps their weight off the receiver's body with their arms. This position creates a snug fit, making the giver's shaft feel larger to their partner.

Also try: The giver will last longer in this position if they switch to shallower thrusts and practice deep breathing.

Hot tip: Givers, less friction means less stimulation—and that can help you last longer. Try using a very slippery silicon-based lubricant, which may allow you to thrust longer before reaching orgasm.

September 19
Squat Press

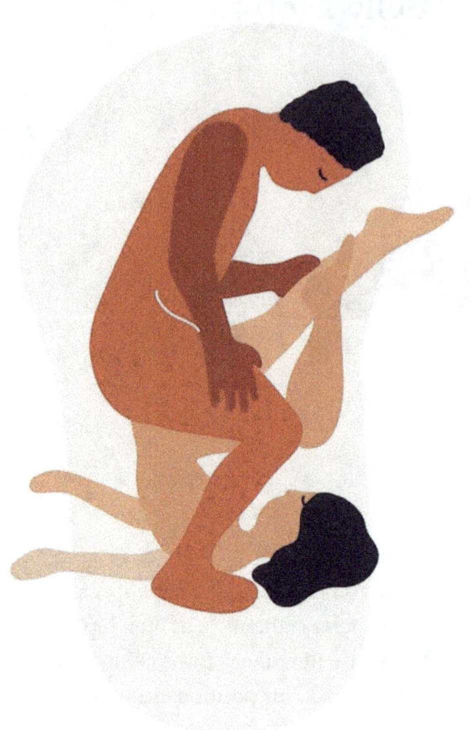

Benefits: An extra rush of blood to the receiver's head to increase their ecstasy.

Technique: The receiver lies on their back with their legs raised over their head. This is not a plain Jane position! The giver squat over them and dips their penis or dildo in and out of them. Penetrating partners, be extra careful to thrust lightly to avoid stressing their neck. This position could potentially result in a neck injury.

Hot tip: Novelty ignites passion by increasing your brain's levels of dopamine, a neurotransmitter linked to romance and sex drive, sayr qualifies for novelty, but you don't need to go to such extremes to sustain romance. Anything that's new and different will do the trick.

September 20
Ballet Dancer

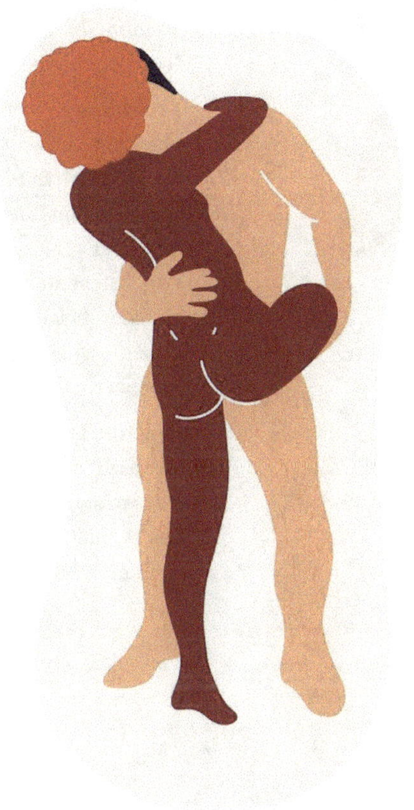

Benefits: Erotic move for quickies in tight quarters. Good option for outdoor sex. Allows for easier penetration. The receiver has control of thrusting, depth, and angle.

Technique: You stand facing one another. The receiving partner raises one of their legs, wraps it around the giver's buttocks or thigh, and pulls the giver into them.

Also try: If that wrapped leg gets tired, the giver can cradle it with their arm. If your mate's very flexible, lift their leg over your shoulder.

Hot tip: Try this standing position in a hot shower. During the steamy foreplay, rub each other's bodies with a coarse salt scrub to stimulate nerve endings and blood flow.

September 21
Iron Chef

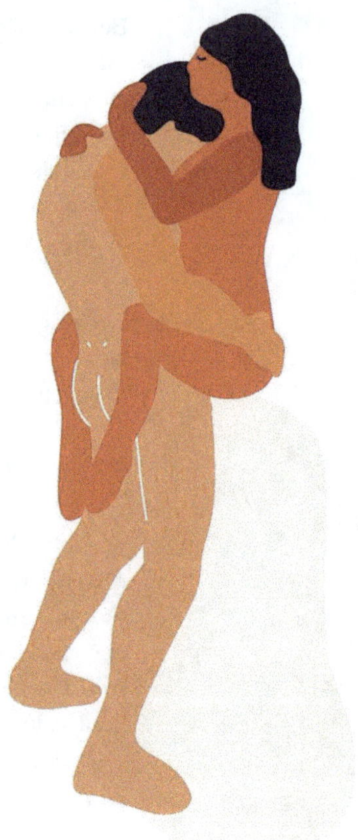

Also known as: Kitchen Confidential

Benefits: Good sex position for a quickie with deep penetration.

Technique: A variation of The Ballet Dancer in which the receiver raises their legs up and wraps them around the giver's butt or thighs. Your kitchen counter is the perfect height for this standing-to-seated appetizer.

Hot tip: The giver can pull the receiver's hips towards them to aid in thrusting (just don't pull them off the counter).

September 22
H2Ohh Yeah

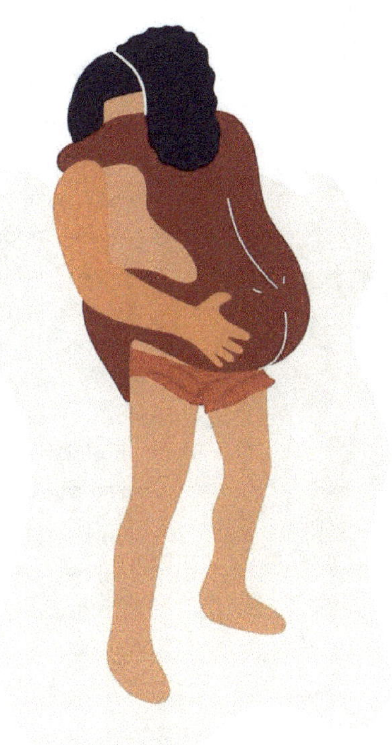

Also known as: Aquaman's Delight

Benefits: Good for an outdoor quickie, while still avoiding prying eyes.

Technique: Another variation of The Ballet Dancer. The receiver's buoyancy in the water makes this sex position easier to hold. And all you need to do is shift some bathing suit material out of the way of certain body parts; the lifeguards will be none the wiser.

Hot tip: Water washes away the body's natural lubrication, so this position might be best for external stimulation.

September 23

The Hoover Maneuver

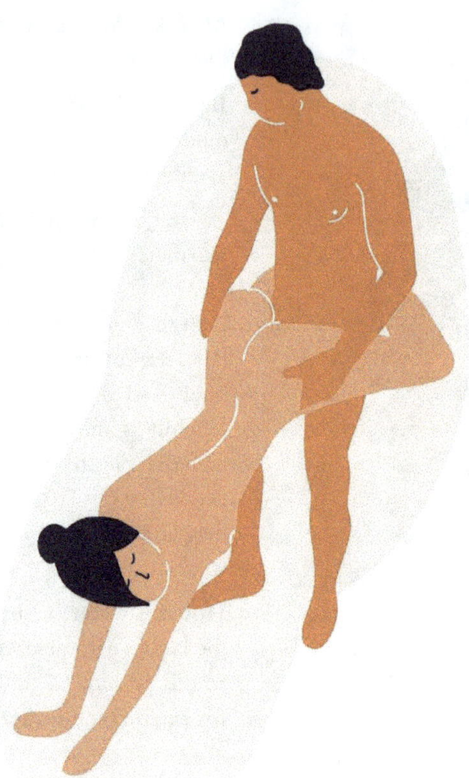

Benefits: Calorie burner because it's so athletic. You can stroll around the house in this position, but draw the shades first.

Technique: The giver enters their partner as they would in a standing, rear entry position, but instead, the giver lifts the receiver up by the pelvis. The receiver then grips the giver's waist with their legs. Summer camp wheelbarrow races were never this much fun!

Hot tip: The receiver can rhythmically squeeze their PC muscles to help them climax.

September 24

Seated Wheelbarrow

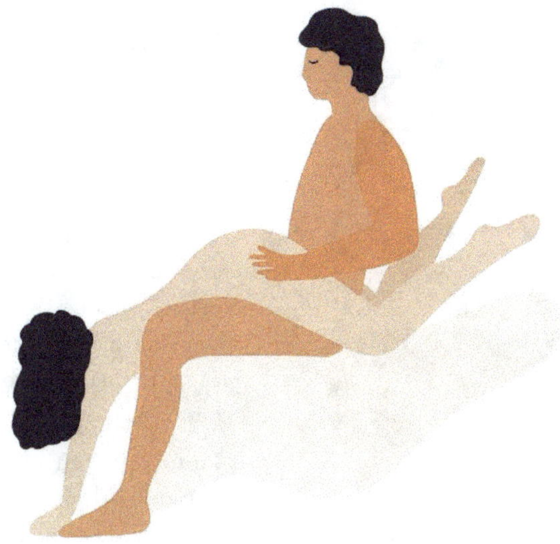

Benefits: Less strenuous than the standing varieties of this sex position, while still offering intense sensation.

Also try: Try the wheelbarrow with the giver sitting on the edge of a bed or chair. Movement is limited, but penetration is deep.

Hot tip: Make some noise. Explore the deeper sexual response and energy by letting loose with powerful sounds—a roar, perhaps?

25

The Standing Dragon

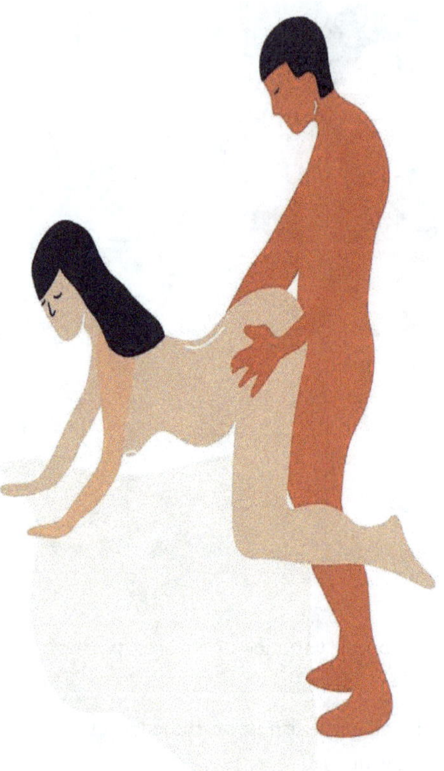

Benefits: An ideal position for G-spot stimulation—and if you're the giver, seeing the curves of your partner's rear can be highly erotic.

Technique: The giver stands and enters the receiver from behind as they pose on all fours on the edge of the bed and arch their back to lift their buttocks.

Hot tip: With their legs outside of their partners, givers can use their thighs to squeeze their partner's knees together, which tightens the receiver's vagina around the giver's penis or dildo.

September 26

Restroom Attendant

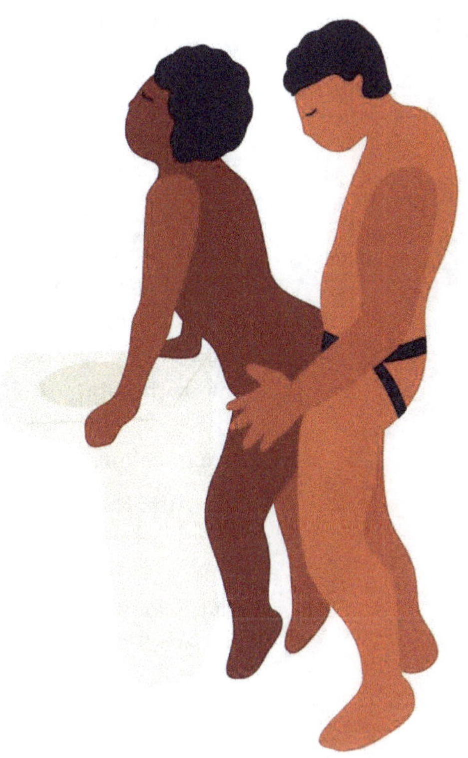

Also known as: Don't Get Caught

Benefits: Good for a quickie at a party.

Technique: After slipping into a bathroom, the receiver looks into the mirror while the giver enters them from behind. This position lets you both have eye contact during this rear-entry sex position.

Hot tip: If the receiver likes to be dominated, pull their hair.

September 27
Couch Surfer

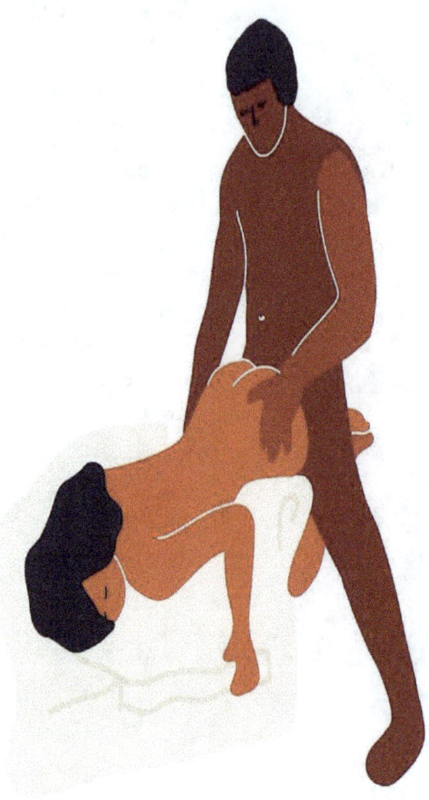

Also known as: The Lazy Susan

Benefits: Convenient for a quickie and adds spice outside the bedroom.

Technique: The receiving partner bends their body over the arm of a couch as the giver enters them from behind. The receiver can grind on the firm but cushy arm for multiple forms of stimulation with minimal effort.

Hot tip: Have the receiver cross their ankles. This will squeeze their pelvic floor and gluteal muscles tightly around the giver's penis or dildo.

September 28
Quickie-Fix

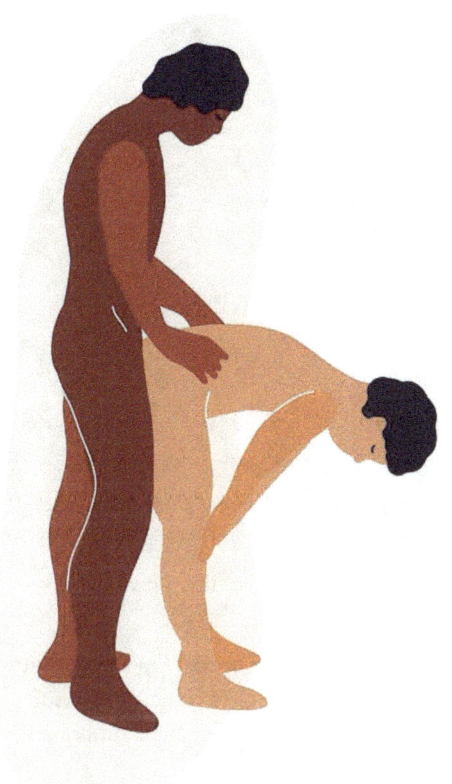

Also known as: The Bends

Benefits: Greater thrusting power, and good for quickie sex in your kitchen, especially if the receiving partner is wearing a skirt.

Technique: The receiver bends at the waist and rests their hands on a piece of furniture, their knees, or the floor for support. The giver enters them from behind and holds their hips for support while thrusting.

Also try: The giver can reach below to caress the receiver's clitoris or penis for extra stimulation.

Hot tip: The giver can also massage the receiver's shoulders or stimulate their breasts by bending over them.

September 29
Mountain Climber

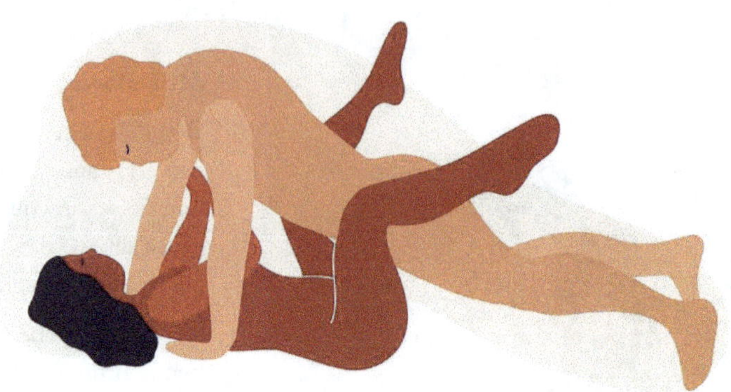

Also known as: The Pushup

Benefits: Creates great eye-to-eye contact. Keeps the giver's weight off the receiver's bod.

Technique: The mountain climber position shows off the giver's strength. While between their partner's legs, the giver assumes the standard "pushup" sex position.

Also try: The giver can lower themselves to kiss their partner teasingly while thrusting with their shoulders as well as their pelvis.

Hot tip: The giver can also tease the receiver with a series of moves: by entering with just the tip; thrusting just halfway in; then out; and stroking the outside with their member. The receiver can reach down and grab the giver's shaft and rub their clitoris with it.

September 30
The Quicker Picker Upper

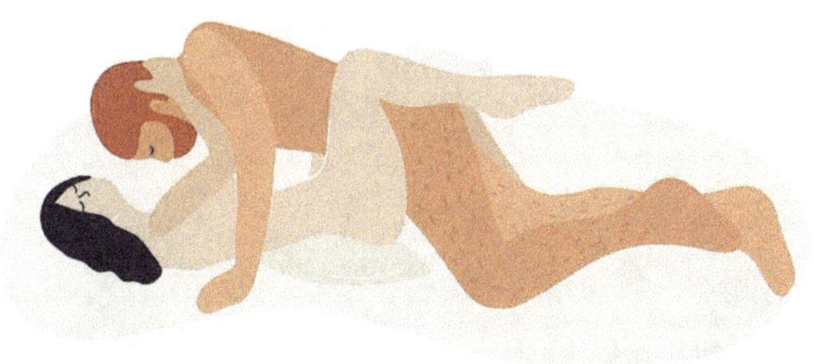

Also known as: The Pillow Driver

Benefits: A little bit of variety if missionary begins to feel stale; good upper body exercise.

Technique: Place a pillow under the small of the receiver's back or their buttocks to tilt their pelvis and change the angle of penetration for different sensations. The giver then braces their body with their hands on the bed in a pushup position, taking their weight off the receiver's body.

Hot tip: For more stability, try using a firm positioning pillow that's specifically designed for sex.

October

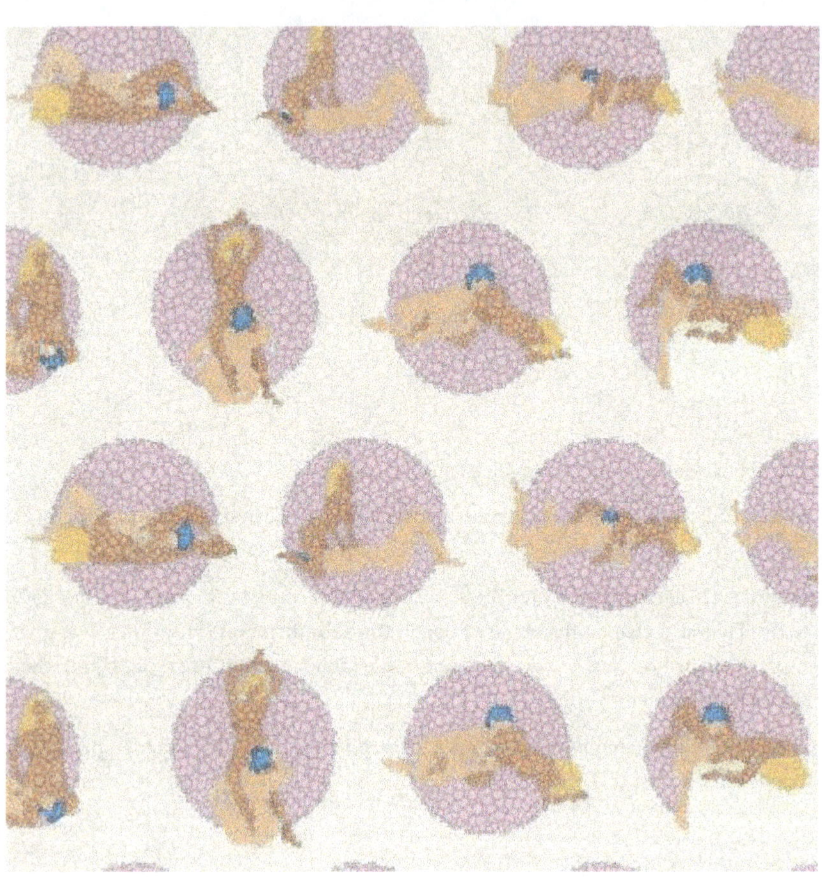

Sexiest Cities Around the World

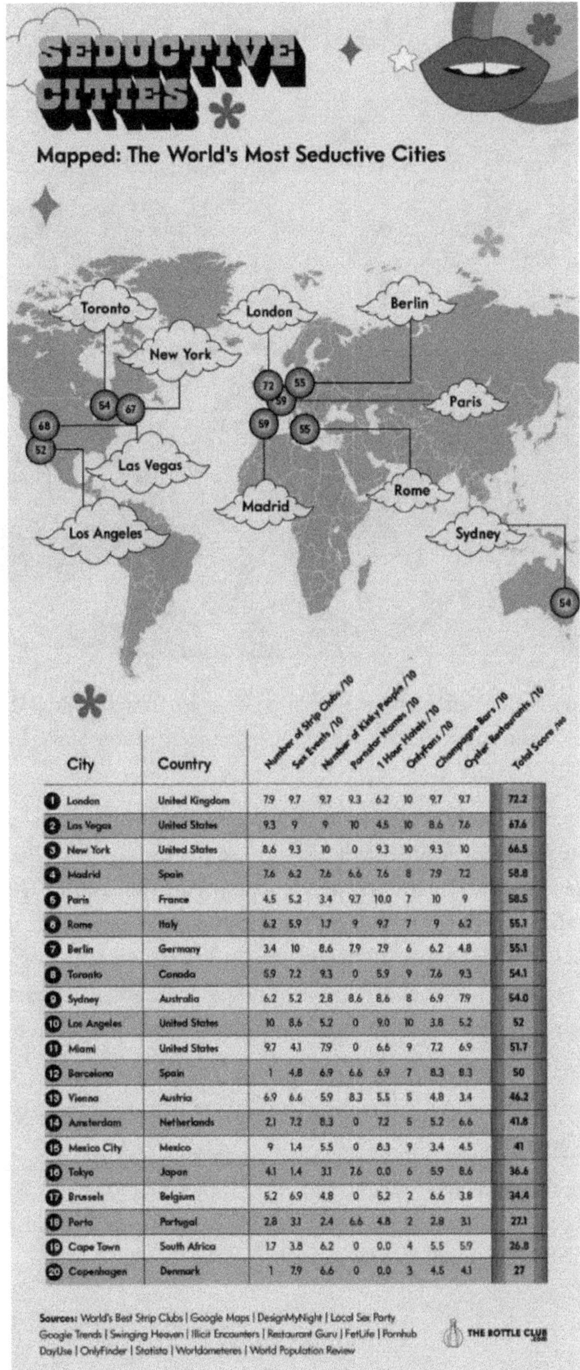

#	City	Country	Number of Strip Clubs /10	Sex Events /10	Number of Kinky People /10	Pornstar Names /10	1 Hour Hotels /10	OnlyFans /10	Champagne Bars /10	Oyster Restaurants /10	Total Score Ave
1	London	United Kingdom	7.9	9.7	9.7	9.3	6.2	10	9.7	9.7	72.2
2	Las Vegas	United States	9.3	9	9	10	4.5	10	8.6	7.6	67.6
3	New York	United States	8.6	9.3	10	0	9.3	10	9.3	10	66.5
4	Madrid	Spain	7.6	6.2	7.6	6.6	7.6	8	7.9	7.2	58.8
5	Paris	France	4.5	5.2	3.4	9.7	10.0	7	10	9	58.5
6	Rome	Italy	6.2	5.9	1.7	9	9.7	7	9	6.2	55.1
7	Berlin	Germany	3.4	10	8.6	7.9	7.9	6	6.2	4.8	55.1
8	Toronto	Canada	5.9	7.2	9.3	0	5.9	9	7.6	9.3	54.1
9	Sydney	Australia	6.2	5.2	2.8	8.6	8.6	8	6.9	7.9	54.0
10	Los Angeles	United States	10	8.6	5.2	0	9.0	10	3.8	5.2	52
11	Miami	United States	9.7	4.1	7.9	0	6.6	9	7.2	6.9	51.7
12	Barcelona	Spain	1	4.8	6.9	6.6	6.9	7	8.3	8.3	50
13	Vienna	Austria	6.9	6.6	5.9	8.3	5.5	5	4.8	3.4	46.2
14	Amsterdam	Netherlands	2.1	7.2	8.3	0	7.2	5	5.2	6.6	41.8
15	Mexico City	Mexico	9	1.4	5.5	0	8.3	9	3.4	4.5	41
16	Tokyo	Japan	4.1	1.4	3.1	7.6	0.0	6	5.9	8.6	36.6
17	Brussels	Belgium	5.2	6.9	4.8	0	5.2	2	6.6	3.8	34.4
18	Porto	Portugal	2.8	3.1	2.4	6.6	4.8	2	2.8	3.1	27.1
19	Cape Town	South Africa	1.7	3.8	6.2	0	0.0	4	5.5	5.9	26.8
20	Copenhagen	Denmark	1	7.9	6.6	0	0.0	3	4.5	4.1	27

October 1

Missionary

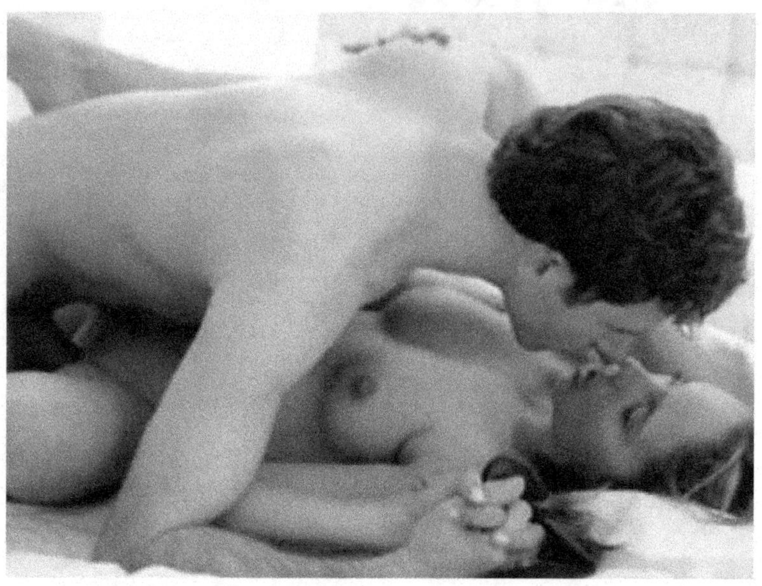

Benefits: We know this one isn't necessarily new to lots of guys, but there's something sort of kinky about doin' it in the most vanilla position of all. Plus, you get lots of eye and body contact.

Technique: The most commonly used position in the world, missionary is an especially intimate position because it allows for face-to-face contact. The giver likes it because they can control penetration depth and speed of thrusting. The receiving partner enjoys feeling the giver's weight on their body and the maximum skin-to-skin contact. Note that this position can make it more difficult to hold off ejaculation because of the intense friction and deep thrusting. To lengthen lovemaking, start there, then switch to a position that maintains clitoral pressure without so much pelvic back and forth.

Also try: The giver can push up to create space and sneak a small vibrator on top of the receiver's mound.

Hot tip: If you're the giver, raise the receiver's left leg so their knee is level with your right shoulder. Keep their other leg flat on the bed. Thrust toward the inner thigh of their raised leg. This adjustment creates more clitoral pressure.

October 2

The Sleeper Hold

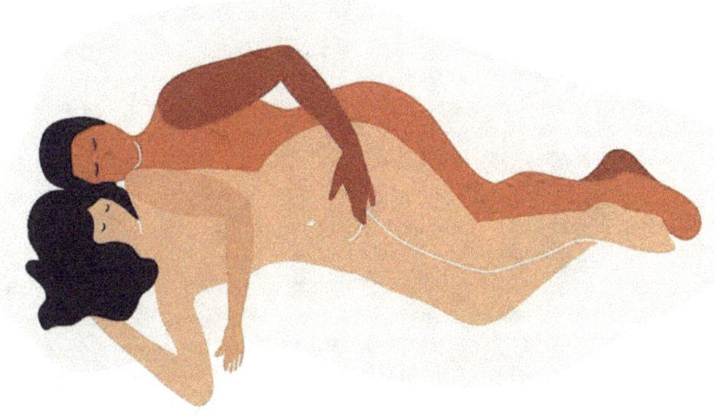

Benefits: Comfortable sex position if a partner is pregnant or if one or both partners have bigger bellies. Good one for falling asleep afterward.

Technique: You both lie on your sides facing the same direction, with the giver in back. The receiving partner bends their knees and pushes their rear back toward the giver for easier access to their vagina or anus. Adjusting the lean of your bodies will vary the angle of entry and help with rocking and thrusting.

Also try: Synchronize your breathing. One of you takes the lead and the other follows so that you inhale and exhale together. The coordinated rhythm opens an unspoken dialogue of intimacy.

Hot tip: To give the receiver the sensation of greater girth inside them, have them bend and lift their top leg to their chest. Adjust your position so you are more on top of them top hip than behind them.

October 3

Open-Legged Spoon

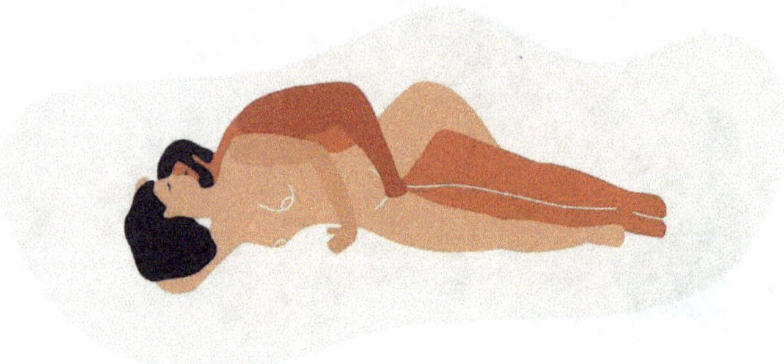

Benefits: It's everything you love about the classic spoon position, with the added opportunity for clit access.

Technique: From the Spoon position above, the receiving partner lifts their top leg and drapes it backward over the penetrating partner's hips.

Hot tip: The open-legged element of this position means the partner in back can reach around and play with their partner's penis or clitoris—either with their hands or a vibrator.

October 4

The Cutlery Combo

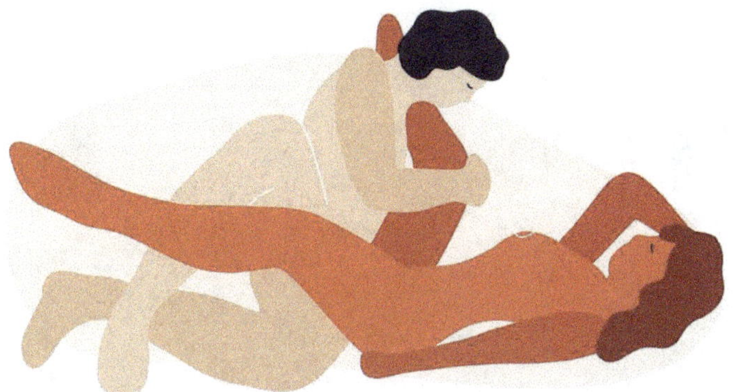

Benefits: Offers a natural bridge to more creative positions.

Technique: The receiver lies on their back and raises their right leg so the giver can position their body between their legs at a 90-degree angle and enter. The receiver's legs will form the tines of a spork. They can do this with the giver facing them or facing their back.

Also try: If the receiver is limber, lift their left leg up to increase the depth of penetration.

Hot tip: From the Spork position, the receiver can lift their top leg and let the giver support it by resting it on their shoulder. From here, the receiver can easily stimulate their clitoris using their fingers while the giver is inside them.

October 5

Th Horny Mantis

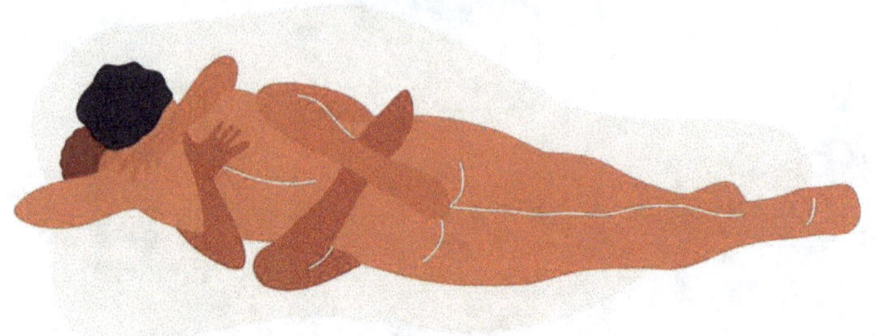

Benefits: Relaxing position with deeper penetration and increased intimacy.

Technique: Both of you lie on your sides facing one another. The receiving partner bends, spreads their legs, and angles their vagina or anus toward the giver. The giver lifts their legs, wraps them around the receiver's back, and enters them.

Hot tip: The receiver can use their legs and feet to pull the giver close during thrusts for deeper penetration.

October 6

Facing Spoon

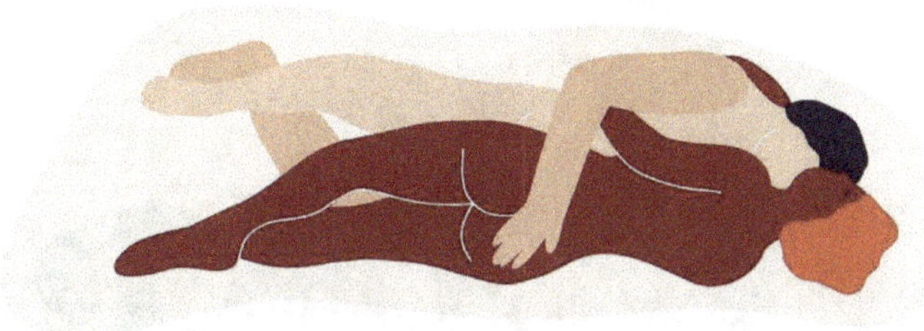

Also known as: Sidewinder

Benefits: A very intimate face-to-face position that encourages hugging and kissing.

Technique: This is an ideal position for pregnant partners and partners with knee injuries because it keeps weight off the body. To get into the position, begin by lying on your sides and facing one another. The receiving partner spreads their legs slightly to allow the penetrating partner to enter them, then closes their legs so the part of the giver's shaft that's outside can press against their clitoris. It's easy to kiss from this intimate face-to-face position.

Also try: Because thrusting is more difficult in this position, use different techniques such as grinding, circular, and up-and-down motions for added stimulation.

Hot tip: Hug each other for 20 seconds before getting busy. Hugging raises your levels of oxytocin, a bonding hormone your body produces naturally, and that will enhance your connection.

October 7

The X Position

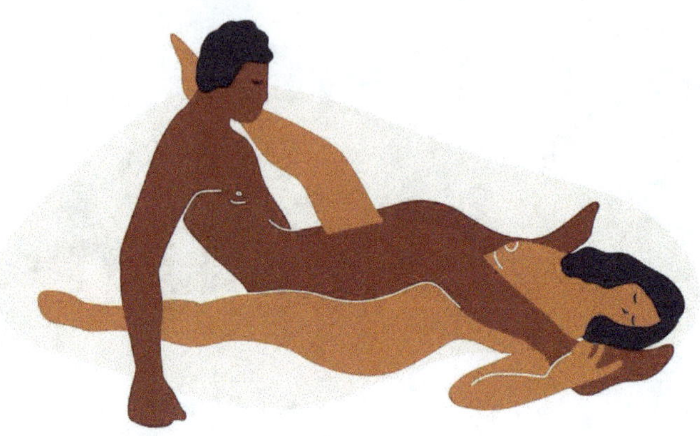

Also known as: Crisscross

Benefits: Prolonged, slow sex to build arousal. Shallow thrusts stimulate the nerve endings in the head of the giver's penis.

Technique: Sit on the bed facing each other with legs forward. The giver should lift their right leg over the receiver's left leg, and the receiver should lift their right leg over the giver's left leg. Come together so the giver can enter. Now both of you lie back, with your legs forming an X. Slow, leisurely gyrations replace thrusting.

Hot tip: Reach out and hold hands to pull together for pelvic thrusting. Also, take turns alternatively sitting up and lying back without changing the rhythm.

October 8

Snow Plow

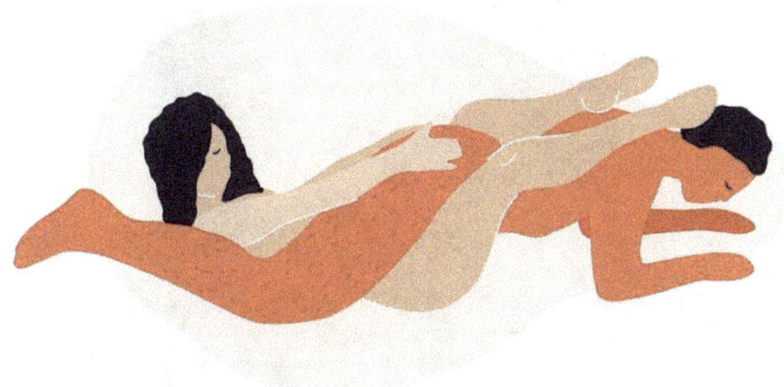

Benefits: The receiving partner gets a prime view of the giver's derriere.

Technique: This is challenging: The receiver lies on their back while the giver straddles them, facing away. The receiver lifts their legs and wraps them around the giver's back to elevate their pelvis so the giver can enter. Then the receiver grabs the giver's butt to help the giver slide up and back. They can add a little massage action to their grip also.

Hot tip: The giver can spin around into missionary style to face the receiver while trying to stay inserted. Then switch positions, this time with the receiver on top and facing away.

October 9

The Fusion

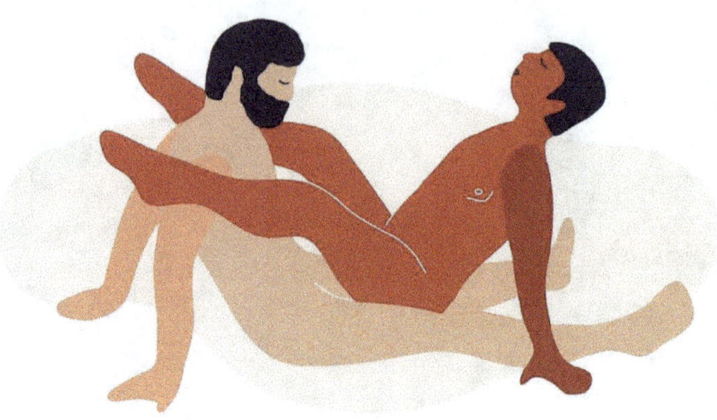

Also known as: Getting a Leg Up

Benefits: Quicker orgasms for the receiver; easier motions.

Technique: From The Spider, the receiver can lift their legs onto the giver's shoulders, which increases the muscular tension that advances the orgasm sequence. By elevating their butt off the bed, it'll be easier for them to thrust and grind in circles.

Hot tip: The giver can lean against a headboard or wall and use their hands to support the receiver's lower back.

October 10

The Tarantula

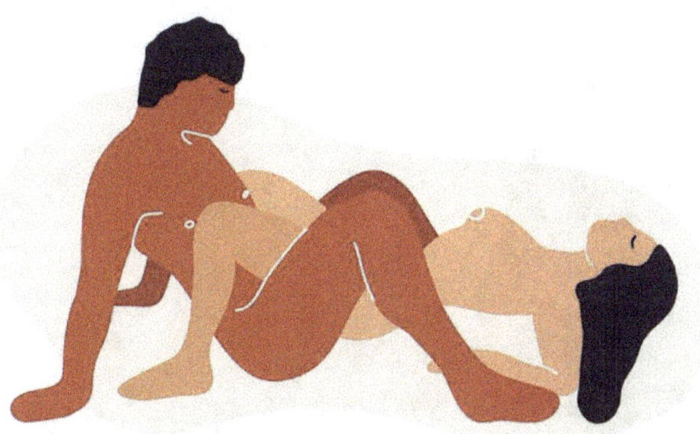

Benefits: You both can still maintain eye contact while viewing the action at center stage.

Technique: Both of you begin seated on the bed with legs toward one another, arms back to support yourselves. Then the receiver moves onto the giver. The receiver's hips will be between the giver's spread legs, their knees bent and feet outside of the giver's hips and flat on the bed. Now rock back and forth.

Hot tip: The receiver can grab the giver's hands and pull themselves up into a squatting position while the giver lies back. Or the giver can remain seated upright and pull the receiver against their chest into the Lazy Man position.

October 11

The Hovering Bradley

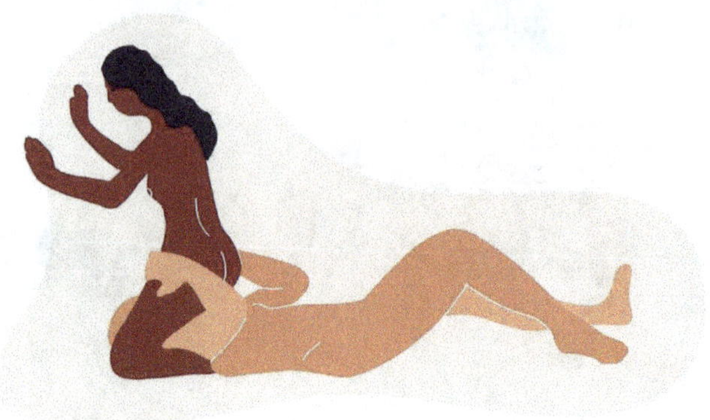

Benefits: The receiver can direct the position of the giver's tongue and the pressure against them by rising up or pressing down.

Technique: The receiver straddles the giver, placing their knees at the giver's ears. They can hold onto a wall or headboard for support. While the giver is doing their thing, the receiver can use their fingers to graze their nipples or rub the top of their vulva.

Also try: The giver can hold their tongue firm as the receiver gyrates their hips, pressing their clitoris against it.

Hot tip: If you have the right equipment and a mutual interest in kink, the receiver can have their hands cuffed over their head.

October 12

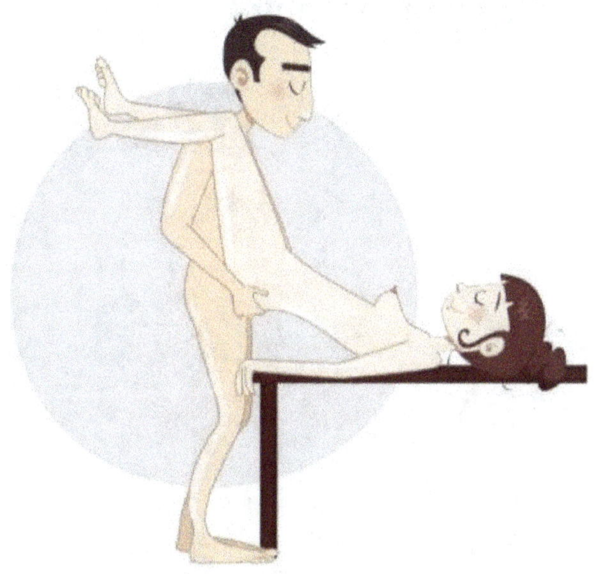

The Butterfly

The Butterfly

Difficulty level: Moderate

Special features: Tabletop position, man standing

Similar to the Mermaid, the Butterfly position involves having sex while the woman lays on a relatively low table with her bottom right on the edge. The man stands and helps her raise her hips with his hands. He penetrates her while she rests her legs on his shoulders.

October 13

The Hovering Housefly

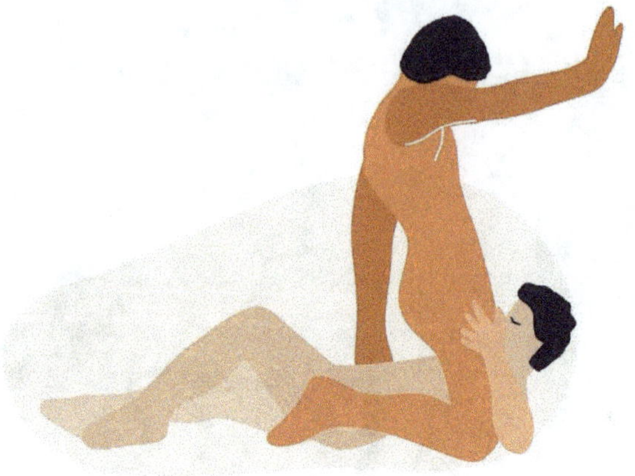

Benefits: A comfortable position for the receiving partner and an erotic one for the giver.

Technique: Rest a pillow behind the giver's head. Then the receiver should straddle their shoulders and support their body by holding the bed's headboard or the wall.

Hot tip: If the giver's mouth becomes dry after a while, they can add some mint- or fruit-flavored lube to the receiver's genitals.

October 14
The Bees Knees

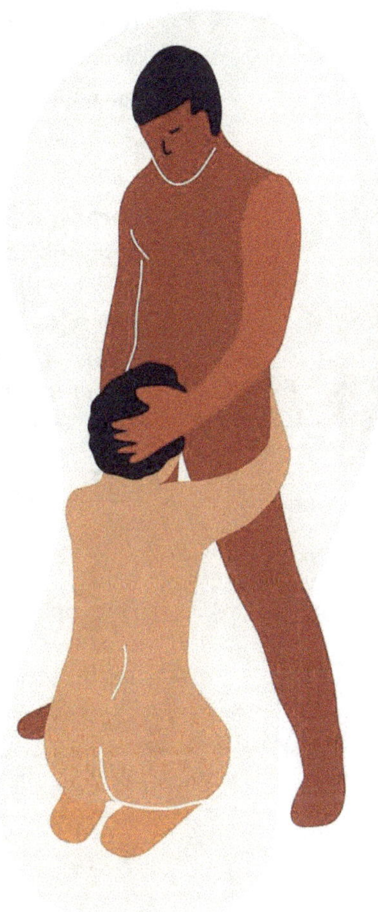

Benefits: Great for out-of-bedroom fellatio.

Technique: The giver kneels in front of the receiver, covering their teeth with their lips and encircling the receiver's glans with their mouth. Then the giver should slowly piston their lips up and down on the receiver's shaft, alternating speeds and occasionally stopping to move their tongue over and around the receiver's head.

Also try: Lean a dressing mirror against a wall to the side of your body so the receiver can enjoy the view of their partner going down on them from the side.

Hot tip: For variation, the giver can take one of the receiver's testicles into their mouth as they stroke the shaft with their hand.

October 15

Swiss Ball Blitz

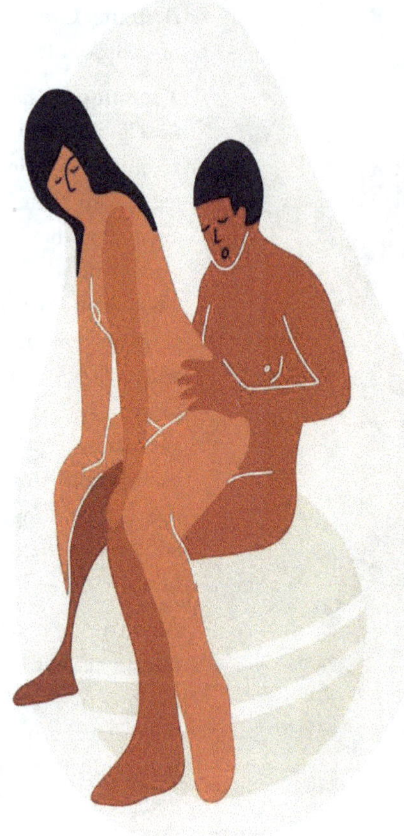

Also known as: Romper Room

Benefits: See The Hot Seat. Also, adds bounce to your thrusts.

Technique: Have a ball in your workout room? Use a stability ball to add some bounce to The Hot Seat. The giver sits on the ball with their feet on the floor. Then the receiver backs up onto the giver, sitting between their legs. Roll and bounce to it.

Hot tip: The giver can lean their back against a wall for additional stability.

October 16

The Rock Climber

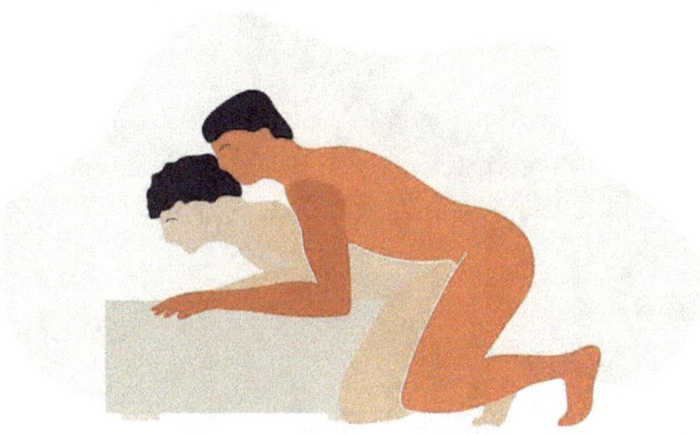

Benefits: Think the deep penetration of Doggy, with the closeness of Flatiron

Technique: Find a low-lying piece of furniture, like an ottoman or a bed. Kneel over it so it provides a bend at the waist (this can also be done with a stack of pillows on the bed). The giver kneels behind the receiver, entering from behind. They then form their body to that of the receivers.

Hot tip: Slow. It. Down. Instead of quick thrusting, aim for a slow and steady flow.

October 17

The Onramp

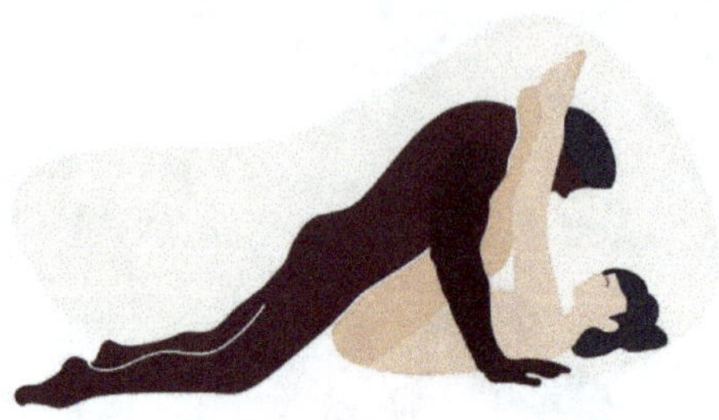

Benefits: This position will provide just about the deepest penetration you can get in a forward-facing position.

Technique: You'll need some flexibility for this one. The seashell is very similar to Happy Baby, except a bit more... folded. Start in missionary, and have the receiver bring both their legs up by their head. The giver then enters facing them, leaning into the receiver's legs.

Also try: If the stretch becomes a bit too much for the receiver, take a break with Happy Baby—where they bend their knees up to 90 degrees. You will both still get the deep penetration that Seashell provides, without the receiver feeling like they're tearing up their hamstrings.

Hot tip: Place a pillow underneath the receiver's hips for more lift—it'll make the bend for the receiving partner a bit more comfortable.

October 18

Bandoleer

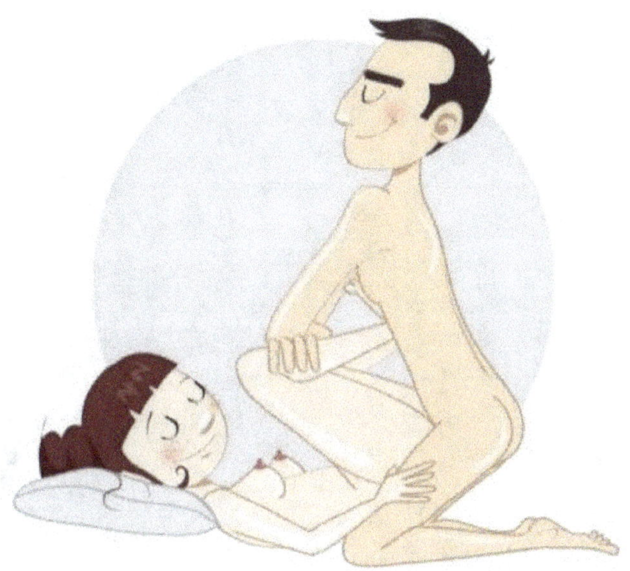

Difficulty level: Easy

Special features: Deep penetration

While the woman lies on her back and lifts both knees up towards her chest, the man kneels facing her. She can then rest her feet on his chest, while he places his forearms on her knees. The woman can then grab the man's thighs and pull him closer for deeper penetration. The more he presses down on her knees, the greater the pleasure for her.

A relatively simple sex position, which doesn't require too much flexibility.

October 19

The Grip

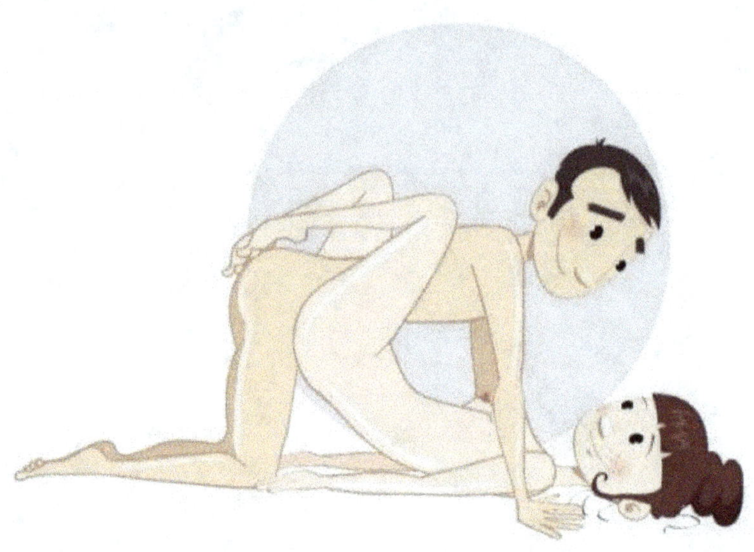

Difficulty level: Easy

Special features: Woman in control

Similar to the missionary position, the grip requires the woman to lay on her back and raise her hips slightly (it may be more comfortable to place a cushion under the woman's bottom). The man then places himself between her legs, while she moves her pelvis side to side.

Simple and good if you're not feeling too energetic.

October 20

The Midnight Snack

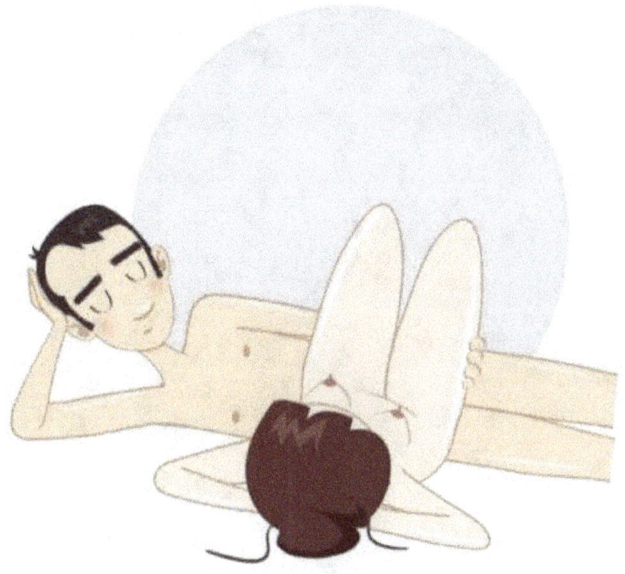

Difficulty level: Easy

Special features: Reclining

The man lays on his side, while the woman lays on her back at a right angle to her partner. She puts her knees over his hip to allow easy penetration.

Extremely easy and perfect for a lazy Sunday afternoon or if you need to slow it down a bit during a long sex session.

October 21

The Bus Driver

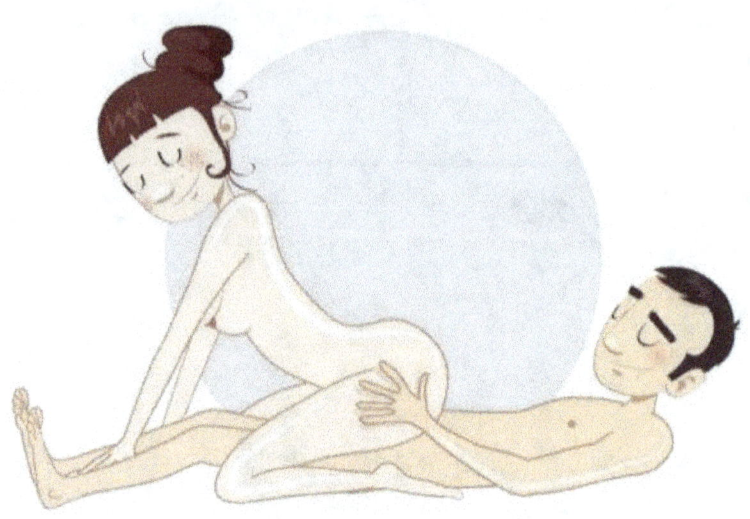

Difficulty level: Easy

Special features: Woman in control, frees up both individuals' hands

Similar to reverse cowgirl, the rider involves the woman straddling the man while facing away from him. She then leans forward and while balancing herself on his knees slides up and down. The man can also control penetration by holding onto the woman's waist.

Not too much flexibility required and both sets of hands are free and well place for extra stimulation.

October 22

The Bird of Prey

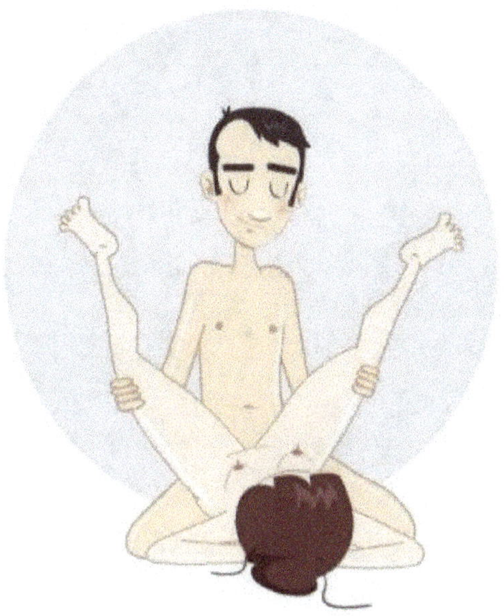

Difficulty level: Easy

Special features: Deep penetration

The woman lays on her back with her legs in the air and knees slightly bent (she may need a cushion under her bottom to make it more comfortable). The man then kneels between her legs and holds onto her ankles while he enters her.

Relatively easy and deep penetration.

October 22

The Midnight Caller

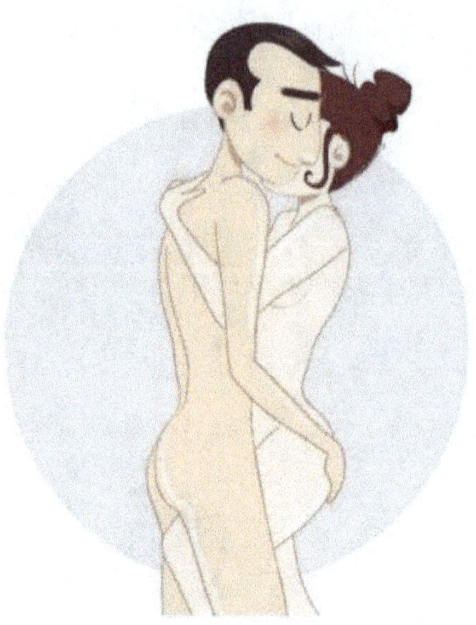

Difficulty level: Easy

Special features: Woman in control

This position is ideal for an impromptu sex session. The man and the woman stand face to face and he stimulates her genitals with his penis before penetrating her.

An easy position if the woman is a similar height to the man (or wearing heels), but if not a table or work surface will help!

October 23

The Slippery Sleeper

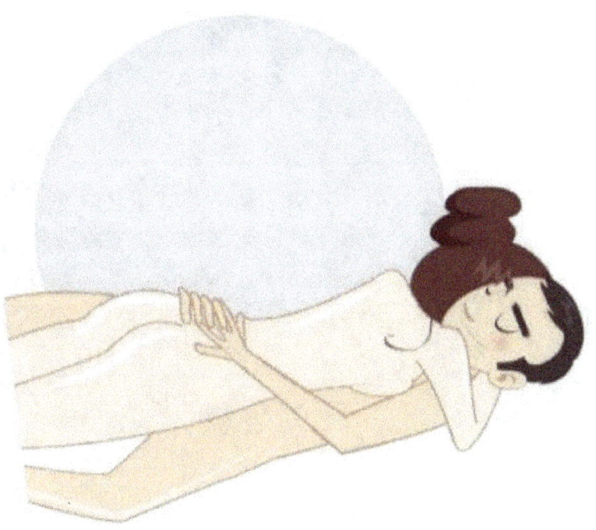

Difficulty level: Easy

Special features: Increased friction

An easy sex position which requires minimal effort and increases tightness.

The man lies flat on his back, while the woman lies on top of him with her legs together. He is then able to penetrate her as she slides up and down on his body.

And try this top tip: keeping your socks on could increase your chances of having an orgasm.

October 24

The Clasp

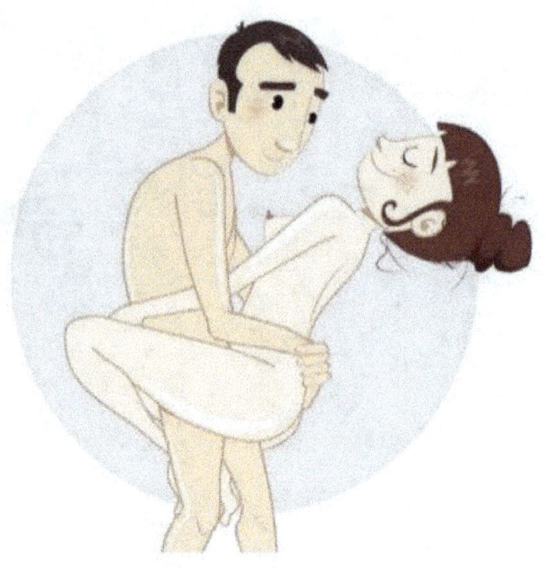

Difficulty level: Moderate

Special features: Requires some upper body strength

He stands and she wraps her legs around his waist while he supports her by holding her bottom and back. For more support and deeper penetration she can rest her back against a wall.

Ideal for anytime/anywhere sex, but does require a certain degree of strength and energy from both the man and woman.

October 25

The Tominagi

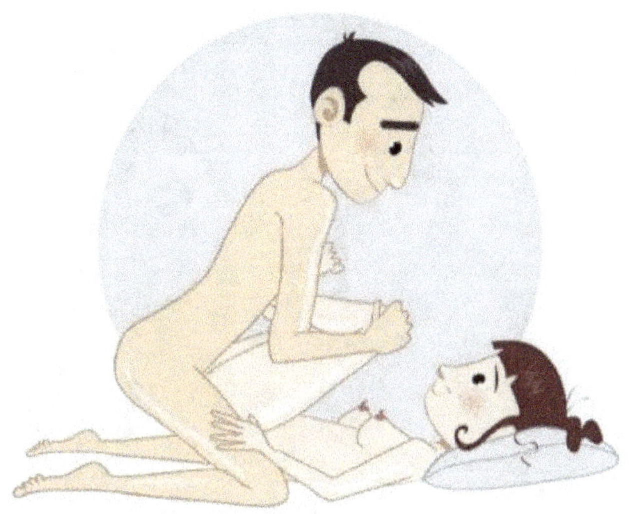

Difficulty level: Easy

Special features: Good for men of varying sizes, man in control

October 26

Seated Ball

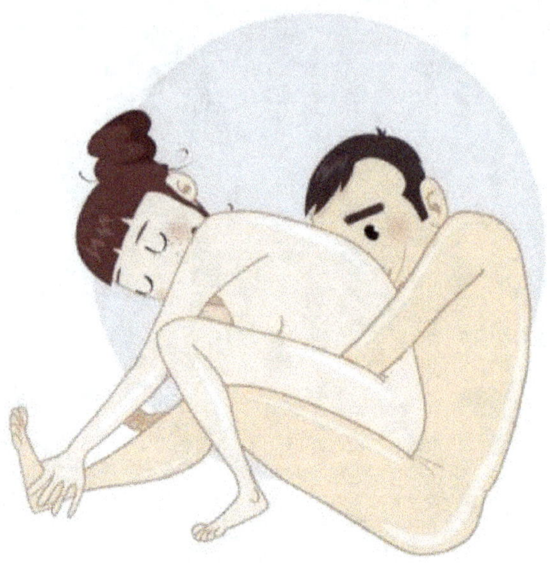

Difficulty level: Moderate

Special features: Woman in control

This position requires quite a lot of strength and flexibility.

The woman crouches down onto the man's lap, while she controls the penetration by rocking back and forth on her heels.

October 27

The Curled Angel

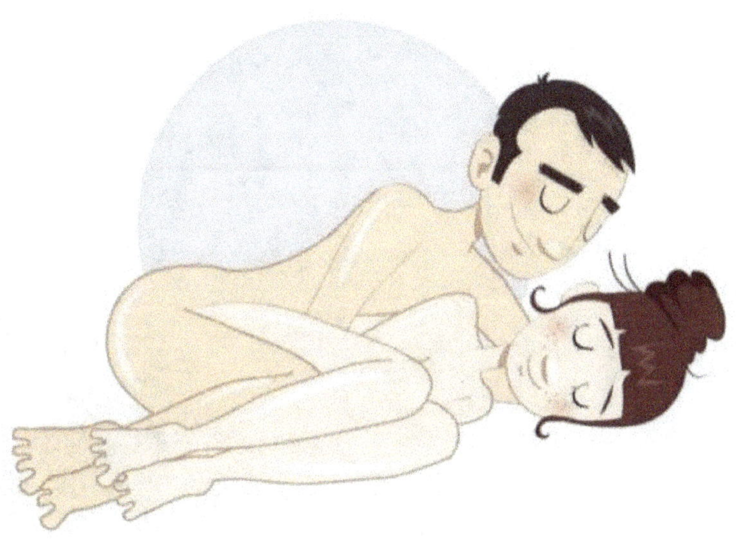

Difficulty level: Easy

Special features: Less energetic, good during pregnancy

The woman curls up into a ball with her knees drawn up to her chest, while the man spoons her from behind. This position is ideal if you're feeling lazy and it is also great for pregnant women too – the woman simply needs to lower her legs to accommodate her growing bump.

October 28

The Glowing Juniper

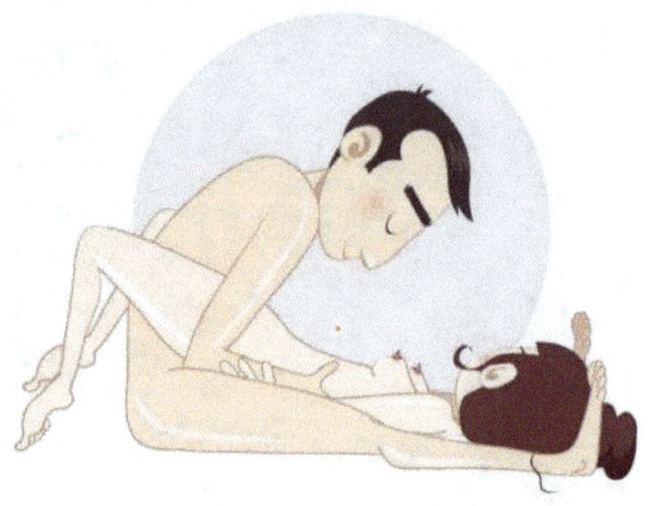

Difficulty level: Easy

Special features: Woman reclining

Perfect for when you're feeling a little bit lazy - the woman lies on her back with her legs parted and knees slightly bent. The man sits between her legs with his legs stretched either side of her. He can then lift her hips for easier penetration while she lays back and enjoys!

October 29

The Cross

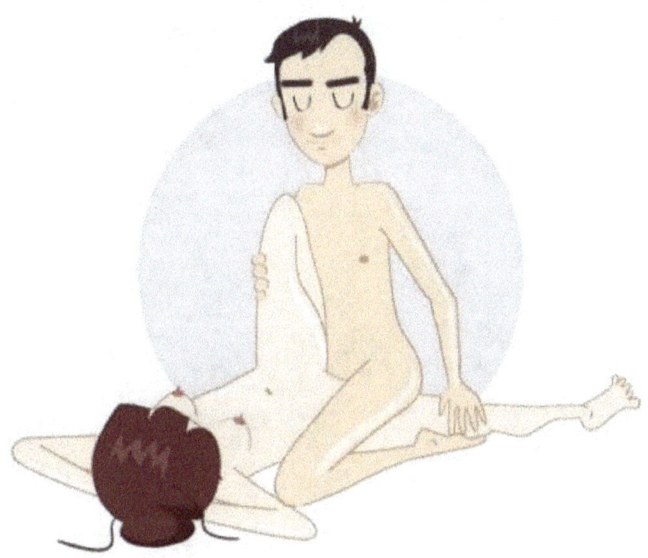

Difficulty level: Easy

Special features: Woman reclining

The woman lies on her back with one leg extended and the other raised in the air, but bent in half. The man then straddles the woman's extended leg, while holding onto her other leg to control penetration.

Relatively easy and good if the woman is tired.

October 30

The Perch

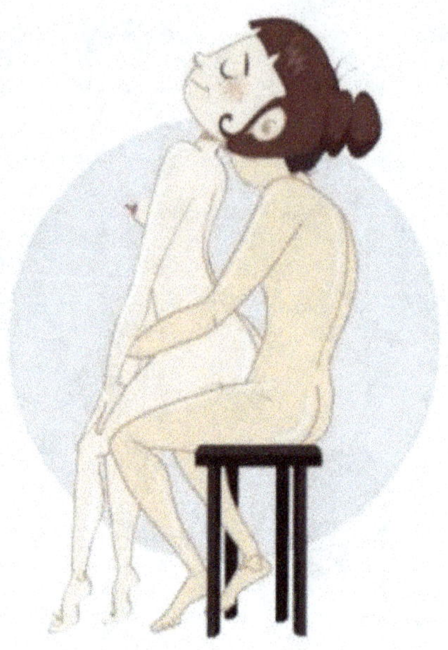

Difficulty level: Easy

Special features: Chair position, woman in control, man's hands free

The man sits on a chair or stool and the woman sits on his lap. With her back to him she can control the penetration by rocking back and forth on her heels. His hands are then free to play with her clitoris and breasts.

A good position for pregnant women and tired men.

October 31
The Toad

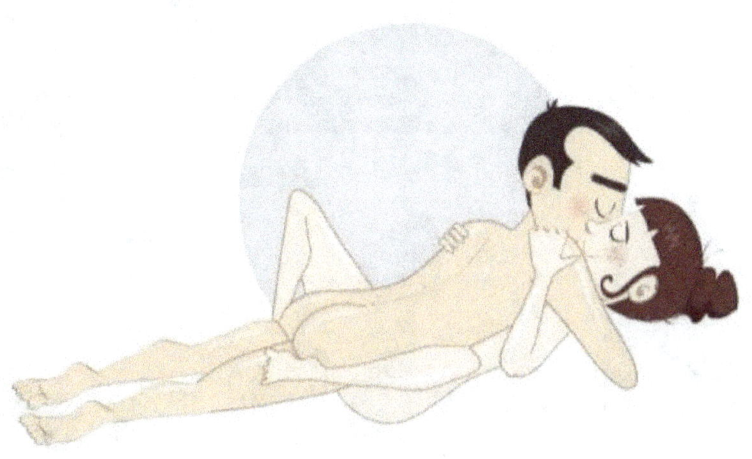

Difficulty level: Easy

Special features: Leisurely

The woman lies back with her legs open, while the man lies between her legs and slowly penetrates her. For greater intimacy, she can wrap her legs around him and control the pressure of his grinding by gently pressing on his buttocks with her feet.

Simple and an ideal sex position for a slower pace of lovemaking.

November

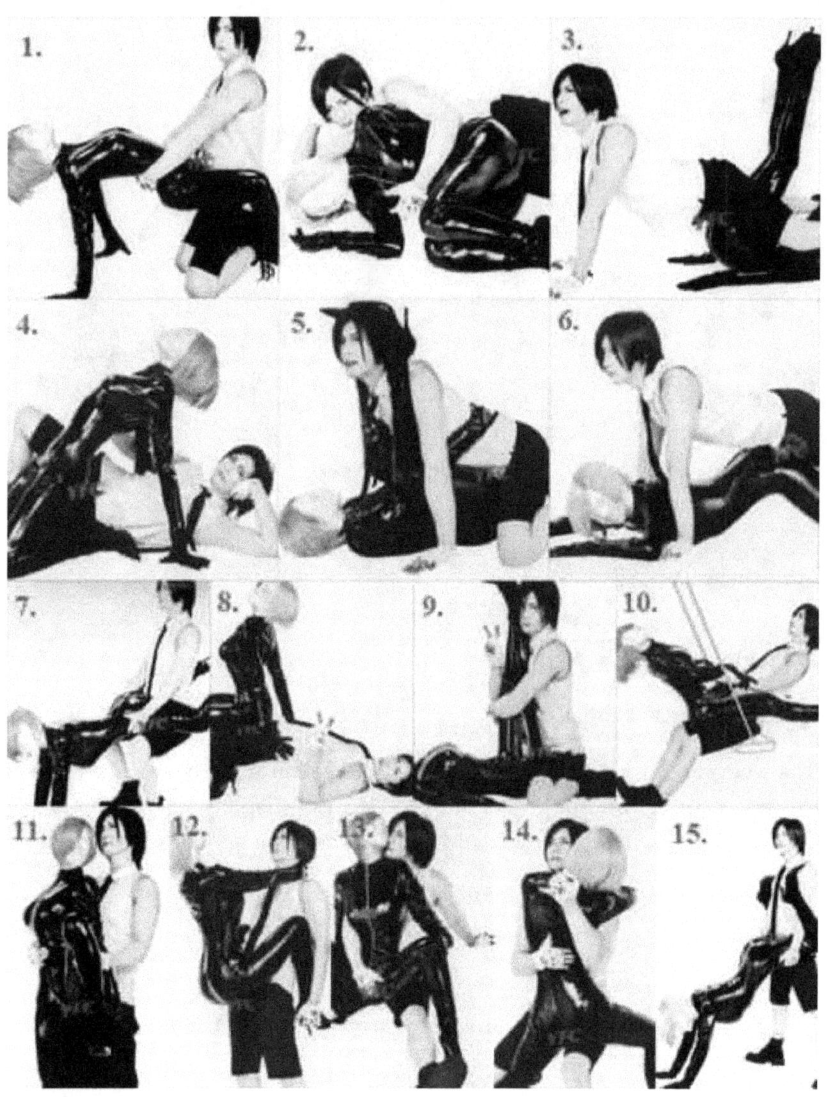

Dirty Talk is Not Just for the Bedroom

The best part about dirty talk is that it can be done anywhere. Sending your partner dirty text messages at work is a great way to build up anticipation for when you both get off of work and get off at home.

Some great places to squeeze in a little dirty talk other than the bedroom:

> **Text messages throughout the day**

Example: "I wish you were here. I want someone to pull my hair and choke me."

Or if that's not your speed, then something like, "Doing laundry and I found that little black dress you peeled off of me the other night. How hot was that?"

> **Leave a handwritten note where you know they'll find it.** I love this!

Example: "I laid out some lingerie on the bed for you to wear tonight. Looking forward to throwing you down on the bed and ripping it off of you later."

> **A choice whisper in the middle of a crowded public place.**

Example: Cup your hand to his ear and whisper, "God, I can't wait to get you home so I can start bouncing on your fucking dick."

> **Fun Fact: Dirty talk doesn't always have to be dirty.**

Example: "I'm doing laundry and I found that red dress you peeled off of me the other night.

Example: "Just got out of the shower and thinking about you."

Read the full Dirty Talk Guide in Allison Eden's *Sexy Game.*

November 1

The Plough

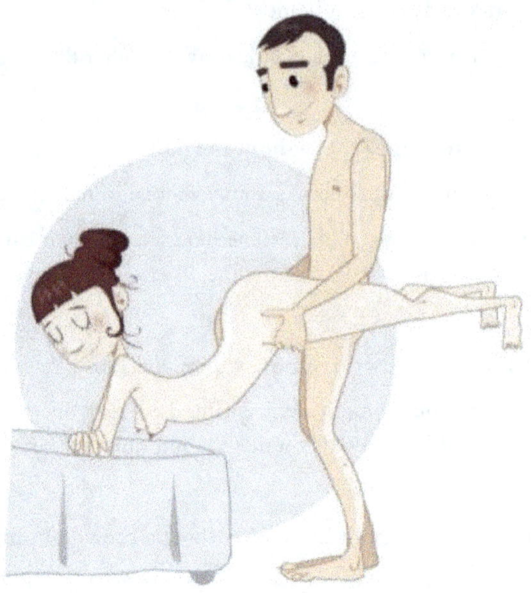

Difficulty level: Advanced

Special features: Requires upper body strength

The woman lays on the edge of the bed with her legs hanging off. The man then positions himself between her legs and lifts her hips and thighs to allow penetration, while she supports herself on her elbows.

This position requires a great deal of strength and flexibility.

November 2
The Hero

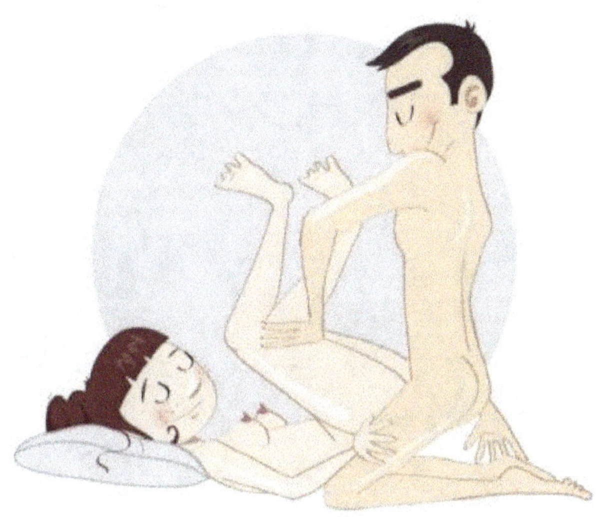

Difficulty level: Moderate

Special features: Requires some flexibility

The woman lies on her back, with her knees pulled up to her chest and her feet pointing up to the ceiling. The man kneels and rests his things under her bum while penetrating her.

An easy (ish) position but the woman may tire faster than the man as she has to hold her legs in the air.

November 3
The Peg

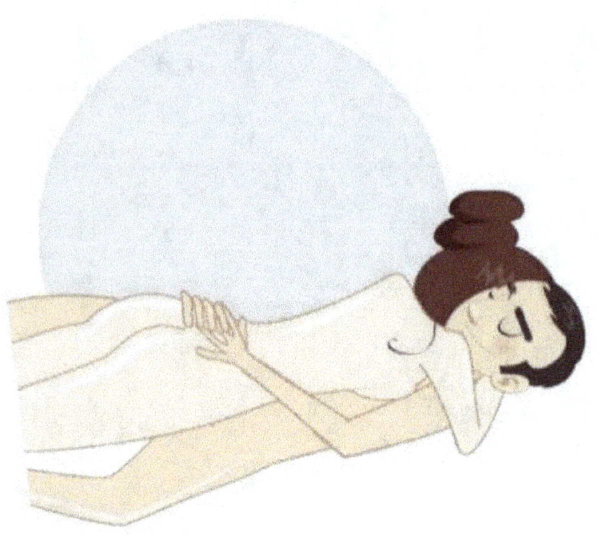

Difficulty level: Easy

Special features: Woman in control, romantic, good with man with larger penis

The man lies on his back with his legs stretched out and parted. The woman lies on top of him with her legs closed and stretched out.

This is a good sex position for well endowed partners as the man can't penetrate too deeply, as the woman's legs are closed. Also good for intimacy as you are face to face.

November 4
The Classic

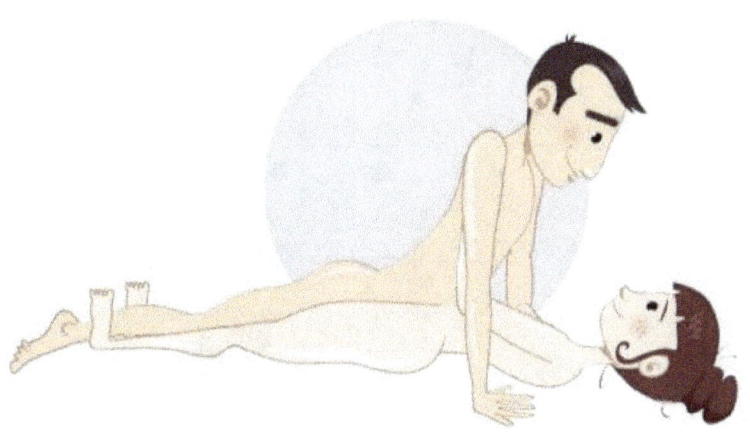

Difficulty level: Easy

Special features: Tried and true with slight modifications, deep penetration

While similar to the missionary, the classic position involves the woman laying on her back with a cushion under her bottom. This slight tilt of the pelvis allows for deeper penetration as the man places himself between her legs and enters her.

Why not treat yourself to some lubricant to add a tingle to your lovemaking? Durex do a three-pack that's available here at Amazon.

November 5

The Fan

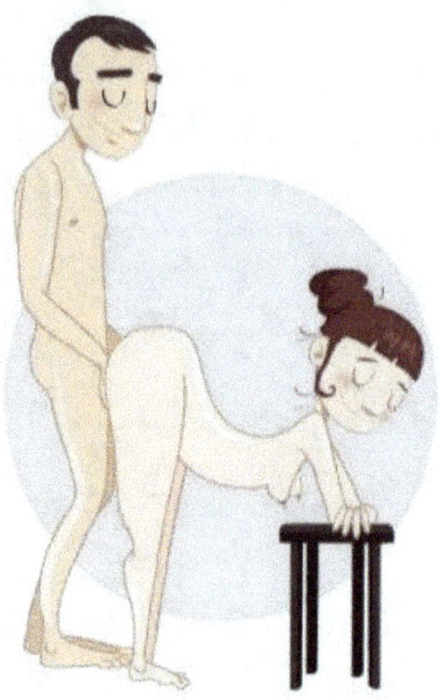

Difficulty level: Moderate

Special features: Uses a chair, good for anal sex, man in control

With her back to her partner, the woman bends over, crosses her arms and rests her elbows on a chair for support. Then man then enters her from behind (ideal for anal sex) and can control the depth and pressure by holding the top of her thighs.

November 6
The Snail

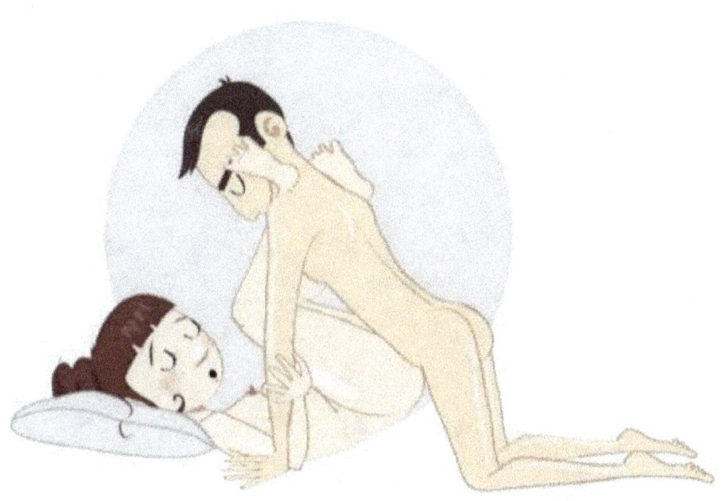

Difficulty level: Moderate

Special features: Very deep penetration

The woman lies on her back and pulls her knees up to her chest. The man kneels down and enters her. She can then rest her feet on his shoulders, while he supports himself with his hands either side of her shoulders.

The penetration is very deep in his sex position, so be careful not to go too fast as it may cause pain for the woman.

November 7
The Slip

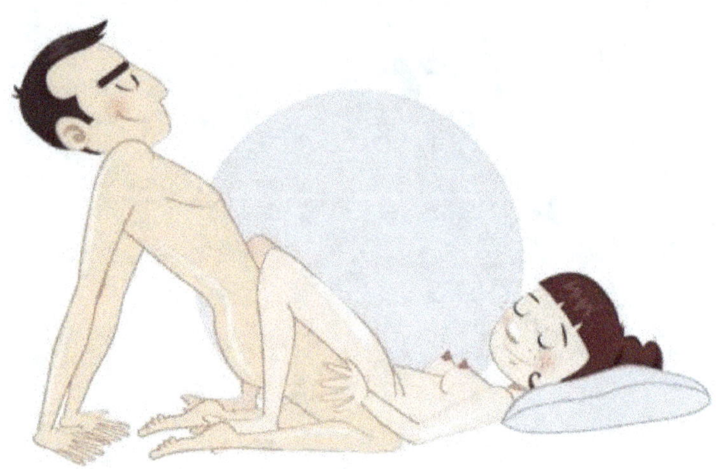

Difficulty level: Easy

Special features: Deep penetration

The man kneels down and leans back, supporting himself with his hands behind him, while the woman lies flat on her back. She then tilts her hips towards him to aid penetration, while positioning her legs either side of his hips.

This is a relatively easy position, which is highly erotic with deep penetration.

November 8

The Hound

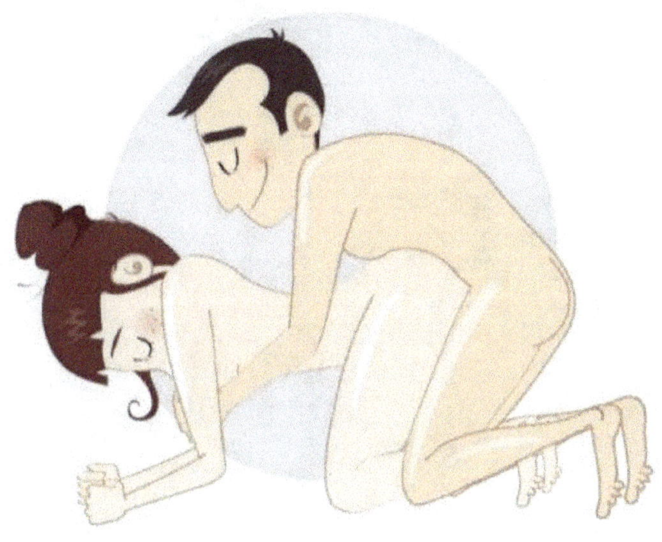

Difficulty level: Easy

Special features: Man's hands free, doggy style

Similar to doggy style, but instead of being on all fours, the woman lowers herself onto her forearms while the man penetrates her from behind. He can also lean forward and as his hands are free he can caress her body at the same time.

November 9

The Crouching Tiger

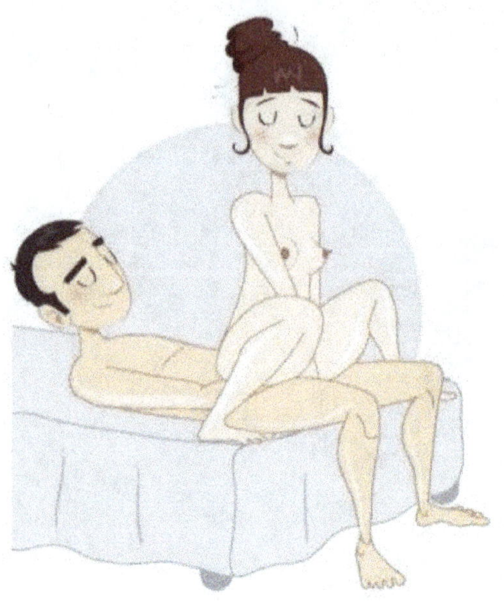

Difficulty level: Moderate

Special features: Woman in control, bed position

While the man lays on the bed with his knees off the edge, the woman squats over him facing away. She is fully in control of depth and pace of penetration.

While this sex position is easy for the man, it requires some decent thigh muscles from the woman and be careful not to lose your balance and fall off the bed.

November 10

The Hinge

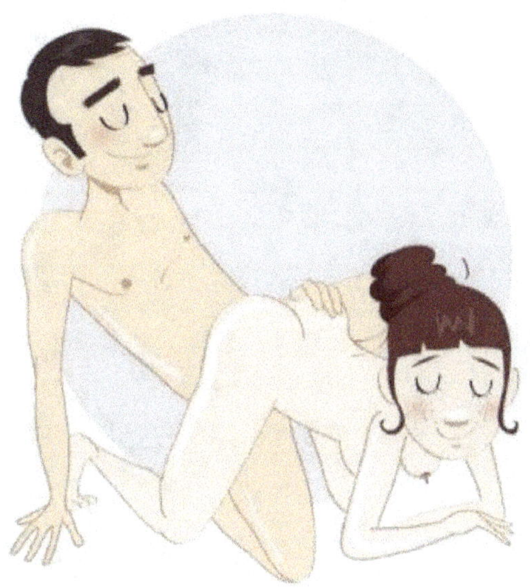

Difficulty level: Moderate

Special features: Man one hand free

This position requires good balance, but once in the rhythm it's great for depth control.

The man kneels behind the woman and while leaning backwards uses one arm to support himself. The women kneels in front of him and supports herself on her elbows, allowing her to thrust back onto him. He can then use his spare hand to touch her.

November 11

The Ship

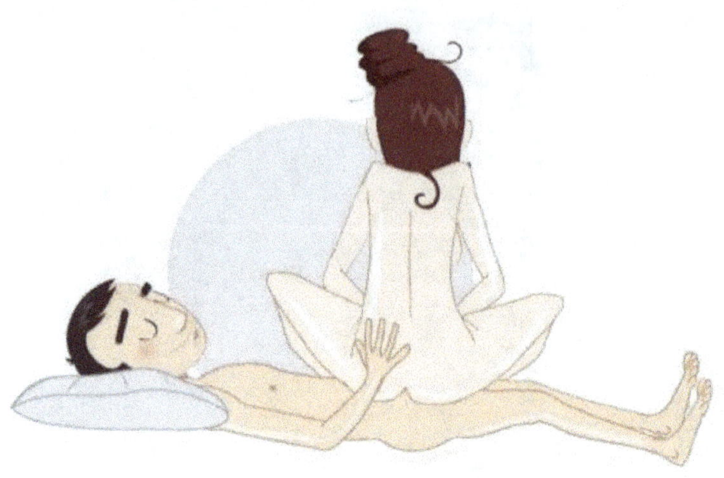

Difficulty level: Easy

Special features: Woman in control, man reclining

While the man lies flat on his back, the woman simply sits on top of him with both legs to one side. The woman is in complete control. Ideal when the man is feeling tired/lazy.

Have a hand-held stimulator can also add another dimension, we like this G-spot vibrator that's available here at Amazon.

November 12
From Behind

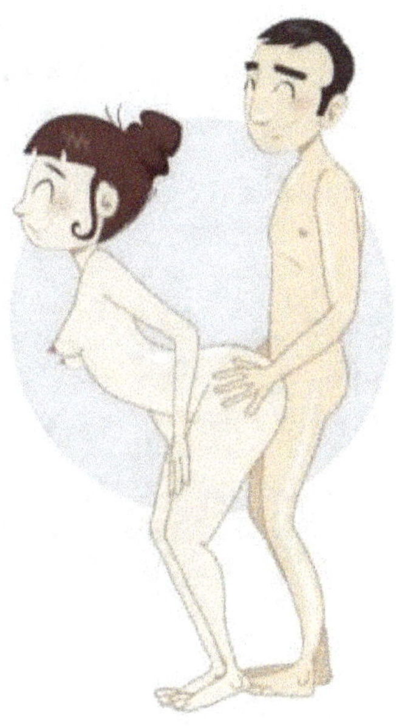

Difficulty level: Easy

Special features: Man in control

The man stands behind the woman and enters her. He's in control of the thrusts. She may find it easier to balance with a wall to lean against.

This sex position is easy for some, but doesn't work so well if you're not similar heights.

November 13

Balancing Act

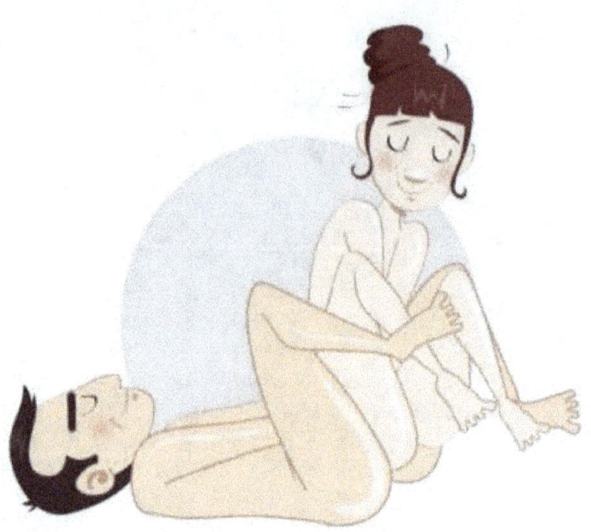

Difficulty level: Moderate

Special features: Woman in control

The man lies on his back with his legs apart while the woman sits down between his thighs. The woman must then curl her body up into a ball while the man supports her. Her hands are free to touch herself or touch his perineum.

This position requires a certain degree of strength from both parties.

November 14

Splitting Bamboo

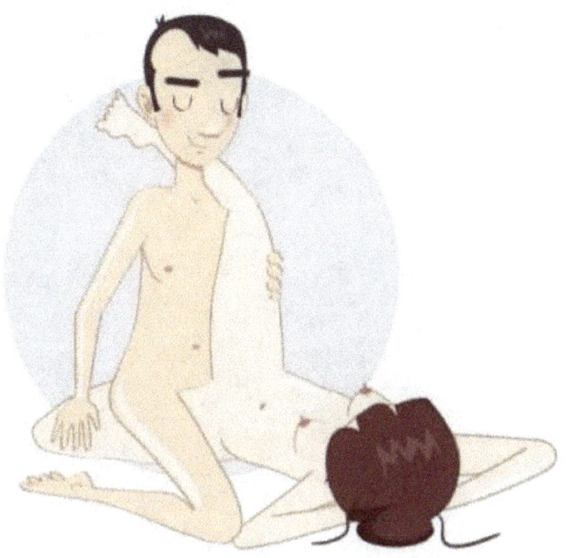

Difficulty level: Easy

Special features: Woman reclining, woman's hands free, good to try during pregnancy

The woman lays on her back with one leg stretched out and the other resting on her partner's shoulder. The man straddles her thigh, while holding on to her elevated leg to balance himself.

A relatively easy position which leaves both of the woman's hands free to fondle herself or her partner.

November 15

The Frog

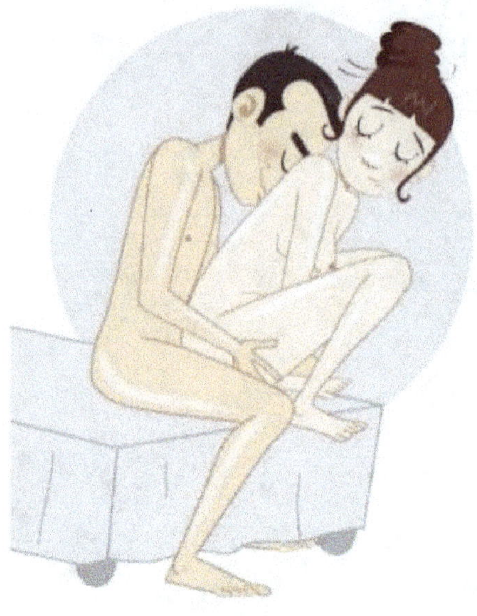

Special features: Woman in control, edge of bed

The man sits on the edge of the bed with his feet on the floor while the woman crouches (like a frog) on his lap. She can then move up and down to control the penetration, while pressing on his thighs for support.

An easy position for the man, but requires strength and balance from the woman.

November 16
The Column

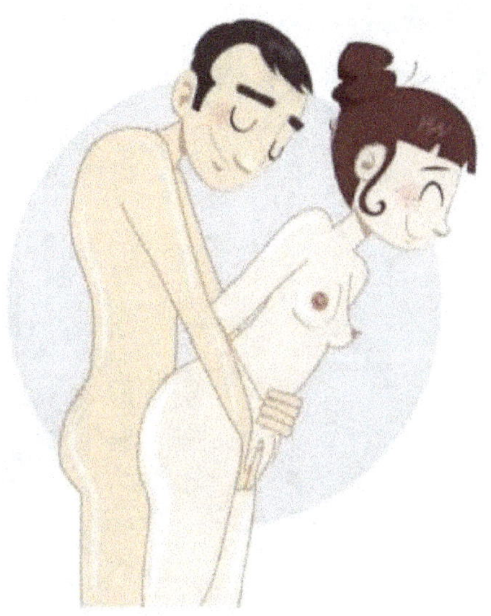

Difficulty level: Easy

Special features: Standing

The woman stands in front of the man with her back to him and their arms intertwined. The man can then penetrate the woman from behind. The woman may find it easier to lean on a table.

November 17

The Candle

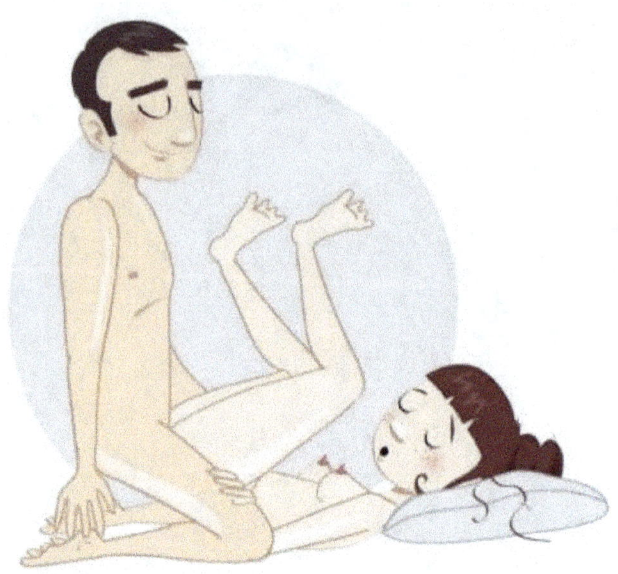

Difficulty level: Moderate

Special features: Woman reclining, deep penetration, man's hands free

The woman lies on her back with one cushion under her head and another under her bottom. She then pulls her knees up to her chest and lifts her legs in the air. The man kneels down with his legs either side of her and enters her hips.

Great for deep penetration and his hands are also free, which is an added bonus.

November 18

The Basket

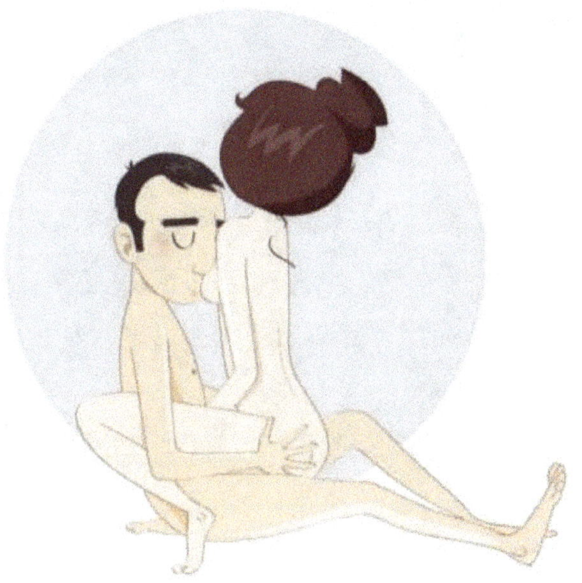

Difficulty level: Easy

Special features: Woman on top

The man sits with one leg stretched out and the other leg bent at the knee to help him balance. The woman sits on his lap. While she can control most of the movement, he also has some control with his hands on her hips. He is also in the ideal position to kiss and suck her nipples while having sex.

November 19

The Galley

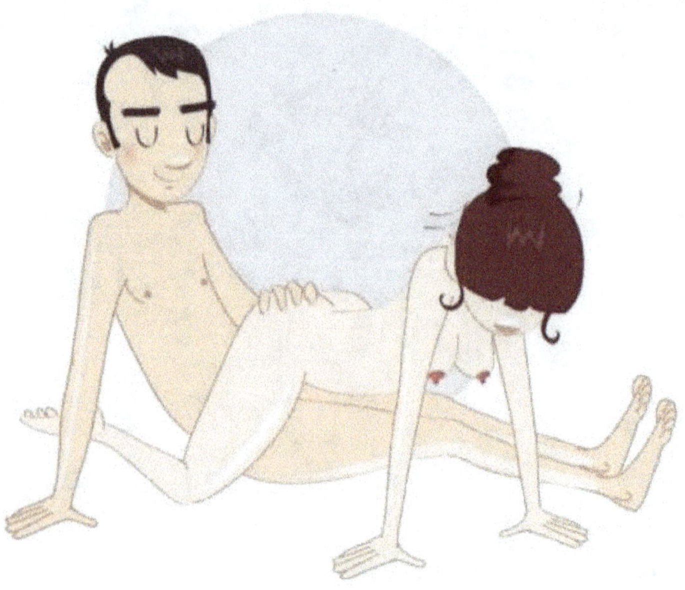

Difficulty level: Easy

Special features: Woman in control

The man sits with his weight on one arm (the other is free to fondle) and his legs stretched out. The woman sits on top of him and leans forward. She can then support herself with her arms, while being in full control of the movement and penetration.

A good position for a tired man and an energetic woman.

November 20
The Clip

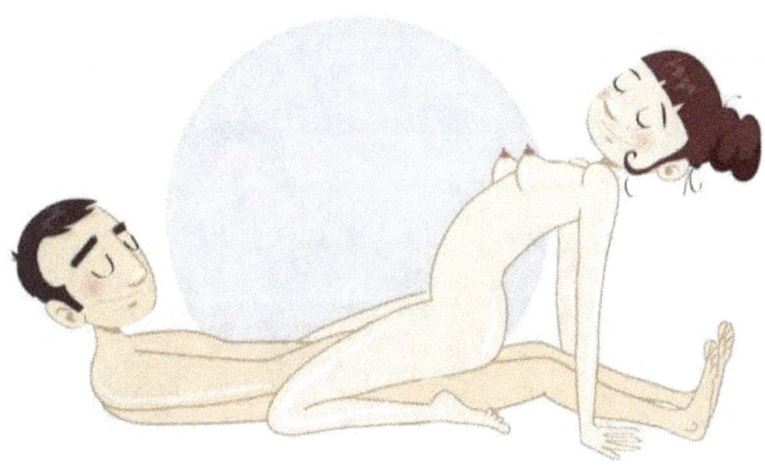

Difficulty level: Easy

Special features: Woman in control, man reclining

The man lies on his back and closes his legs while the woman sits astride him and leans back supporting herself on her arms. She can then grind on to him while he lays back and enjoys himself.

November 21

The Whisper

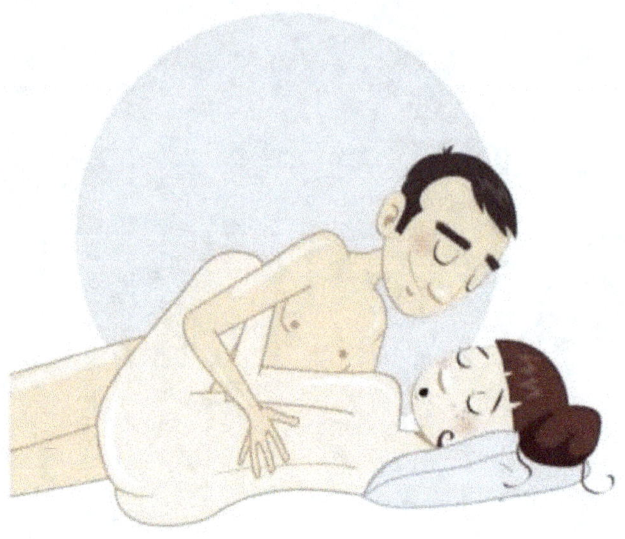

Difficulty level: Easy

Special features: Man in control, reclining

The man lies on his side while the woman wraps her legs around his waist and crosses her ankles. He is then free to thrust in and out.

November 22

The Challenge

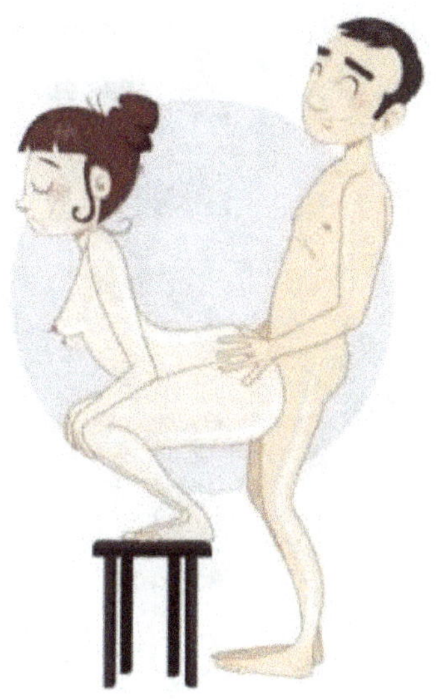

Difficulty level: Advanced

Special features: Man in control

This position requires a sturdy chair/stool and a great deal of balance. The woman crouches on the stool while the man enters her from behind. He will need to hold firmly onto her waist to stop her toppling over.

November 23

The Kneel

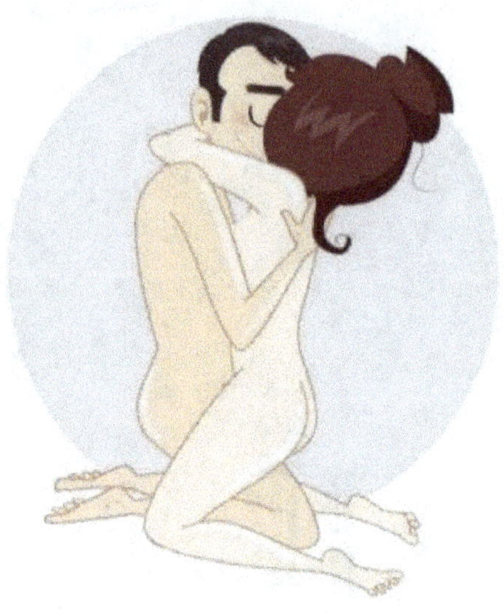

Difficulty level: Easy

Special features: Romantic

In this sex position the woman and the man both kneel. The woman puts her legs either side of the man's so he can penetrate her. They can both wrap their arms around each other.

A relatively easy, and yet extremely passionate position.

November 24
The Standing Wheelbarrow

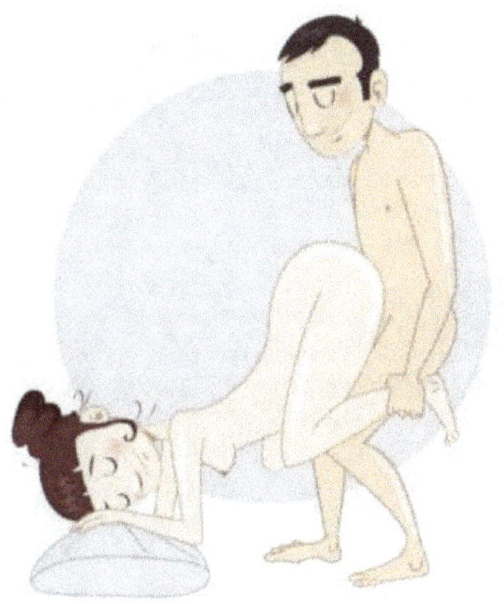

Difficulty level: Advanced

Special features: Requires upper body strength, deep penetration

Another challenging position, which requires a great deal of skill and balance.

The woman starts on all fours, she can rest her elbows on a pillow if that's more comfortable. The man kneels behind the woman and enters her. Once he has penetrated the woman he can slowly lift her off the ground by holding onto her ankles.

November 25

The Kneeling Wheelbarrow

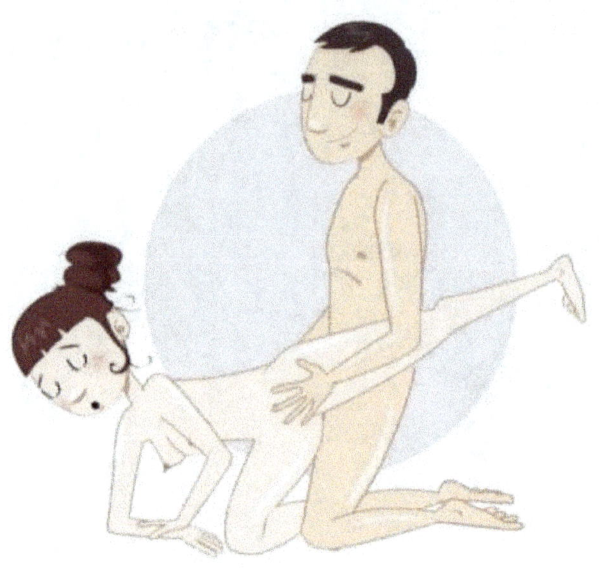

Difficulty level: Moderate

Special features: Energetic

The Kneeling Wheelbarrow is a slightly easier variation of the standing wheelbarrow. The woman kneels on one leg with her other leg stretched out. She then leans on the opposite elbow to the leg she is kneeling on while her partner kneels behind her. The man can hold the woman's hips to help her balance while he enters her.

Be warned, it's a very tiring position for the woman so make sure you don't overdo it!

November 26

The Spider

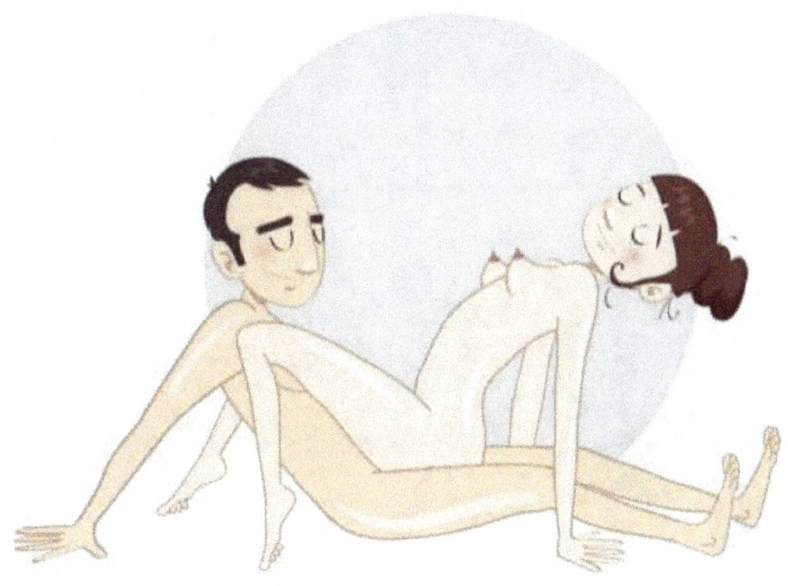

Difficulty level: Easy

Special features: Woman in control

The man sits with his legs stretched out and leans back on his hands. The woman sits astride him facing the man. She also leans back on her hands and can use them to help her rock back and forth.

November 27

The Fold

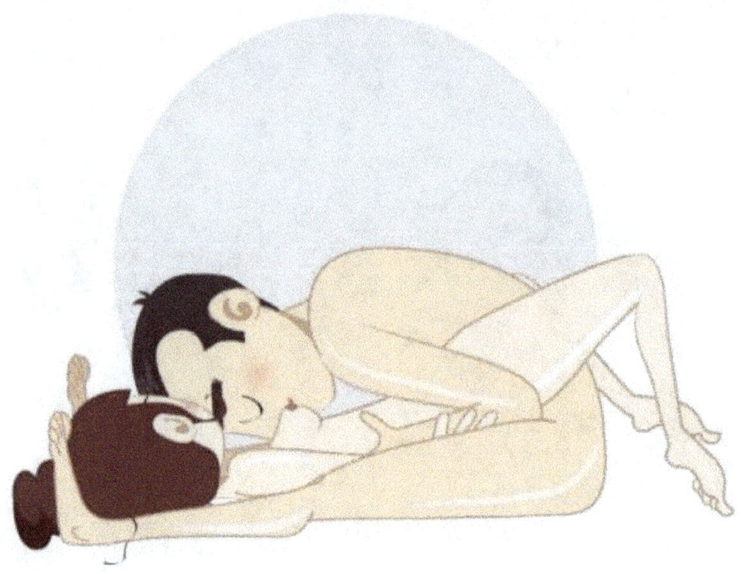

Difficulty level: Easy

Special features: Relaxed

The woman lies on her back with a cushion under her bottom to raise her hips. The man sits with his legs stretched out either side of her, while she lets her legs hang behind his back.

An ideal sex position if you're both lacking in energy.

November 28

The Sphinx

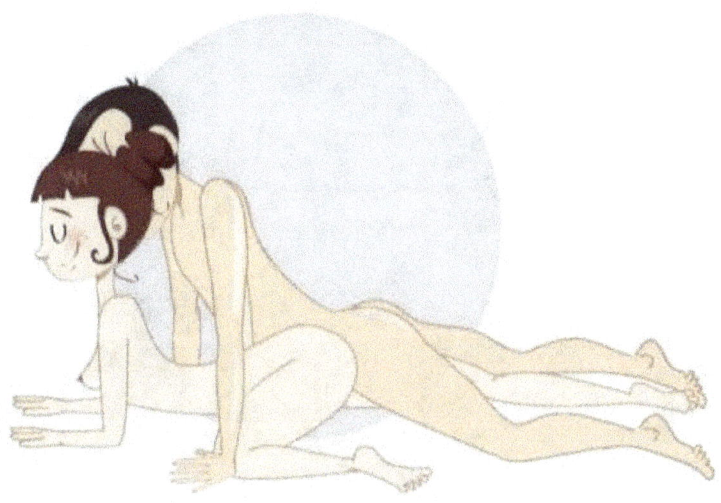

Difficulty level: Moderate

Special features: Energetic for the man

The woman lies on her front with her weight on her elbows. She stretches one leg out and bends the other to the side. The man lays on top and can penetrate from behind while leaning on his hands for support.

A tiring position for the man, but worth it for the woman as the pressure of his body on her pelvis helps her to climax.

November 29

The Deckchair

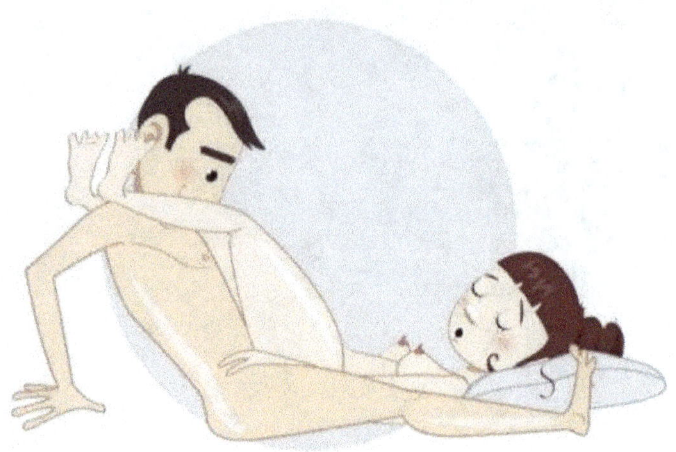

Difficulty level: Easy

Special features: Woman reclining, deep penetration

The man sits with his legs stretched out and leans back on his hands. The woman lays on her back facing him and with a pillow under her bottom she can comfortably rest her feet on his shoulders.

This is a good sex position for deep penetration.

November 30

The Waterfall

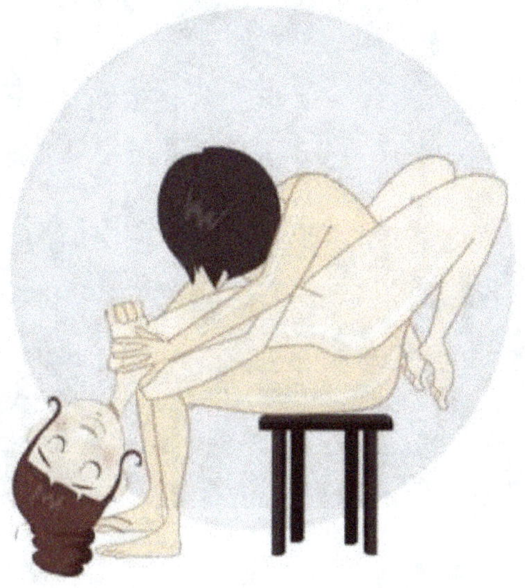

Difficulty level: Advanced

Special features: Chair position, man in control

The man sits on a chair or a stool while the women sits on his lap. Once he is penetrating her she leans right back (if necessary she can rest her head on a cushion on the floor) while he takes full control of all the movement.

Not for the faint-hearted! This sex position requires a lot of strength and flexibility.

December

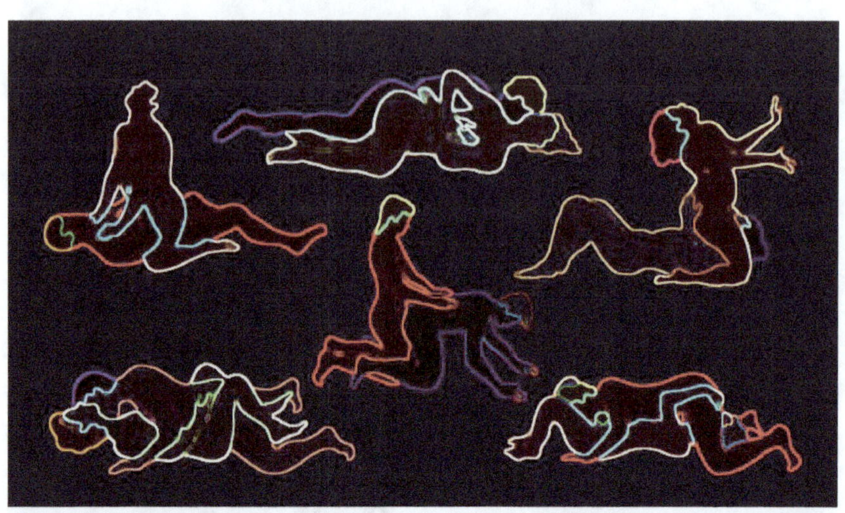

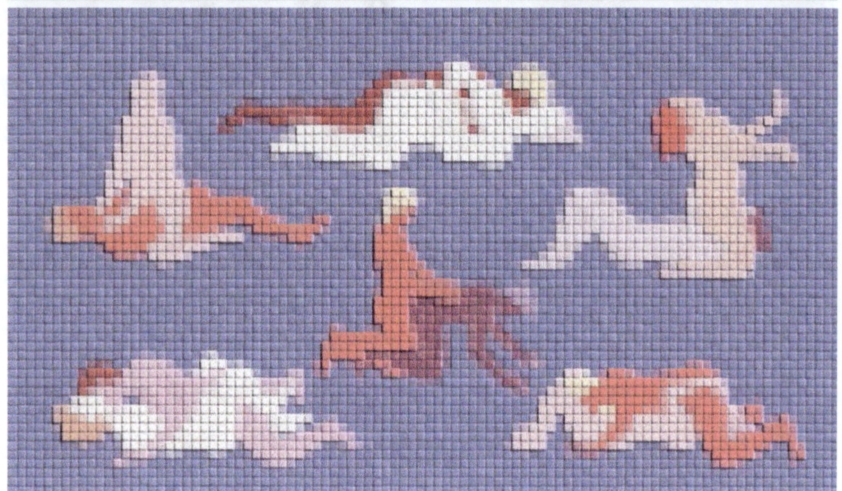

Most Common Kinks

Here is a list of some of the most common kinks. They're actually a lot more common then you might think.

If you'd like to consider exploring some of these, I go in-depth about each kink and fetish (and the difference between the two) in my book, *Sexy Games.*

<table>
<tr><td>BDSM</td><td>Financial domination</td></tr>
<tr><td>Sadism and masochism</td><td>Auralism</td></tr>
<tr><td>Ropes and Bondage</td><td>Age play</td></tr>
<tr><td>Hosiery</td><td>Orgasm control</td></tr>
<tr><td>Voyeurism</td><td>Impact play</td></tr>
<tr><td>Exhibitionism</td><td>Consensual Nonconsent</td></tr>
<tr><td>Roleplay</td><td>Gags</td></tr>
<tr><td>Dirty talk</td><td>Praise kink</td></tr>
<tr><td>Urophilia</td><td>Degradation kink</td></tr>
<tr><td>Nipple play</td><td>Blood play</td></tr>
<tr><td>Humiliation</td><td>Autoplushophilia (furries)</td></tr>
<tr><td>Cuckolding</td><td>Mummification</td></tr>
<tr><td>Female-led relationships</td><td></td></tr>
</table>

December 1
The Double Decker

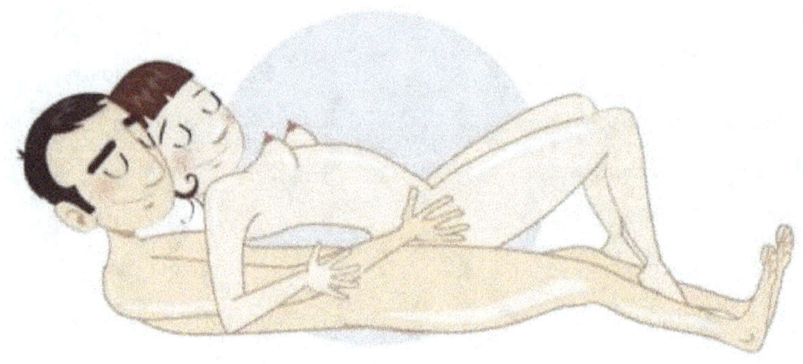

Difficulty level: Easy

Special features: Reclining

The double decker is the perfect sex position for when you are transitioning between other positions.

While the man lies on his back, the woman lies on top of him with her back to him. She supports herself on her elbows, either side of the man's waist and to help her balance she puts her feet on the man's knees.

December 2
The Dolphin

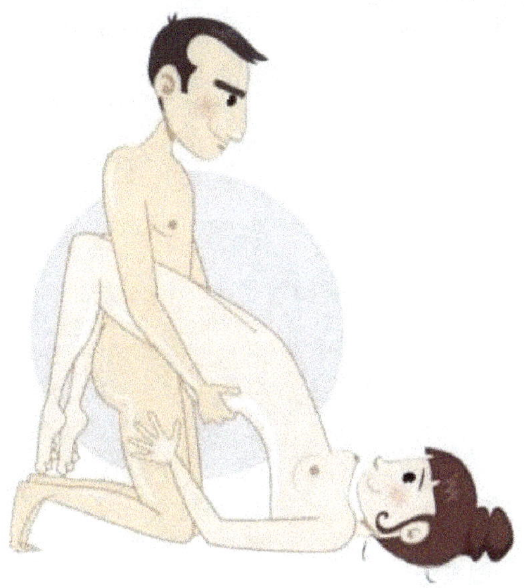

Difficulty level: Advanced

Special features: Upper body strength for the man

The woman lies down on her back and the man places himself between her legs. He then lifts her up by the waist so all of her weight is on her head and shoulders.

A moderately easy sex position, but it may be hard to maintain for a long time as the woman may get uncomfortable.

December 3

The Cherry Blossom

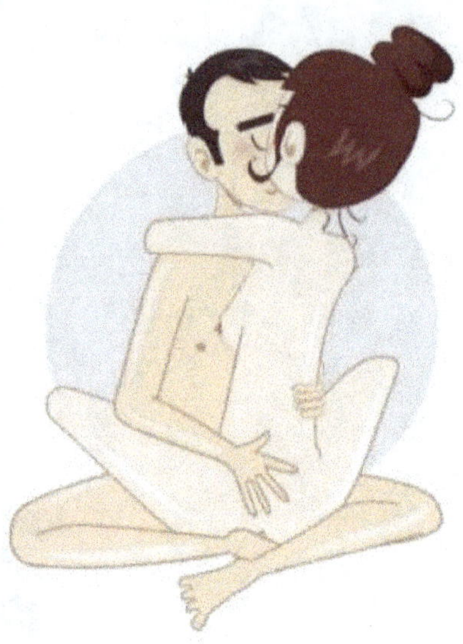

Difficulty level: Easy

Special features: Romantic

The man sits with his legs crossed while the woman sits on his lap with her legs wrapped around his waist.

An easy, intimate sex position if you are relatively flexible.

Face-to-face intimacy and either partner can take over when one of you gets tired.

December 4

The Amazon

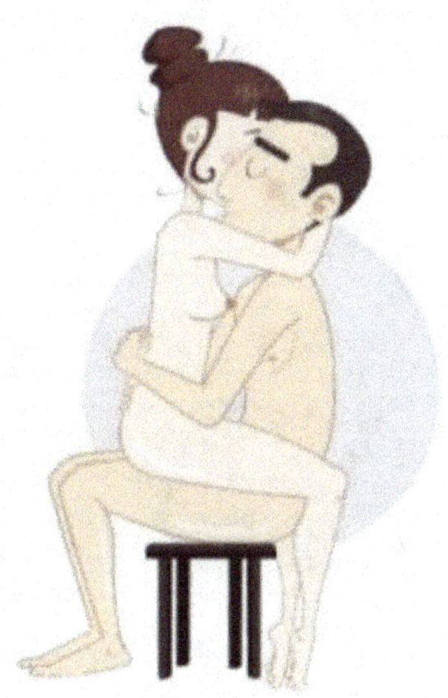

Difficulty level: Easy

Special features: Chair position, somewhat tiring for the woman

The man sits on a chair – ideally the chair won't be too high as the woman's feet need to touch the ground. The woman sits on his lap facing him and uses her feet to bounce up and down.

Enjoy giving your thighs a good work out with this sex position!

December 5
The Close-Up

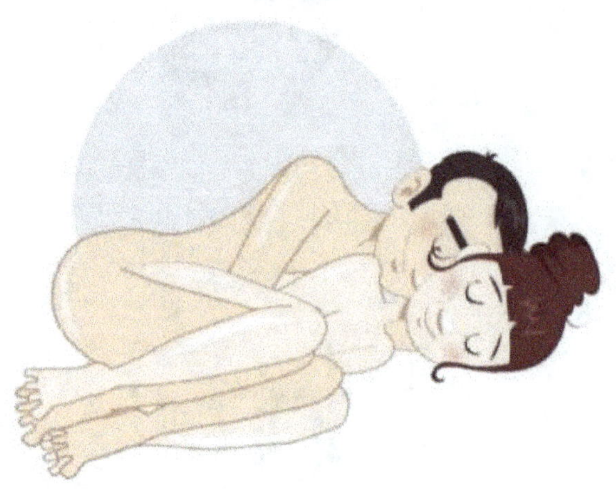

Difficulty level: Easy

Special features: Romantic, reclining

The man and woman both lie on their sides with their legs pulled up to their chests. The woman faces away from the man and pushes her hips down into his crotch.

A very easy, gentle sex position, which can be extremely intimate too.

December 6
The Star

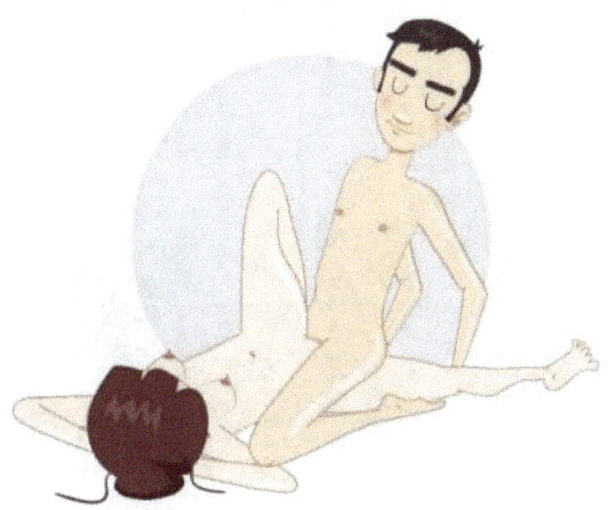

Difficulty level: Easy

Special features: Woman reclining

The woman lies on her back with one leg stretched out and the other bent up. The man slides in between her legs and pushes one of his legs underneath her to raise her hips. To help his balance the man leans back on his hands.

December 7

The Indian Handstand

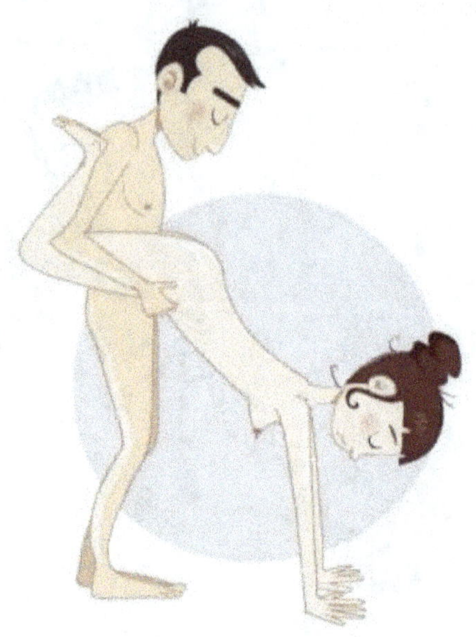

Difficulty level: Advanced

Special features: Upper body strength for the woman

This position is quite challenging; it requires a great deal of strength and balance from the woman.

The man stands while the woman does a headstand. The man enters the woman from behind and helps her to balance by holding onto her hips.

December 8
The Rocking Horse

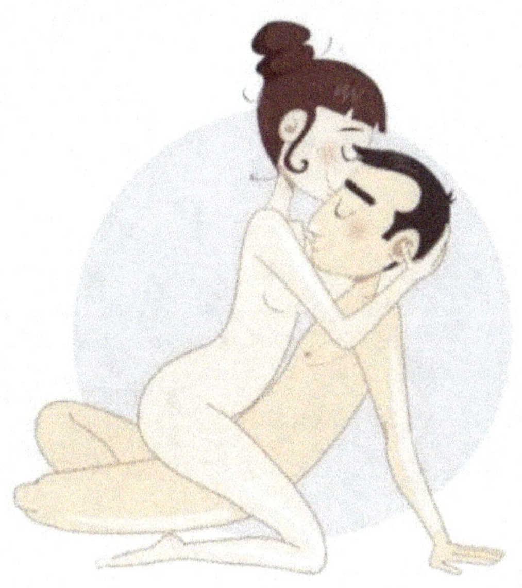

Difficulty level: Easy

Special features: Woman in control

The man sits with his legs crossed and leans back supporting himself with his arms. The woman sits astride him with her knees bent either side of his waist. The woman can then rock back and forth in a rocking horse motion.

December 9

The Super 8

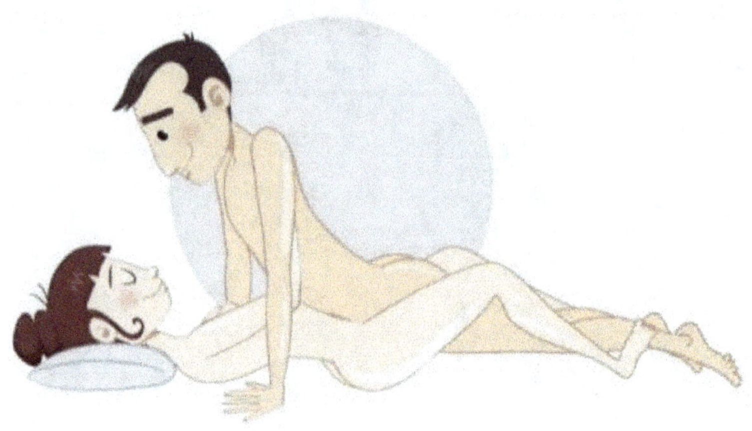

Difficulty level: Easy

Special features: Woman reclining

The woman lies flat on her back with a small cushion under her bottom to raise her hips. The man lies between her legs and supports himself on his arms. Both the man and the woman are free to move in rhythm with each other.

December 10

Ascent to Desire

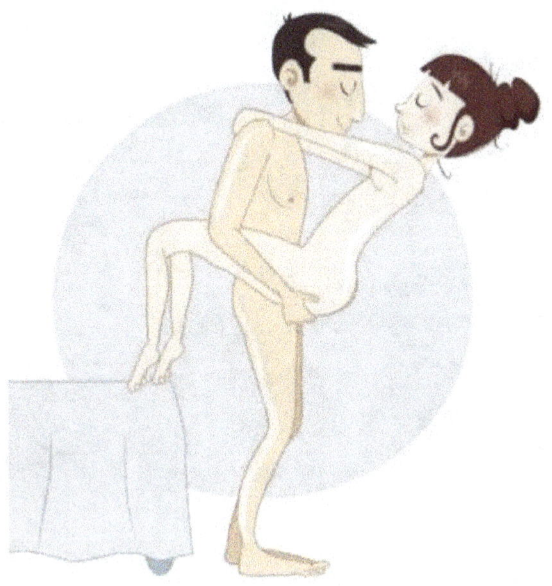

Difficulty level: Easy

Special features: Standing, requires upper body strength

The man stands with his knees ever so slightly bent and the woman stands facing him. He then lifts her off the ground and she wraps her legs around his waist and her arms around his neck while he penetrates her.

It maybe easier to start with the man sitting and once in position he can stand.

December 11

The Glowing Triangle

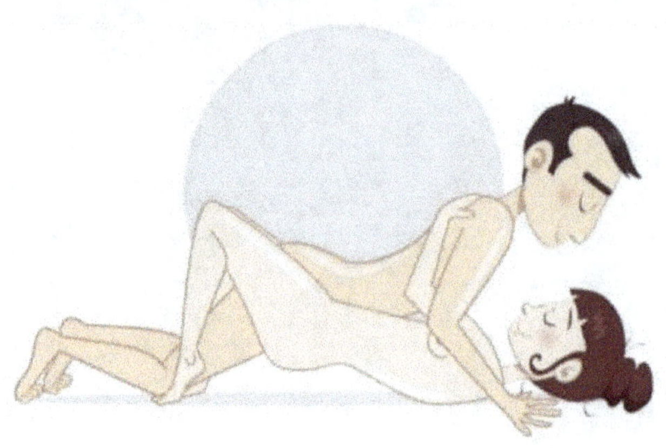

Difficulty level: Easy

Special features: Woman reclining, woman in control

The glowing triangle position is a simple, yet extremely effective, twist on the classic missionary position.

The woman lays on her back, while the man moves on top of her. But instead of laying on top of her, he gets onto all fours and she has to raise her pelvis so he can penetrate her. He then stays still and she does all the work.

December 12

The Nirvana

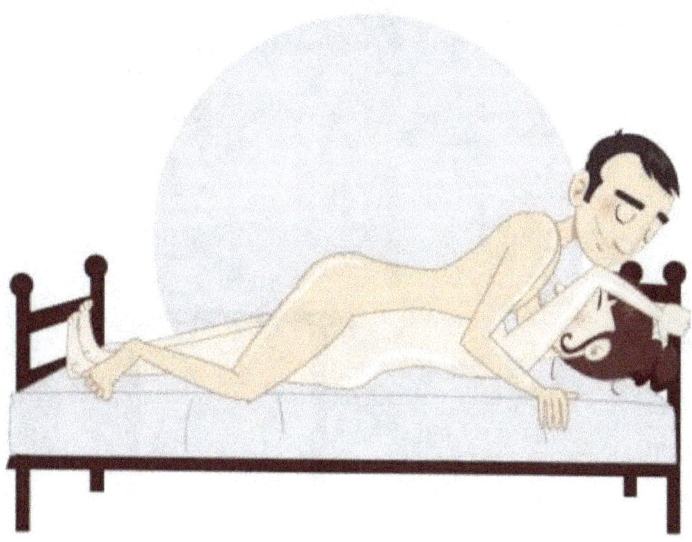

Difficulty level: Easy

Special features: Increased friction, reclining

In this kamasutra sex position the woman lies flat on her back with her legs closed and her arms stretched out holding the bedposts (if possible).

The man lays on top of her with his legs either side of hers. He slowly penetrates her while her legs remain shut.

December 13

The Padlock

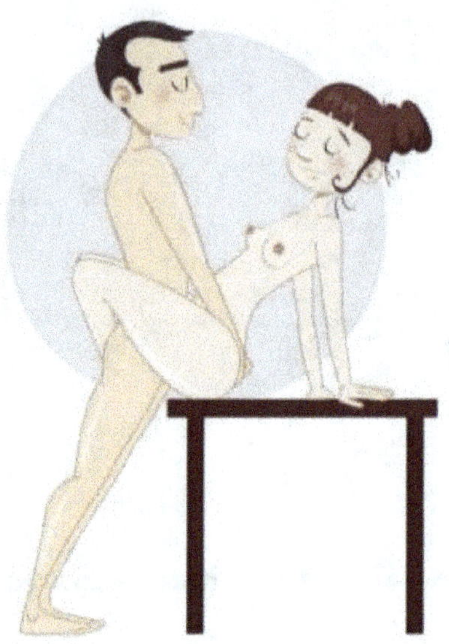

Difficulty level: Easy

Special features: Tabletop position

In this sutra sex position, the woman sits on the edge of a high piece of furniture, for example a table or a washing machine. She leans back and supports herself with her arms. The man stands in front of her. She can wrap her legs around his waist as he enters her.

December 14

The Rock 'n' Roller

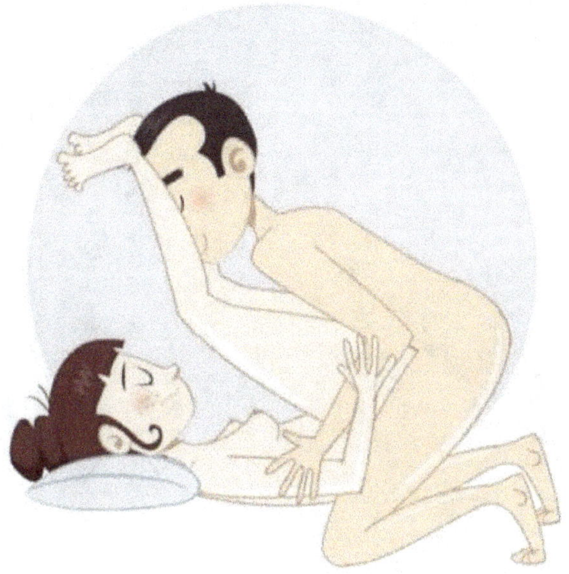

Difficulty level: Moderate

Special features: Requires flexibility for the woman

As the couple are making love, the woman lies on her back with a pillow behind her head. She then lifts her legs in the air and rocks back - like she's going to do a backwards roll. The man kneels behind her and keeps her hips elevated on his thighs while entering her.

December 15

The Backward Slide

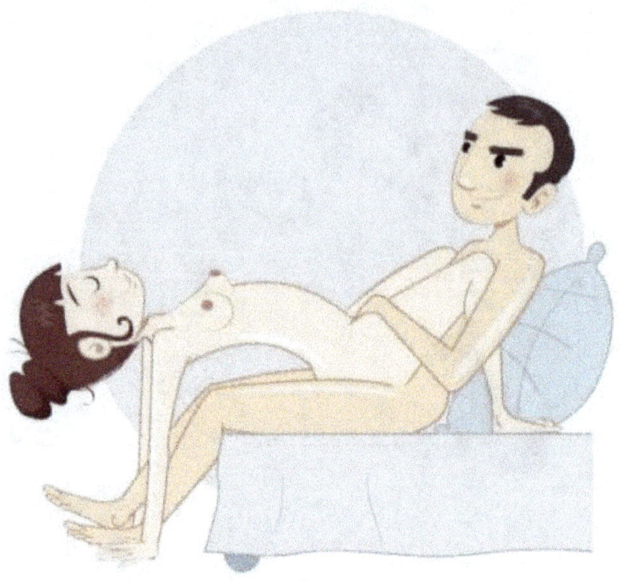

Difficulty level: Moderate

Special features: Edge of bed, requires flexbility from the woman

The man sits on the edge of the bed with his legs hanging down and a cushion behind his back for support. The woman sits astride him and bends her legs so her knees are level with his shoulders. She then carefully leans back and rests her hands on the floor, either side of his feet, to balance.

December 16
The Crossed Keys

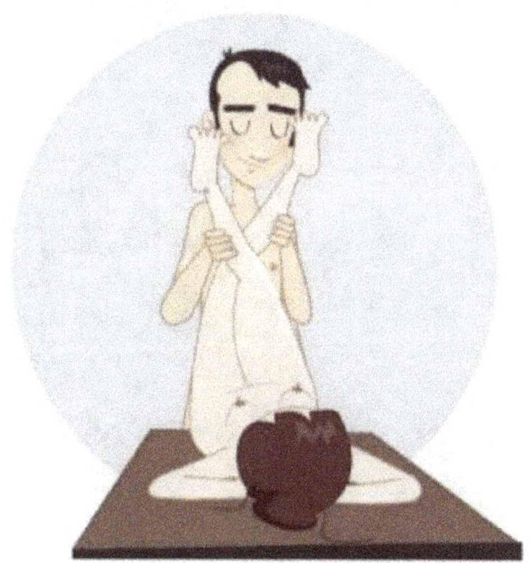

Difficulty level: Easy

Special features: Edge of bed, man standing

One of the easier kamasutra sexual positions, the woman lies on her back with her legs in the air. Her bottom needs to be at the edge of the bed and her legs must be crossed. The man stands facing her and holds onto her legs while he penetrates her.

An easy sex position.

December 17

The Ape

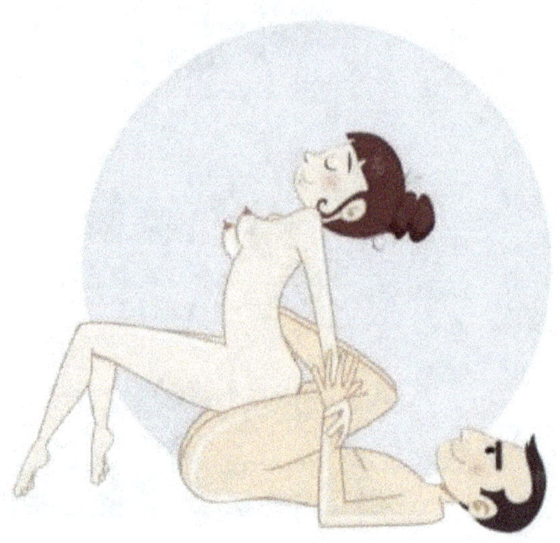

Difficulty level: Advanced

Special features: Woman in control, deep penetration

If you fancy something a little bit different give this position a try.

The man lies on his back and brings his knees up to his chest. The woman sits down on her partner facing away from him while he rests his feet on her back and penetrates her. The woman uses her feet to balance and control the motion.

Great for deep penetration.

December 18
The Reclining Lotus

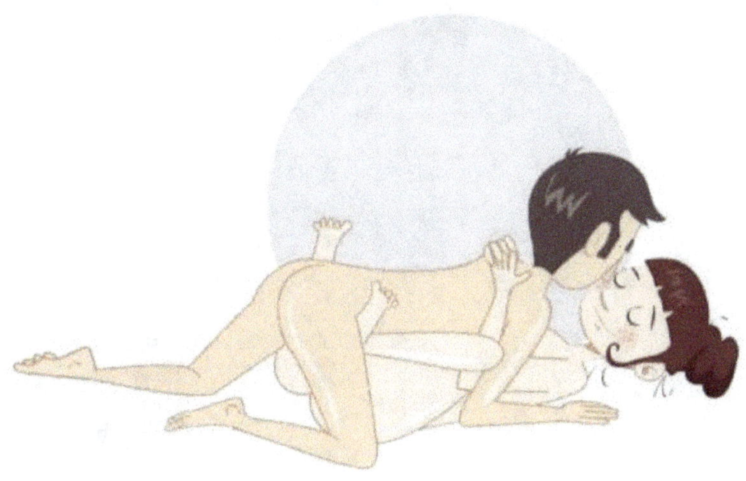

Difficulty level: Moderate

Special features: Requires flexibility from the woman

This position requires a great deal of flexibility from the woman, who lays on her back with her legs crossed.

The man lays on top and uses his arms to balance as he penetrates her.

December 19
Wide Opened

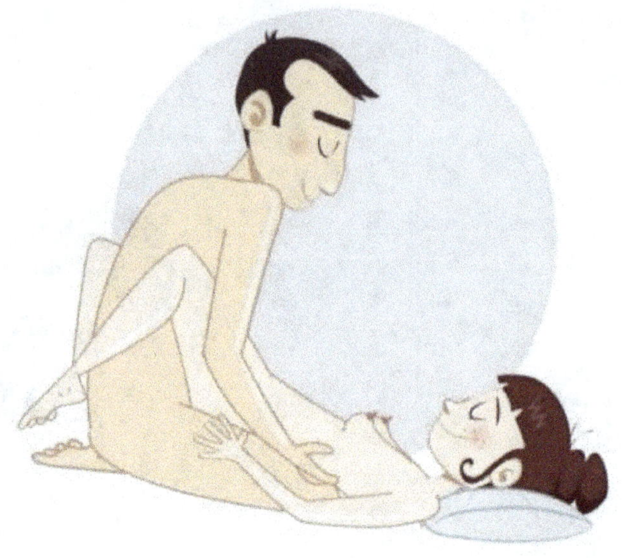

Difficulty level: Easy

Special features: Woman reclining, good during pregnancy

The woman lays on her back with a pillow under her head. The man kneels between

December 20

Indrani

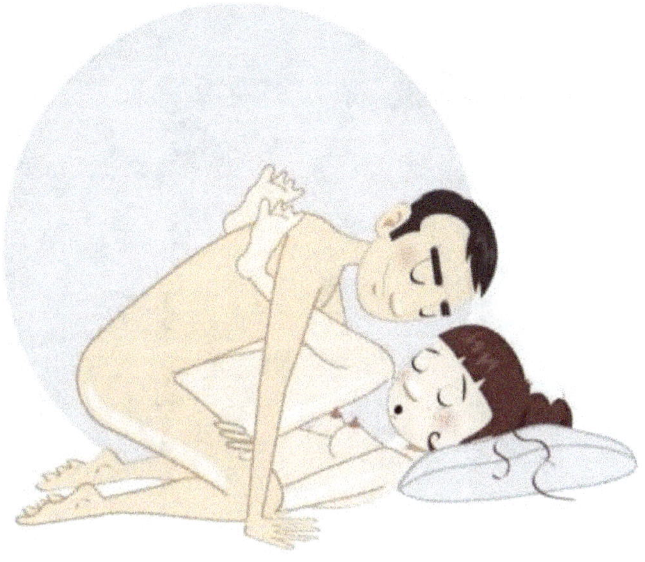

Difficulty level: Moderate

Special features: Woman in control, hands free for women

The woman lies on her back with a pillow under her head. She pulls her knees up to her chest while the man slides between her legs. The woman has her hands free to pull the man towards her and control penetration.

December 21

Suspended Congress

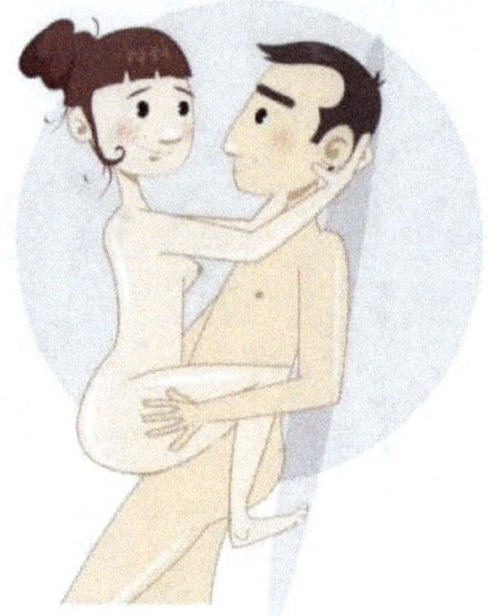

Difficulty level: Advanced

Special features: Standing, requires strength

The man leans against a wall while lifting the woman off the floor and supporting her with his hands under her bottom. The woman can grip the man's waist with her thighs.

Requires strength from both parties, but well worth the effort.

December 22

The Suspended Scissors

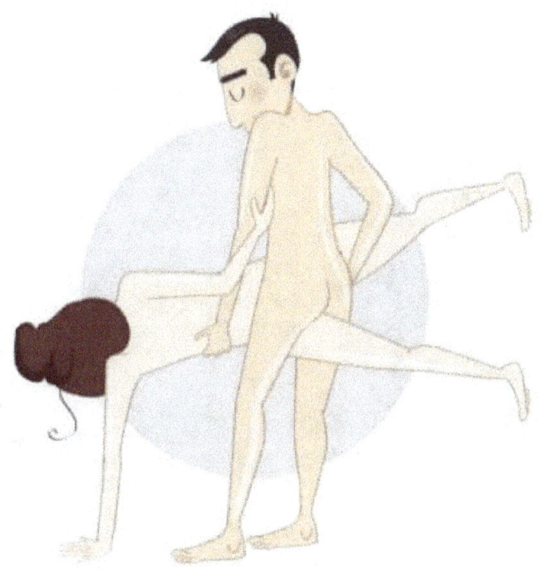

Difficulty level: Advanced

Special features: Requires upper body strength

Warning: this position requires lots of strength and plenty of balance.

The woman lies right on the edge of the bed with just her feet touching the mattress for support. She then balances on the floor with her left arm. The man stands astride her left leg and raises her right leg with his hands.

A bit tricky, but not so difficult once you're in position.

This vibrator by Tracy's Dog caused a sensation last year, read more about it here! You can also buy it at Amazon.

December 23

The Propeller

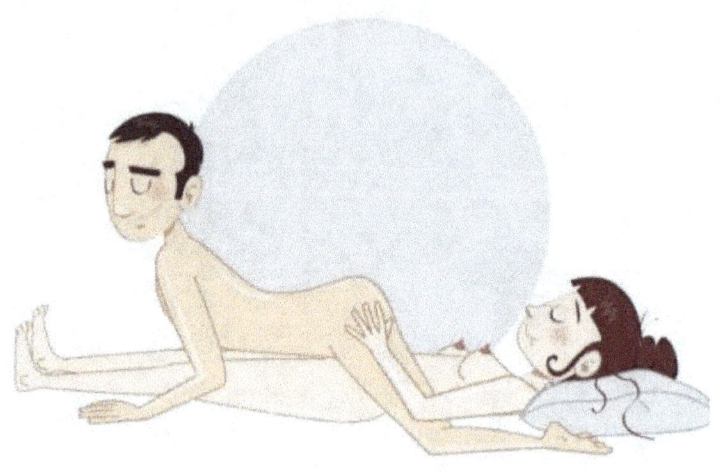

Difficulty level: Advanced

Special features: Good with man with a large penis

This one definitely won't work for everyone. In fact it will only work if the man is extremely well endowed.

The woman lies flat on her back with her legs closed. The man lies on top of her facing the opposite direction. Once inside her he can slowly move his hips in a circular motion.

December 24
The Prone Tiger

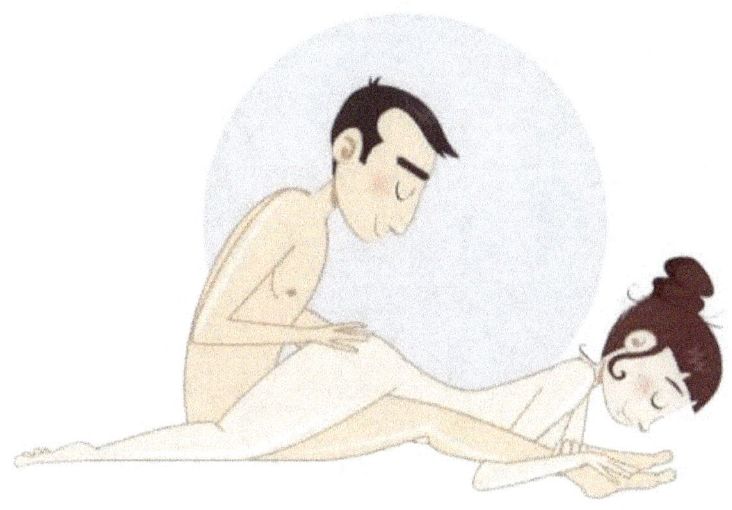

Difficulty level: Moderate

Special features: Man seated

The man sits on the bed with his legs stretched out in front of him. The woman lays on her front, parts her legs and slowly backs into him, lowering herself onto his penis. The woman's legs should be stretched out behind the man.

December 25

The Crisscross

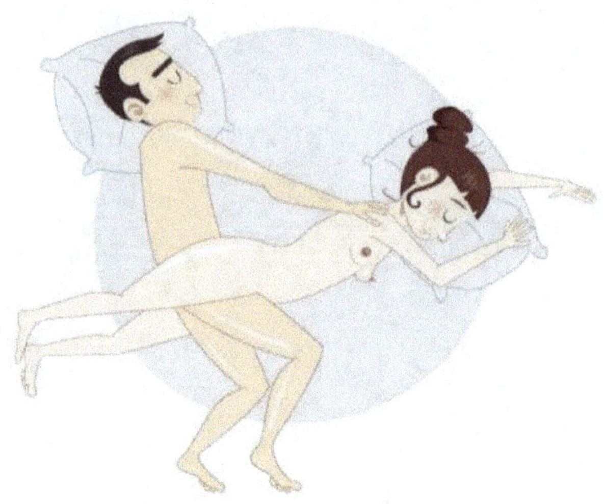

Difficulty level: Advanced

Special features: Woman in control

The woman lays on her side facing away from the man with her legs slightly parted. The man also lays on his side, but at a right angle to the woman, and slides in between her legs to enter her.

December 26

The Erotic V

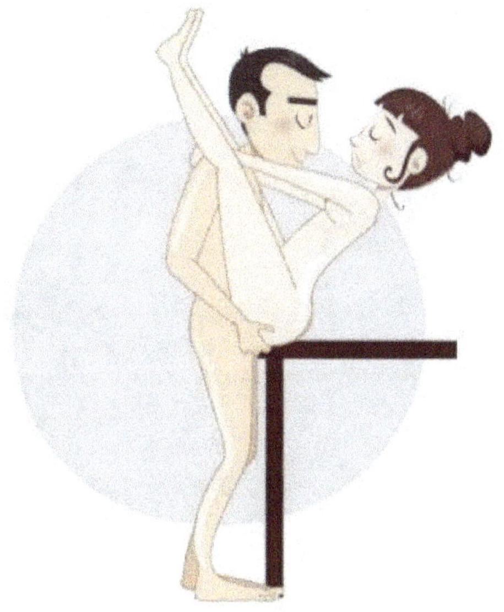

Difficulty level: Advanced

Special features: Tabletop position, requires flexibility for the woman

The woman sits on the edge of a table and the man stands in front of her. The woman needs to lift her legs right up and rest the back of her knees on the man's shoulders. She can also wrap her arms around his neck for support, while he can grip her bottom to help control the motion.

December 27
The Catherine Wheel

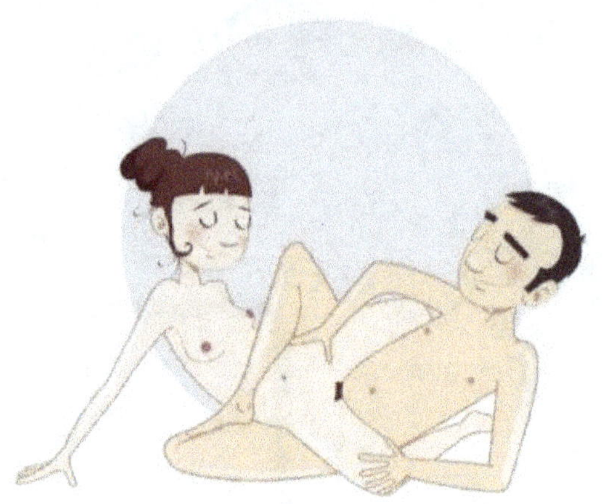

Difficulty level: Advanced

Special features: Requires flexibility

This one's a bit bendy! The man and woman sit down facing each other. She wraps her legs around his waist while he enters her. He then wraps one of his legs over her waist. To maintain balance the woman can lean on her arms, while the man rests on his elbows.

Quite a tricky sex position to master.

December 28
The Triumph Arch

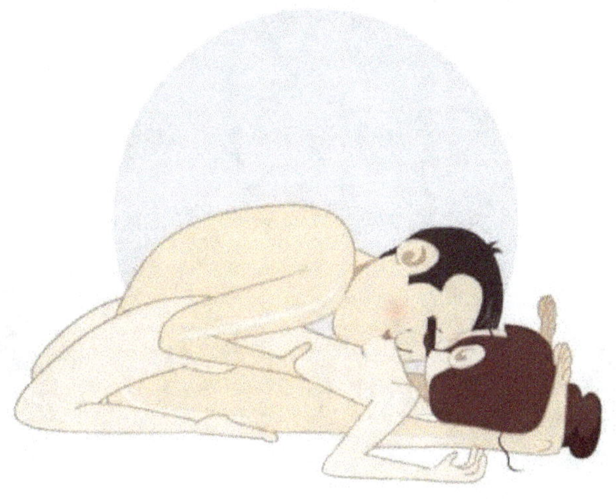

Difficulty level: Advanced

Special features: Requires flexibility from the woman

This position requires an extremely supple woman as she needs to lie flat on her back with her legs bent underneath her. The man then slides in between her legs with his legs stretched out so they are either side of her head.

December 29
The X-Rated

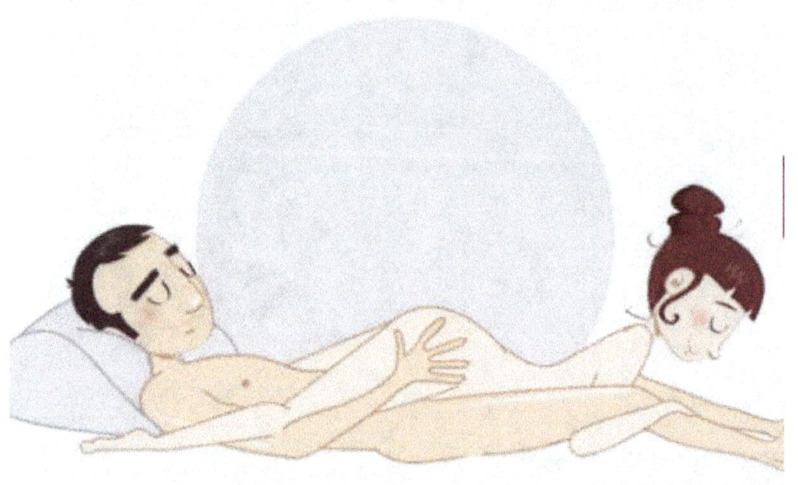

Difficulty level: Moderate

Special features: Reclining for both, woman in control

The man lies flat on his back with a pillow under his head. The woman lies on top of him facing away from him with her legs either side of his waist and her arms wrapped around his legs. She is in the perfect position to slide up and down, while he has an x-rated view.

December 30

The Shoulder Stand

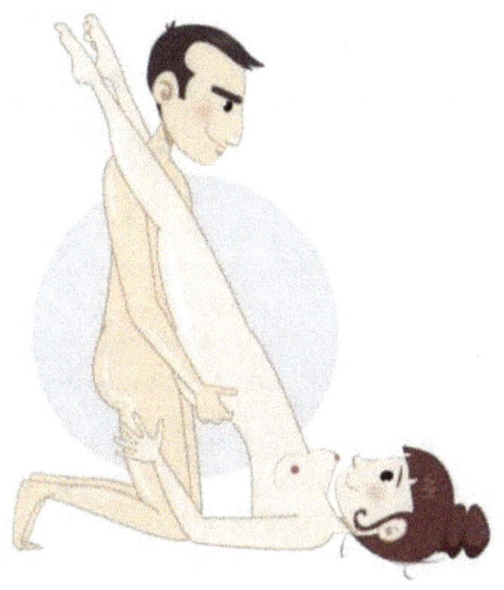

Difficulty level: Advanced

Special features: Requires strength and flexibility

The woman lays on her back and lifts her legs and entire torso in the air, with help from the man. The man kneels behind her and enters her while she rests her legs on his shoulders.

This sex position is best if you go slow.

December 31

The Rowing Boat

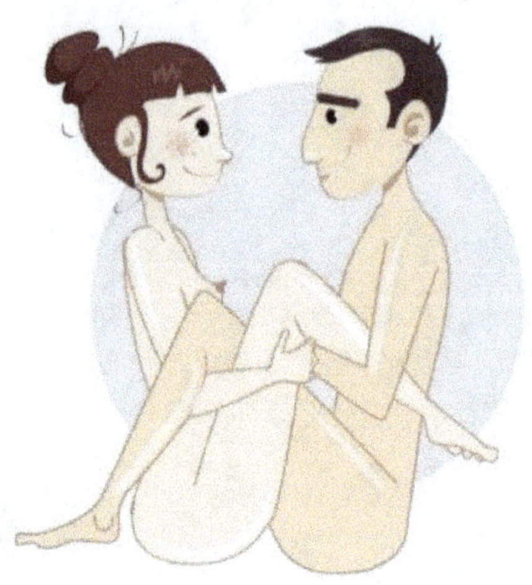

Difficulty level: Moderate

Special features: Requires flexibility, seated

The best way to start this position is with the man laying back and the woman sitting astride him. Once he is penetrating her the man can slowly sit up, so they are facing each other with their legs intertwined. For added comfort they can both slip their arms under each other's knees.

Bonus Sex Position

I snuck in these extra sex positions just because I felt bad about using some of the same positions twice in the calendar. It was not easy getting people to let me take pictures of them having sex, so I had to use all the pictures (Jan – June)!

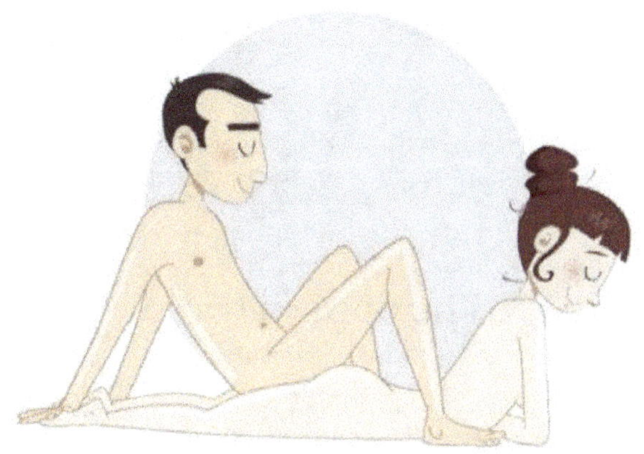

The Landslide

Difficulty level: Advanced

Special features: Good with men with a large penis

Because of the angles, this position is best suited to a well endowed man.

The woman lies on her stomach, with her legs stretched out and raises her torso by resting on her elbows. The man sits between her legs, facing the back of her head, with his legs parted either side of her waist. He tilts his body at a slight angle to enter her and while doing so supports himself with his hands propped up behind him.

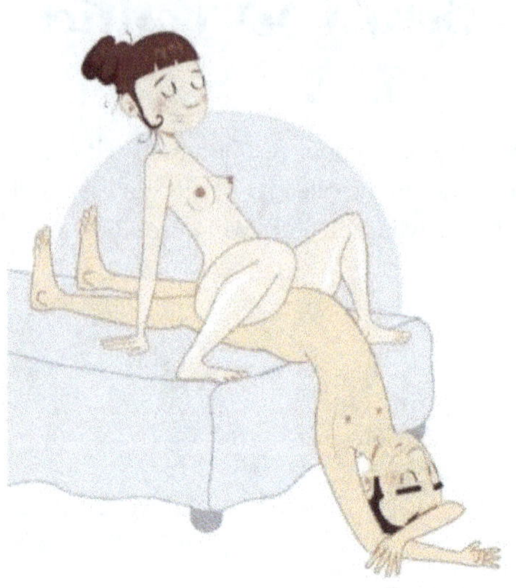

The Supernova

Difficulty level: Advanced

Special features: Requires flexibility and strength

This sex position is a slight variation of the classic woman-on-top, but this time the man lays with the top half of his body handing off the edge of the bed, while the woman sits astride him and leans back onto her arms for support.

Careful not to topple over the edge of the bed.

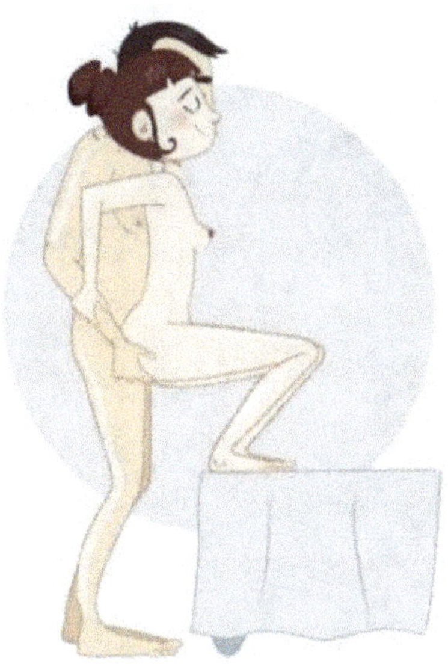

The Squat Balance

Difficulty level: Advanced

Special features: Beside position

The woman stands on the bed with the man standing behind her. He places his hands on her bottom and she slowly lowers herself onto him. He can then penetrate her while she uses his arms to balance.

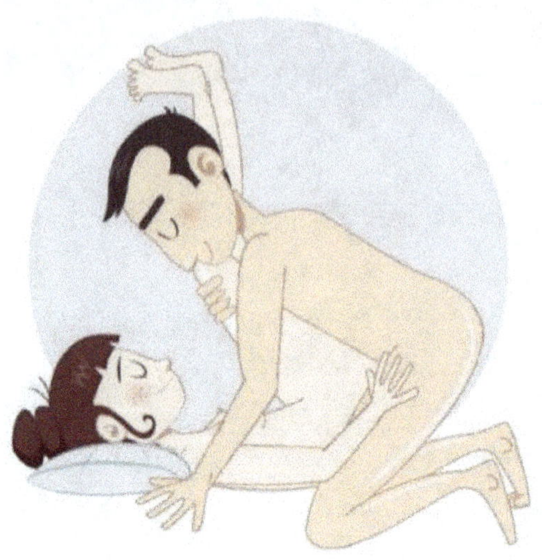

The Shoulder Holder

86/103

The Shoulder Holder

Difficulty level: Moderate

Special features: Deep penetration

The woman lies on her back with a pillow under her head and her legs straight up in the air. The man kneels to penetrate her, while gripping her legs and resting them against one of his shoulders. He can use his other hand for support.

Ideal for deep penetration.

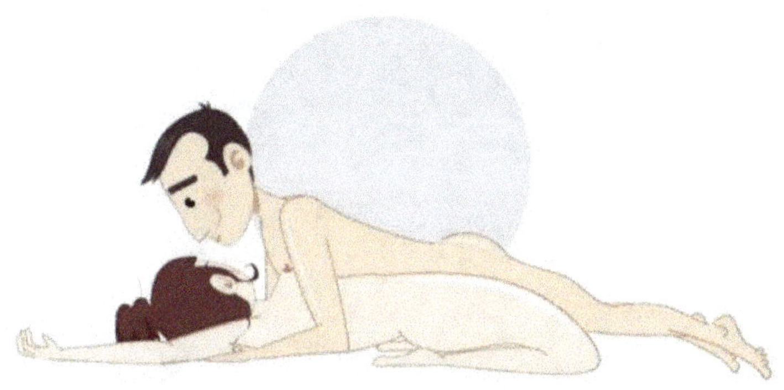

The Seduction

Difficulty level: Advanced

Special features: Requires flexibility from the woman

The woman lies on her back with her legs bent underneath her body – only attempt this if you are quite flexible and don't have knee trouble. The man then lays on top of the woman to penetrate her.

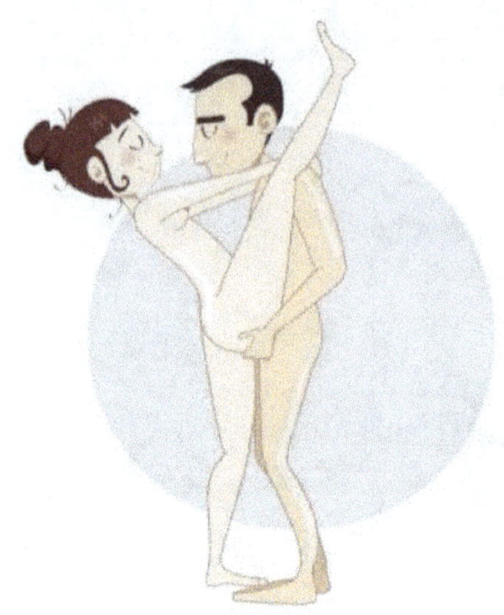

The Lustful Leg

Difficulty level: Advanced

Special features: Standing, requires flexibility and strength

Another position which requires a great deal of flexibility.

The man and the woman both stand facing each other. The woman starts by placing her leg on the bed so the man can enter her. Once inside he can slowly help her to raise her leg onto his shoulder.

Careful not to lose your balance and topple over!

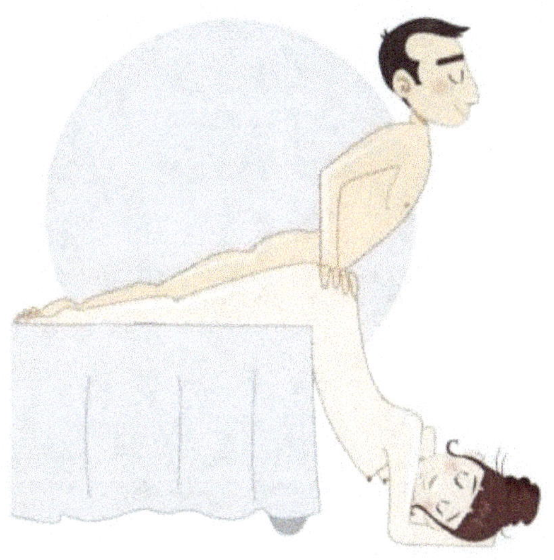

The Y Curve

Difficulty level: Moderate

Special features: Requires strength and balance from the man

This is quite a tricky position.

The woman lays face down on the bed and lets the top half of her body hang off the edge. She may need a pillow to rest her head on. The man lays between her legs to penetrate her and pushes his body up so he isn't laying on her back.

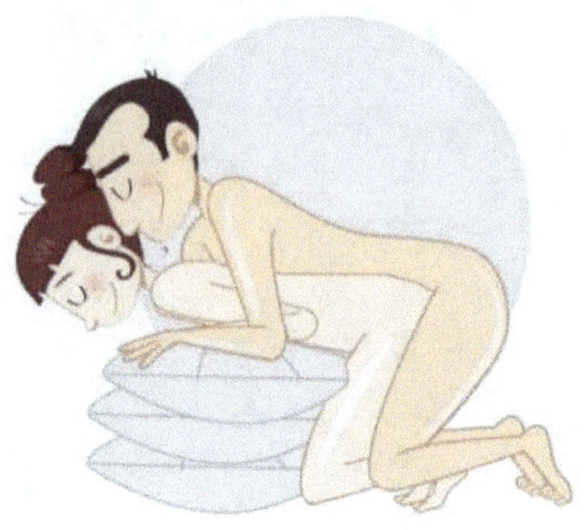

The Magic Mountain

Difficulty level: Easy

Special features: Romantic, uses pillows/cushions, deep penetration

First you need to stack a pile of firm pillows to form your 'mountain'. Then the woman kneels down and bends over the pillows, so her chest is flat on the cushions. The man kneels behind her and with his legs either side of her, penetrates her deeply.

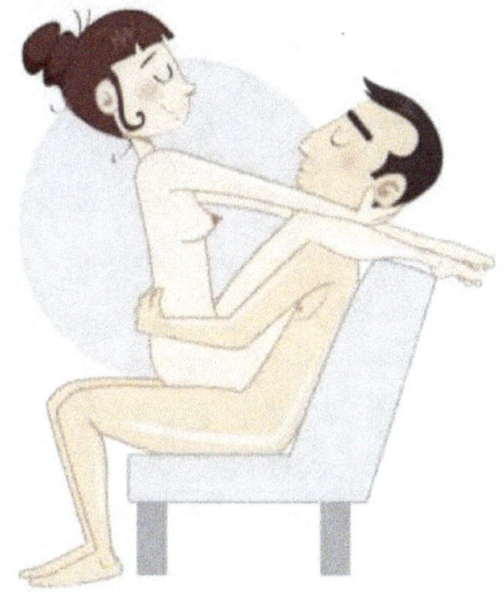

The Lap Top

Difficulty level: Advanced

Special features: Chair position, requires flexibility from the woman

A twist on the classic chair position: The man sits on a chair with a pillow under his knees to elevate them. The woman sits on his lap and raises her legs so they are wrapped around his neck. The woman can then rock back and forth on his penis while he supports her back with his hands.

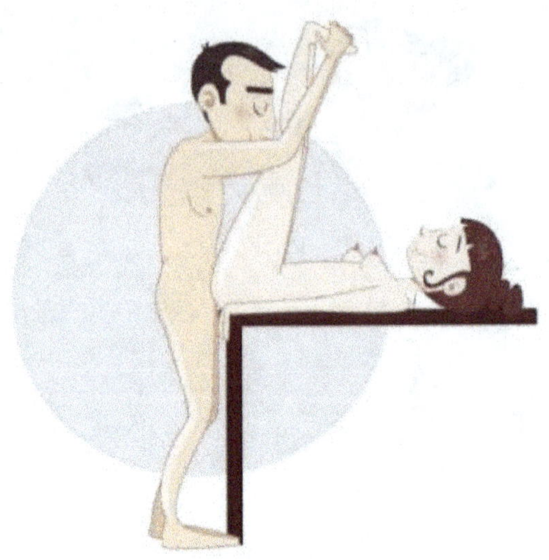

The Mermaid

The Mermaid

Difficulty level: Moderate

Special features: Tabletop position

The woman lies on a table with her bottom right at the edge. She then lifts both legs in the air (she can place a pillow under her bottom if it's more comfortable) while the man stands and penetrates her. For extra stability he can steady himself by holding her feet.

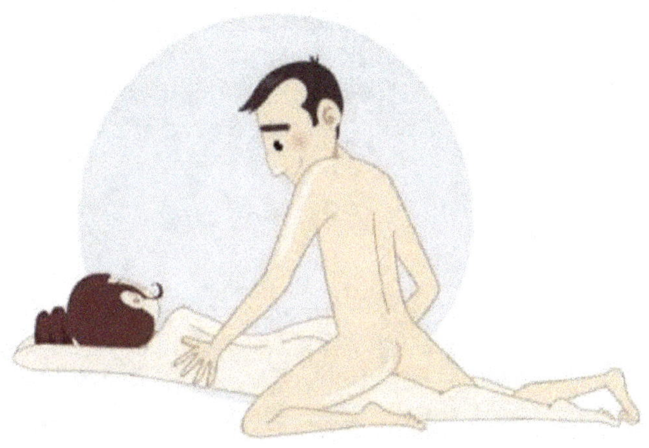

The Sidekick

Difficulty level: Easy

Special features: Woman reclining

The woman lies on her side with her back to the man. He kneels behind her, facing towards her head and straddles her leg while entering her. She then stretches out her top leg to allow him more room to maneuver.

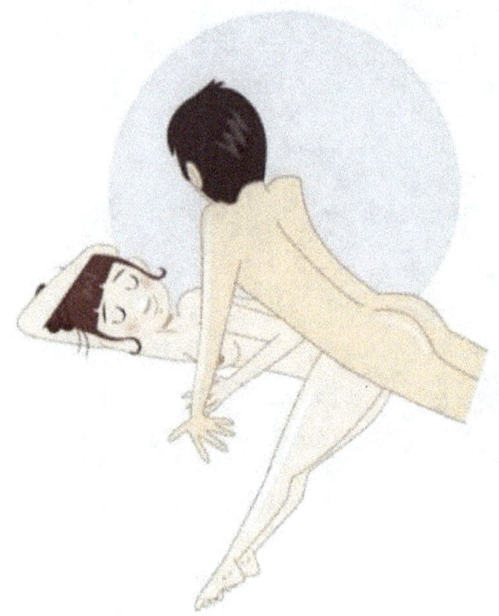

The Sideways Samba

Difficulty level: Advanced

Special features: Requires flexbility from woman, upper body strength from man

The woman lays on her side with her legs stretched out in front of her at a 90' degree angle. She needs to tilt her pelvis inwards, while the man lays behind her and raises his torso with an arm either side of waist for support as he penetrates her.

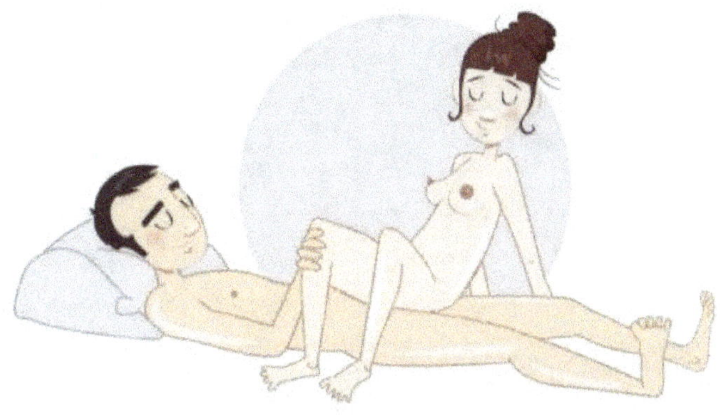

The Side Saddle

Difficulty level: Easy

Special features: Man reclining

An easy sex position and great if you fancy trying some a little bit different, which doesn't require too much effort.

The man lays on his back, with a pillow behind his head and his legs stretched out. The woman sits across him with her legs on one side of his waist and her hands on the other, supporting her weight. As he penetrates her she can slowly open and close her legs, while making swivelling motions to drive him wild.

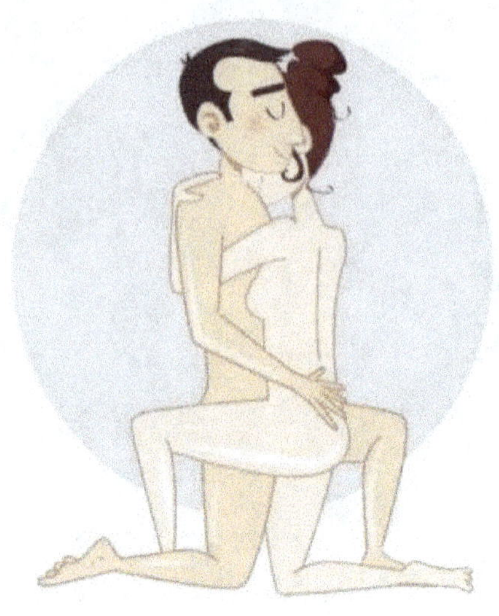

The Proposal

Difficulty level: Easy

Special features: Romantic

Both the man and the woman kneel facing each other (it helps if you are similar heights). He puts one foot on the ground (as if he were proposing) and she puts the opposite foot on the ground ready for penetration to begin.

You may need to wiggle around a little bit to get into a comfortable.

A relatively easy sex position and good if you want to try something new.

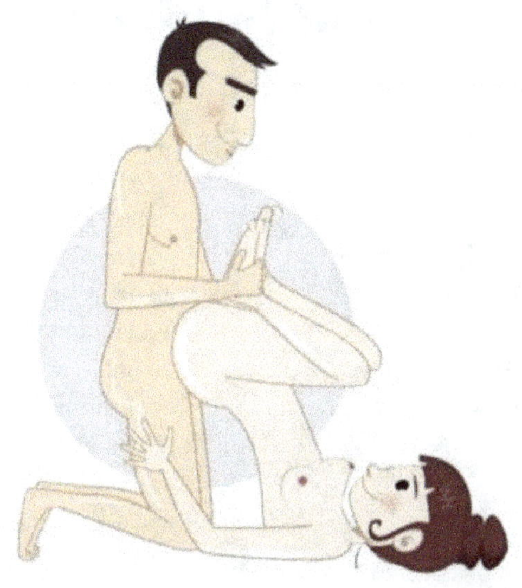

The G-Force

The G-Force sex position

Difficulty level: Advanced

Special features: Requires balance

In this sex position the woman lays on her back and pulls her knees right up to her chest. The man kneels behind her and lifts her torso off the ground so her back is parallel to his thighs. She can help herself balance by holding onto his legs, while he holds onto her feet and penetrates her.

About the Author

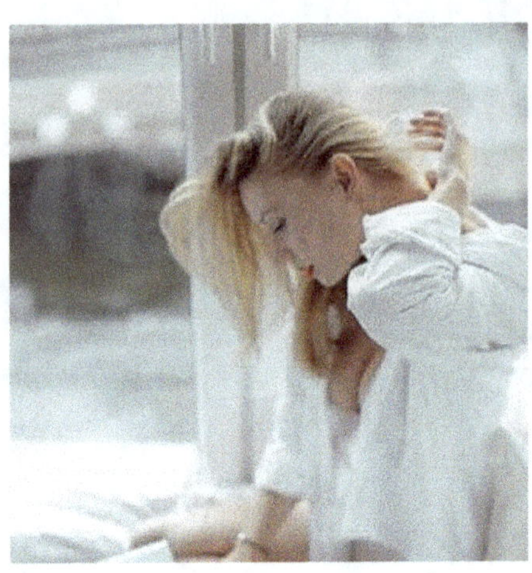

Writing is therapeutic for Allison Eden, who channels her daddy issues into her erotic romance novels (OUT NOW!). She identifies as a submissive before a writer, but her insatiable dirty thoughts were enough to write 8 books in the "A Very Polyamory" series, as well as her bestselling Sexy Games book, which is updated annually with writing partner Ryan Stabile and Words Are Swords Publishing.

You can also read about Allison's further sexploits in the "Festival Hookup Nightmares" column at Festival Drip.

Allison is a part of the Los Angeles fetish and kink community and does her best writing while sitting by the bay windows overlooking the street in her birthday suit

The easiest way to stalk her is by following her on Amazon for updates on her latest books:

https://www.amazon.com/stores/Allison-Eden/author/B08LK6KP18

Other Books by Allison Eden

- The Exhibitionist Bingo Challenge
- Sexy Games 10 Year Anniversary Edition.
- Downright Dirty: A Raunchtastic Adult Coloring Book